Clinical Pharmacology for the Oral and Maxillofacial Surgeon

Editor

HARRY DYM

ORAL AND MAXILLOFACIAL SURGERY CLINICS OF NORTH AMERICA

www.oralmaxsurgery.theclinics.com

Consulting Editor
RUI P. FERNANDES

February 2022 • Volume 34 • Number 1

ELSEVIER

1600 John F. Kennedy Boulevard • Suite 1800 • Philadelphia, Pennsylvania, 19103-2899

http://www.oralmaxsurgery.theclinics.com

ORAL AND MAXILLOFACIAL SURGERY CLINICS OF NORTH AMERICA Volume 34, Number 1
February 2022 ISSN 1042-3699, ISBN-13: 978-0-323-89720-4

Editor: John Vassallo; j.vassallo@elsevier.com
Developmental Editor: Jessica Nicole B. Cañaberal

Oral and Maxillofacial Surgery Clinics of North America (ISSN 1042-3699) is published quarterly by Elsevier Inc., 360 Park Avenue South, New York, NY 10010-1710. Months of issue are February, May, August, and November. Business and Editorial Offices: 1600 John F. Kennedy Blvd., Suite 1800, Philadelphia, PA 19103-2899. Periodicals postage paid at New York, NY and additional mailing offices. Subscription prices are $405.00 per year for US individuals, $961.00 per year for US institutions, $100.00 per year for US students/residents, $478.00 per year for Canadian individuals, $990.00 per year for Canadian institutions, $100.00 per year for Canadian students/residents, $530.00 per year for international individuals, $990.00 per year for international institutions and $235.00 per year for international students/residents. To receive student/resident rate, orders must be accompanied by name or affiliated institution, date of term, and the *signature* of program/residency coordinator on institution letterhead. Orders will be billed at individual rate until proof of status is received. Foreign air speed delivery is included in all *Clinics* subscription prices. All prices are subject to change without notice. **POSTMASTER:** Send address changes to *Oral and Maxillofacial Surgery Clinics of North America,* Elsevier Periodicals **Customer Service, 11830 Westline Industrial Drive, St. Louis, MO 63146. Tel: 1-800-654-2452 (U.S. and Canada); 314-447-8871 (outside U.S. and Canada). Fax: 314-447-8029. E-mail: journalscustomerservice-usa@elsevier.com (for print support); journalsonlinesupport-usa@elsevier.com (for online support).**

Reprints. For copies of 100 or more, of articles in this publication, please contact the Commercial Reprints Department, Elsevier Inc., 360 Park Avenue South, New York, NY 10010-1710. Tel.: 212-633-3874; Fax: 212-633-3820; Email: reprints@elsevier.com.

Oral and Maxillofacial Surgery Clinics of North America is covered in *MEDLINE/PubMed* (*Index Medicus*), *Science Citation Index Expanded (SciSearch®)*, *Journal Citation Reports/Science Edition*, and *Current Contents®/Clinical Medicine*.

Contributors

CONSULTING EDITOR

RUI P. FERNANDES, MD, DMD, FACS, FRCS(Ed)
Clinical Professor and Chief, Division of Head and Neck Surgery, Program Director, Head and Neck Oncologic Surgery and Microvascular Reconstruction Fellowship, Departments of Oral and Maxillofacial Surgery, Neurosurgery, and Orthopaedic Surgery and Rehabilitation, University of Florida Health Science Center, University of Florida College of Medicine, Jacksonville, Florida

EDITOR

HARRY DYM, DDS, FACS
Chairman, Department of Dentistry and Oral and Maxillofacial Surgery, Program Director, Oral and Maxillofacial Surgery Residency Program, The Brooklyn Hospital Center, Senior Attending, Woodhull Hospital, Attending, Brooklyn VA Medical Center, Brooklyn, New York; Clinical Professor, Oral and Maxillofacial Surgery, Columbia University College of Dental Medicine, New York, New York

AUTHORS

SHELLY ABRAMOWICZ, DMD, MPH, FACS
Associate Professor, Division of Oral and Maxillofacial Surgery, Chief, Section of Oral and Maxillofacial Surgery, Department of Surgery, Emory University School of Medicine, Children's Healthcare of Atlanta, Emory University, Atlanta, Georgia

DAVID R. ADAMS, DDS, FICD
Associate Professor, Clinic Chief, Oral and Maxillofacial Surgery, University of Utah, School of Dentistry, Salt Lake City, Utah

AMANDA ANDRE, DDS
Oral and Maxillofacial Surgery Resident, The Brooklyn Hospital Center, Brooklyn, New York

GUILLERMO PUIG ARROYO, DMD
Department of Oral and Maxillofacial Surgery, Woodhull Medical Center, Brooklyn, New York

MICHAEL BENICHOU, DMD
Resident, Oral and Maxillofacial Surgery, The Brooklyn Hospital Center, Brooklyn, New York

NATASHA BHALLA, DDS
Resident, Oral and Maxillofacial Surgery, The Brooklyn Hospital Center, Brooklyn, New York

SAM R. CARUSO, DMD
Resident, Department of Oral and Maxillofacial Surgery, Broward Health Medical Center, Nova Southeastern University College of Dental Medicine, Fort Lauderdale, Florida

PETER CHEN, DDS, MS
Resident, Oral and Maxillofacial Surgery, NYC Health + Hospitals/Woodhull, Brooklyn, New York

MICHAEL H. CHAN, DDS
Director, Oral and Maxillofacial Surgery, Department of Veterans Affairs, New York Harbor Healthcare Care System (Brooklyn Campus), Senior Attending, Oral and Maxillofacial Surgery, Department of Oral and Maxillofacial Surgery, The Brooklyn Hospital Center, Brooklyn, New York

EARL CLARKSON, DDS
Chairman, Oral and Maxillofacial Surgery, NYC Health + Hospitals/Woodhull, Brooklyn, New York

CHAD DAMMLING, DDS, MD
Resident, Department of Oral and Maxillofacial Surgery, School of Dentistry, The University of Alabama at Birmingham, Birmingham, Alabama

NATALIE DUNLOP, DDS, MD
Resident, Oral and Maxillofacial Surgery, Division of Craniofacial and Surgical Care, The University of North Carolina at Chapel Hill, Chapel Hill, North Carolina

HARRY DYM, DDS, FACS
Chairman, Department of Dentistry and Oral and Maxillofacial Surgery, Program Director, Oral and Maxillofacial Surgery Residency Program, The Brooklyn Hospital Center, Senior Attending, Woodhull Hospital, Attending, Brooklyn VA Medical Center, Brooklyn, New York; Clinical Professor, Oral and Maxillofacial Surgery, Columbia University College of Dental Medicine, New York, New York

HILLEL EPHROS, DMD, MD
Chairman, Department of Dentistry, Program Director of Oral and Maxillofacial Surgery, St. Joseph's University Medical Center, Paterson, New Jersey

YIJIAO FAN, DDS
Department of Oral and Maxillofacial Surgery, The Brooklyn Hospital Center, Brooklyn, New York

ELDA FISHER, MD, FACS
Associate Professor, Division of Oral and Maxillofacial Surgery, Program Director,

Residency Program in Oral and Maxillofacial Surgery, The University of North Carolina at Chapel Hill, Chapel Hill, North Carolina

PAUL GAMMAL, DDS
PGY2, Department of Dentistry/Oral Surgery, Woodhull Hospital and Mental Health Center, Brooklyn, New York

ALLEN GLIED, DDS
Department of Dentistry, St. Barnabas Hospital, Bronx, New York

LESLIE R. HALPERN, DDS, MD, PhD, MPH, FACS, FICD
Professor, Section Head, Oral and Maxillofacial Surgery, University of Utah, School of Dentistry, Salt Lake City, Utah

MONICA HANNA, DMD
Resident, Oral and Maxillofacial Surgery, NYC Health + Hospitals/Woodhull, Brooklyn, New York

ROBERT J. HERROD, DMD
Former Resident, Oral and Maxillofacial Surgery, St. Joseph's University Medical Center, Paterson, New Jersey; Private Practice, St. Petersburg, Florida and Little Falls, New Jersey

JOSEPH KANG, DDS
Oral and Maxillofacial Surgery Resident, The Brooklyn Hospital Center, Brooklyn, New York

BRIAN KINARD, DMD, MD
Assistant Professor, Department of Oral and Maxillofacial Surgery, School of Dentistry, The University of Alabama at Birmingham, Birmingham, Alabama

CHRISTOPHER J. LANE, DDS
Chief, Oral and Maxillofacial Surgery, St. Barnabas Hospital, SBH Health System Bronx, Bronx, New York

ASHLEY LOFTERS, DDS
Department of Oral and Maxillofacial Surgery, Woodhull Medical Center, Brooklyn, New York

JONATHAN MALAKAN, DDS
Oral and Maxillofacial Surgery Intern, The Brooklyn Hospital Center, Brooklyn, New York

JARED MILLER, DDS
Attending, Oral and Maxillofacial Surgery, The Brooklyn Hospital Center, Brooklyn, New York

NABIL MOUSSA, DDS
PGY 4 Resident, Department of Oral and Maxillofacial Surgery, The Brooklyn Hospital Center, New York, New York; Department of Dentistry, Division of Oral and Maxillofacial Surgery, Brooklyn, New York

JUNAID MUNDIYA, DMD
Chief Resident, Department of Dentistry and Oral and Maxillofacial Surgery, The Brooklyn Hospital Center, Brooklyn, New York

YOAV NUDELL, DDS, MS
Chief Resident, Oral and Maxillofacial Surgery, The Brooklyn Hospital Center, Brooklyn, New York

ORRETT E. OGLE, DDS
Attending Surgeon, Department of Oral and Maxillofacial Surgery, The Brooklyn Hospital Center, New York, New York; Department of Dentistry, Division of Oral and Maxillofacial Surgery, Brooklyn, New York

JASON E. PORTNOF, DMD, MD, FACS, FACD, FICD
Adjunct Associate Professor, Department of Oral and Maxillofacial Surgery, Nova Southeastern University College of Dental Medicine, Private Practice, Oral and Maxillofacial Surgery, Surgical Arts of Boca Raton, Boca Raton, Florida

JOEL ROSENFELD, DMD
Resident, Department of Oral and Maxillofacial Surgery, The Brooklyn Hospital Center, Brooklyn, New York

SNEHA SHAH, DMD
Chief Resident, Department of Oral and Maxillofacial Surgery, St. Joseph's University Medical Center, Paterson, New Jersey

FEIYI SUN, DDS
Resident, Oral and Maxillofacial Surgery, The Brooklyn Hospital Center, Brooklyn, New York

JAYKRISHNA P. THAKKAR, DDS
Resident, Oral and Maxillofacial Surgery, The Brooklyn Hospital Center, Brooklyn, New York

EDWARD WOODBINE, DDS
Attending, Department of Dentistry and Oral and Maxillofacial Surgery, The Brooklyn Hospital Center, Brooklyn, New York

ELENA YAMAGUCHI, MD, FACP
Private Practice, Infectious Diseases, Delray Beach, Florida

Contents

> This article illustrates the indications and mechanism of action of core emergency medications as well as emergency medications for intravenous sedation in the oral and maxillofacial surgeon office. The recognition of medical emergencies and comprehensive knowledge of pharmaceutical medical intervention can prevent deterioration in medical emergencies. In addition, this article also reviews common dosages as well as administration techniques that should be regularly reviewed and be fundamental knowledge to the oral surgeon and staff.

> Dental anxiety is a leading cause of postponing treatment and/or complete avoidance of professional oral care. Therefore, effective sedation and pain control are integral components of dental care for the fearful and anxious patient. The application of oral sedation aids the trained practitioner to provide care to the anxious dental patient and remains the safest, most established, and most commonly used route of drug administration. Proper training and understanding of pharmacologic properties allows for safe and effective application of analgesics and sedatives for oral sedation.

> The oral and maxillofacial surgery model of anesthesia delivery is the subject of some controversy. However, a long track record of patient safety provides compelling support for the dual role of the oral and maxillofacial surgeon as proceduralist and anesthetist. Among the elements critical to continued success is a clear understanding of the pharmacology of the agents used to produce sedation and general anesthesia. This review highlights 6 sedation agents used as part of a balanced anesthesia technique in oral and maxillofacial surgery.

> Control of acute pain in oral and maxillofacial surgery is important for patient care and comfort. Oral surgical procedures are associated with tissue injury and inflammation. Acute pain can arise directly from a surgical procedure or from problems such as dental caries, infection, perforation of maxillary sinus, pericoronitis, and jaw fractures. The major factor in acute pain management is deciding on an appropriate intervention and/or analgesics that will provide the best pain relief. Multimodal pain control has taken a leading role in effectively managing acute pain. This article covers the different options available to dental clinicians.

Corticosteroids have been the cornerstone for treatment of many inflammatory and immune disorders with these beneficial effects well recognized by the medical community. It also possesses many undesirable clinical adverse effects that can occur within 2 weeks of use. Moreover, in the past decade, chronic users of corticosteroids have been linked to skeletal (vertebral and hip) osteoporosis/osteonecrosis with some patients requiring adjunctive antiresprotive medications to counteract fracture prevention. Additionally, two case reports have implicated daily prednisone user to cause osteonecrosis of the mandible. This chapter highlights current adrenal suppression classifications, pathophysiology, drug interactions, and perioperative surgical and anesthesia management.

Selective serotonin reuptake inhibitors (SSRIs) have been the cornerstone for the treatment of depression, anxiety, obsessive-compulsive disorder, and panic disorder for a wide spectrum of age groups. Although the beneficial therapeutic properties are well recognized by the medical community, it also possesses many undesirable adverse effects with clinical manifestations. Some of the effects can be severe. This chapter highlights use of SSRIs, the mechanism of action, medication dosages, common drug to drug interactions, and recommendations on management of the oral and maxillofacial surgery patient on SSRIs.

In this chapter, the authors review the benefits of saliva and the destructive consequences of its loss. It is hoped that this will help their colleagues identify and treat patients before development of symptoms. Xerostomia is the subjective complaint of dry mouth or sensation of oral dryness. Hyposalivation is the actual decrease in measured salivary outflow. The authors discuss a compiled list of highly cited medications commonly used today that are linked with xerostomia and hyposalivation. There are numerous treatment modalities that are present, such as saliva substitutes, mouth rinses, sugar-free candy, and pilocarpine among others.

Use of topical and local anesthesia (LA) is the workhorse of all aspects of dentistry. There was a time in the past when dentistry was performed without any local pain control. Owing to this there are patients with dental anxiety and fear of a dental office. The media portraying dentistry as being painful, or showing a dentist with needles, enlists fear and distrust of dentists. In contrast, pain is what brings the patient to the dental office and with local pain control measures a dentist is able to alleviate the patient's cause of pain.

Antibiotic prophylaxis is the use of antibiotics in the perioperative period to prevent surgical site infections from local flora. Specific guidelines and criteria exist to prevent these infections while also practicing antimicrobial stewardship. Most dentoalveolar procedures do not require antibiotic prophylaxis. For nondentoalveolar procedures, the decision to provide antibiotic prophylaxis is based on involvement of the respiratory, oral, or pharyngeal mucosa. Special considerations exist for patients at high risk for infective endocarditis, patients with head and neck cancer, and temporomandibular joint replacement procedures. This article discusses indications for antibiotic prophylaxis during oral and maxillofacial surgical procedures.

This article focuses on the antimicrobial therapy of head and neck infections from odontogenic origin. Odontogenic infections are among the most common infections of the oral cavity. They are sourced primarily from dental caries and periodontal disease (gingivitis and periodontitis). Many odontogenic infections are self-limiting and may drain spontaneously. However, these infections may drain into the anatomic spaces adjacent to the oral cavity and spread along the contiguous facial planes, leading to more serious infections. Antibiotics are an important aspect of care of the patient with an acute odontogenic infection. Antibiotics are not a substitute for definitive surgical management.

Most jaw lesions are treated surgically. Areas of abnormal proliferation or destruction in bone are commonly treated by regional curettage, excision, or resection. However, surgery is invasive and leaves a defect where the lesion was removed. Surgical trauma to adjacent healthy tissue, including vital neurovascular bundles is often unavoidable, and can be especially traumatizing to the pediatric patient. Select jaw lesions with well-studied nonsurgical pharmaceutical treatments are presented here.

The realm of aesthetic medicine is broad, and there are countless medications and topical agents used in the practice of aesthetic medicine. The most commonly used injectable medicines include botulinum toxin for mimetic lines and hyaluronic acid fillers for deeper facial rhytids and volume rejuvenation. Topical aesthetic medicines are useful adjuncts for facial rejuvenation and commonly include tretinoin, hydroquinone, growth factors, and vitamin C, as well as a wide range of chemical peels.

The purpose of this article is to clarify clinically impactful features of the perioperative and postoperative pharmacologic management of pregnant and lactating patients in the maxillofacial or dental setting. Before prescribing any drug to a nursing mother or pregnant patient, the maxillofacial surgeon and other dental and medical providers should consider the available evidence, benefits, and risk for that particular drug. There are many complex factors to consider when prescribing in order to maintain the safety of the pregnant individual, fetus, and infant. This article aims to provide concise, memorable, and actionable information to use in your clinical practice.

ORAL AND MAXILLOFACIAL SURGERY CLINICS OF NORTH AMERICA

SERIES OF RELATED INTEREST

Atlas of the Oral and Maxillofacial Surgery Clinics
www.oralmaxsurgeryatlas.theclinics.com

Dental Clinics
www.dental.theclinics.com

THE CLINICS ARE NOW AVAILABLE ONLINE!
Access your subscription at:
www.theclinics.com

Preface
Appreciation

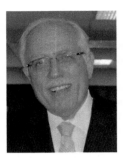

Harry Dym, DDS, FACS
Editor

I am privileged and honored to once again have had the opportunity to edit another issue of *Oral and Maxillofacial Surgery Clinics of North America*. It is truly a pleasure working with Mr John Vassallo, associate publisher of the *Oral and Maxillofacial Surgery Clinics of North America* and *Dental Clinics of North America*, as well as Jessica Canaberal, the very capable developmental editor for *Oral and Maxillofacial Surgery Clinics of North America*. I have worked with John for decades, and what began as a formal and professional relationship has evolved into a strong friendship for which I am truly grateful.

I consider *Oral and Maxillofacial Surgery Clinics of North America* to be an essential text that brings to our oral and maxillofacial surgical community concise, new, and timely scientific information that is both appropriate and meaningful to the everyday clinician in his or her practice. I wish to thank all the contributors to this issue, dedicated to the pharmacology of drugs commonly used in the treatment of maxillofacial and related conditions, for their successful completion of the tasks assigned. In my opinion, the readership will benefit immensely from these well-executed, clearly delineated articles that review old, well-known, existing medications as well as bring to light some new medications that may prove useful to many of the clinicians.

I would be remiss if I were not to address the events of this past year that have touched and impacted everyone in the community, as it certainly did me and my family.

As I write this preface, the COVID-19 crisis, which seemed to be abating and slowly drawing to a close, has once again been revived by the Delta variant. Unfortunately, it continues to leave in its wake serious financial, personal, and communal disruption, the toll of which will not be truly appreciated for many years to come. Many of us in the oral and maxillofacial surgical community were of course directly impacted; a great percentage of our community of surgeons were forced to either completely close or partially close their offices, and many may have lost loved ones to this dreadful illness or lost staff members, friends, and patients.

In my capacity as Chairman of the Department of Dentistry and Oral and Maxillofacial Surgery at The Brooklyn Hospital Center, I and my

Oral Maxillofacial Surg Clin N Am 34 (2022) xiii–xiv
https://doi.org/10.1016/j.coms.2021.08.016

department were certainly in the eye of the COVID storm. COVID-19 landed squarely in our community, and at one time, we had become completely inundated with COVID inpatients and COVID emergency room patients. Many of my oral and maxillofacial surgical residents became sick, but thankfully, all quickly recovered (though one of my residents made the *New York Times* while lying on a gurney due to his COVID infection).

I am humbled by my oral and maxillofacial residents and attendings who braved this virus and continued to directly treat our community's patients' infections, lacerations, and fractures with the same intensity and dedication that they always exhibited prior to this scourge. I and the entire Brooklyn Hospital administration and community at large owe them a debt of gratitude. In fact, this issue is dedicated to my residents, attendings, and the entire administration and medical community of The Brooklyn Hospital Center, who rose to the occasion and truly demonstrated the highest qualities of healers and community doctors.

I would like to take this opportunity again to acknowledge the Chairperson of the Board of Trustees of The Brooklyn Hospital Center, Ms Lizanne Fontaine, who is totally committed to the concept of providing equality of care to all members of our community regardless of their financial abilities. We are fortunate to have her at the helm, and I wish her continued success and only good fortune in the coming years. Mr Gary Terrinoni, our president and CEO, reacted forcefully and adroitly to the complex challenges our institution faced during the height of the COVID crisis. He smartly prioritized and redirected the hospital's mission to deal with the crisis, saving countless many lives. Mr Robert Aulicino, our COO, Dr Vasantha Kondamudi, our CMO, and Ms Judy McLaughlin, our CNO, all worked tirelessly and innovatively helping to coordinate and lead the dedicated physicians, nurses, and employees during this past year.

I am indebted to the following individuals for a lifetime of friendship and mentorship:

Dr Peter Sherman, who has been mentor, colleague, and one of my dearest of friends for over 40 years. He has always been a beacon of optimism, who encouraged me throughout my career and has guided me both professionally and personally. Dr Earl Clarkson and Dr Orett Ogle, wonderful friends and colleagues for almost 40 years, with special thanks to Dr Clarkson for having administered the oral surgery department during a recent medical leave. Dr Elliot Segal, a lifelong friend and colleague, who generously shares life experiences through enjoyable vignettes. Dr Stanley Bodner, another lifelong friend, who has always provided me with insight and clarity. Arthur Blutstein, for his many years of friendship and sound advice. Rabbis Sadowsky and Goldstein, for their spiritual guidance.

To many of my former residents, who call and text often, Dr Larry Brown, Dr Josh Wolf, Dr Gregg Strull, Dr Tom Cerbone, their ongoing contact is most appreciated.

To my dedicated executive assistant Ms Gloria Stallings, Dr Ricardo Boyce, Dr Earl Clarkson, Dr Ed Woodbine, Dr Michael Chan, and Dr Jared Miller, who so ably helped run and coordinate the dental and oral surgery service during my medical leave, much appreciation is owed.

To my children, Yehoshua, Hindy, Daniel, and Akiva and their spouses, as well as my siblings, Steven and Fayge, for their ongoing concern and love.

Finally, recent life events have only reinforced my love, admiration, and respect for my wife Freidy. Hopefully, we will continue to grow old together, watching our grandchildren mature.

"Helping others find meaning and purpose in their lives is the true meaning and purpose of life."

Harry Dym, DDS, FACS
The Brooklyn Hospital Center
121 Dekalb Avenue
Brooklyn, NY 11201, USA

E-mail address:
hdym@tbh.org

Emergency Drugs for the Oral and Maxillofacial Surgeon Office

Joel Rosenfeld, DMD*, Harry Dym, DDS

KEYWORDS

- Emergency drugs • IV sedation • Management of airway emergencies
- Management of sedation emergencies

KEY POINTS

- Oral surgeons and staff should be prepared for perioperative emergencies.
- Prompt recognition and preparedness are the most important factors in managing emergencies in the oral surgery office.
- Emergency drugs along with their mechanism of action, dosages, and preparations should be well known to the oral surgeon and team.

INTRODUCTION

For more than 90 years, office-based anesthesia has been a part of the history, training, and practice of oral and maxillofacial surgery (OMFS).[1,2] There may be a significant component of fear, anxiety, and pain that should be alleviated in order to carry out procedures comfortably for patients.

Every oral surgeon should recognize that medical emergencies may transpire during the course of practice and office-based anesthesia. These emergencies could be connected to surgical management, anesthesia administration, or patient risk factors.[3] Medical emergencies can easily evolve into a life-threatening emergency without prompt recognition and treatment. It is for this reason emergency medications should be present and available in the oral surgery office.

Oral surgeons who use advanced anesthesia, like moderate sedation, in addition to deep sedation/general anesthesia must be skilled in diagnosis and management of emergencies, which may result from their usage.[4] Resuscitative equipment (**Box 1**), oxygen, and other resuscitative medications should be accessible for immediate use.[5,6]

This list is a suggested list of the core emergency drugs and a of suggested emergency medications for those doing advanced anesthesia. Always check with your state dental board for the mandatory emergency medications you must have in your office.[7]

CORE EMERGENCY DRUGS
Oxygen

Oxygen is used for the treatment of hypoxemia, which is common in numerous medical emergencies.[8] This underlines the significance and need for a supplemental oxygen delivery system.[9] Multiple routes are available for delivery. The oral surgery office should also be equipped with a bag-valve mask with full face mask to allow for positive-pressure ventilation.[10]

Nitroglycerin

Nitroglycerin is used for relief of acute chest pain with history of angina, or undiagnosed angina with symptoms of myocardial infarction. It is an antianginal that stimulates cyclic guanosine monophosphate production, which relaxes vascular smooth muscle specifically in the coronary arteries

Department of Oral and Maxillofacial Surgery, The Brooklyn Hospital Center, 121 Dekalb Avenue, Brooklyn, NY 11201, USA
* Corresponding author.
E-mail address: JoelWRosenfeld@Gmail.com

Oral Maxillofacial Surg Clin N Am 34 (2022) 1–7
https://doi.org/10.1016/j.coms.2021.08.007
1042-3699/22/© 2021 Elsevier Inc. All rights reserved.

in the presence of an anginal attack. The usual dose of nitroglycerin is 1 sublingual (0.4 mg) tablet or 1 spray (0.4 mg) from a nitroglycerin spray atomizer every 5 minutes. Common side effects are headaches, dizziness, and flushing. Nitroglycerin is contraindicated for patients with hypotension and should not be given to patients taking medication for erectile dysfunction, such as sildenafil (Viagra), tadalafil (Cialis), and vardenafil (Levitra) because of risk of severe hypotension, tachycardia, and cardiovascular collapse.[11,12]

Aspirin

Aspirin is used for suspected myocardial infarction or ischemia. It is an antiplatelet and works by inhibiting prostaglandin synthesis and irreversibly inhibits platelet aggregation. Dosage is one 325 mg nonenteric-coated aspirin tablet, which is chewed for 30 seconds and swallowed. Aspirin should not be given to people with recent bleeding peptic ulcer or history of aspirin allergy.[13]

Epinephrine 1:1000

Epinephrine 1:1000 is used for anaphylaxis, for bronchospasm, and as a cardiac stimulant during cardiac arrest. It is a sympathomimetic drug that activates alpha- and beta-adrenergic receptors. It increases heart rate and myocardial contractility. It also causes vasoconstriction and bronchial

dilation and stabilizes mast cells. For anaphylaxis, the adult dose of epinephrine is 0.3 mg (1:1000), and the children's dose is 0.15 mg (1:2000) intramuscular (IM) via autoinjector for anaphylaxis. An IM preparation can also be made by drawing up 0.3 mL from a vial of 1 mg/mL (1:1000) into a syringe for use for adults with anaphylaxis (**Fig. 1**). The epinephrine 1:10,000 concentration is designed for intravenous (IV) administration. Caution should be used, as it may cause tachydysrhythmias. It also decreases placental blood flow and may induce premature labor.[14,15]

Albuterol

Albuterol is used for bronchospasm and wheezing secondary to an acute asthmatic episode. It is a bronchodilator that stimulates beta-2 adrenergic receptors, causing bronchodilation. Albuterol is available in a metered-dose inhaler and can be used 2 to 3 times every 1 or 3 minutes as needed.[16]

Aromatic Ammonia

Aromatic ammonia is used for syncope/fainting/loss of consciousness. It is a respiratory stimulant, and when crushed, releases a noxious odor that stimulates the respiratory and vasomotor centers of the medulla. Return to consciousness is typically achieved by placing patients in the Trendelenburg position, with administration of oxygen and by using aromatic ammonia.[17]

Diphenhydramine

Diphenhydramine is used for allergic reactions/anaphylaxis. It is an antihistamine that antagonizes histamine at the H-1 receptor. It causes sedation and has an anticholinergic effect. Diphenhydramine can be given 50 mg IM or IV.[18]

Glucose (Dextrose 50%)

Glucose (dextrose 50%) is used to increase glucose levels in hypoglycemic states. Simple sources may be used, such as orange juice, cola, or granulated sugar, in conscious patients. The oral formulation should not be given to unconscious patients because of risk of aspiration. If patients are unable to swallow, IV access should be obtained, and dextrose 50% in water can be given or by IM injection of glucagon.[19]

Emergency Medications for Advanced Anesthesia

The American Association of Oral and Maxillofacial Surgeons Committee on Anesthesia recommends that the oral surgery office maintain supplies of the following   medications: vasopressors,

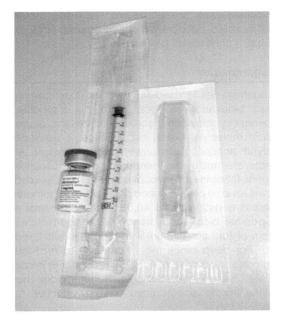

Fig. 1. Preparation of 0.3-mg solution of epinephrine.

corticosteroids, bronchodilators, muscle relaxants, narcotic antagonists, benzodiazepine antagonists, antihistamines, antiarrhythmics, anticholinergics, coronary artery vasodilators, antihypertensives, and drugs for treatment of malignant hyperthermia.[20]

VASOPRESSORS
Ephedrine

Ephedrine is an adrenergic agonist used to manage moderate to severe hypotension when patients are also bradycardic. Ephedrine displays both alpha-1 and beta-1 adrenergic agonism. Ephedrine causes increased peripheral vascular resistance, positive cardiac chronotropy, and positive cardiac inotropy. Ephedrine can be prepared by diluting a 50-mg/mL vial in 9 mL of saline to make a 5-mg/mL solution. Typical dosing is a 5-mg bolus titrated to the desired effect.[21]

Phenylephrine

Phenylephrine is an adrenergic agonist used to manage hypotension when patients have tachycardia or normal heart rate. Phenylephrine is a selective alpha-1 agonist, which results in peripheral vasoconstriction and increased blood pressure. Reflex bradycardia typically accompanies administration. Phenylephrine can be prepared by diluting a 10-mg/mL vial in 9 mL of saline; 9 mL of this solution can be discarded, and an additional 9 mL of saline can be added to create a 0.1-mg/mL

solution. Alternatively, the 10-mg/mL vial can be added to a 100-mL bag of saline to also obtain the desired 0.1-mg/mL solution (**Fig. 2**). Typical dosing is 0.1 mg/mL titrated to the desired effect.[22]

CORTICOSTEROID
Dexamethasone

Dexamethasone is a synthetic adrenal corticosteroid used as an antiemetic and for treatment of severe allergies, pruritus, asthma, bronchospasm, and postoperative edema. It can provide membrane-stabilizing effects, reduce leukotriene formation, and reduce histamine release from mast cells. There is a slow onset of action. A typical dose is 4 to 12 mg IV. Caution should be used for patients with preexisting infection, peptic ulcer, or hyperglycemia.[21]

Hydrocortisone

Hydrocortisone is a corticosteroid with similar indications and anti-inflammatory properties as dexamethasone. It is the preferred corticosteroid for management of acute adrenal insufficiency. The typical dose is 125 mg.[23]

MUSCLE RELAXANTS
Succinylcholine

Succinylcholine is a depolarizing neuromuscular blocker used for management of laryngospasm after other methods have proved unsuccessful. It helps relax the vocal cords and causes general muscle paralysis. It binds directly to postsynaptic acetylcholine receptor endplates, leading to fasciculations followed by muscular paralysis. It has a very rapid onset (45–60 seconds) and short duration of action (4–6 minutes). A typical dose is 0.1 to 0.2 mg/kg or 20 mg IV to break the spasm. It will require ventilation support. There is a lack of fade in train-of-four response. It should not be used whenever hyperkalemia is possible, such as muscular dystrophy or other myotonias, in muscle denervation, cerebral palsy, multiple sclerosis, or burn patients. An increase in potassium from succinylcholine use in hyperkalemic conditions may lead to cardiac arrest. It is a trigger for malignant hyperthermia and can result in prolonged paralysis in patients with pseudocholinesterase deficiency. It has a shelf life of 2 weeks.[24]

Dantrolene

Dantrolene is used for the treatment of malignant hyperthermia crisis. It is required in any clinic that uses known triggers like sevoflurane, isoflurane, desflurane, and succinylcholine. It interferes

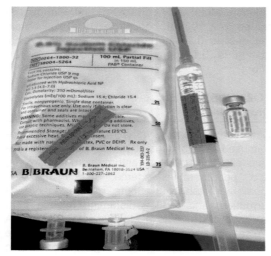

Fig. 2. Preparation of 0.1-mg/mL solution of phenylephrine.

with calcium release from the sarcoplasmic reticulum and leads to muscle relaxation. Triggering agents should be discontinued. The patient should be hyperventilated with 100% oxygen at a 10-L/min flow rate, and then sodium bicarbonate administered, the patient cooled, and diuretics (furosemide) administered. The initial dose is a bolus of 2.5 mg/kg with increments up to 10 mg/kg administered via a large-bore IV catheter. It is formulated in 20 mg per bottle of powder, which needs to be reconstituted in 60 mL sterile water. The Malignant Hyperthermia Association of the United Sates recommends 36 vials be kept on site if a triggering agent is stocked in the clinic.[21]

Ryanodex

Ryanodex is an alternative to the conventional dantrolene sodium formulation, used for the treatment of malignant hyperthermia. It is a ryanodine receptor 1 antagonist. Each vial contains 250 mg of dantrolene and is reconstituted in 5 mL of sterile water to allow rapid administration.[21]

Rocuronium

Rocuronium is a nondepolarizing muscle relaxant. It works by competing for cholinergic receptor at the motor endplate. It has a rapid onset (dose dependent 45–120 seconds) with intermediate duration of action (30–90 minutes). When used in high concentration, it may be considered a substitute for succinylcholine to break laryngospasm. A typical dose is 0.6 to 1.2 mg/kg; a higher dose of 1.2 mg/kg will decrease the onset of action to 45 to 60 seconds. It may require prolonged ventilation support. It does not depend on plasma

cholinesterase for metabolism. Local anesthetics will increase the duration of neuromuscular block. It has a shelf life of 12 weeks.[21]

Sugammadex

Sugammadex is used for reversal of neuromuscular blockade from rocuronium. It is a modified gamma cyclodextrin that encapsulates the rocuronium molecule. Unlike neostigmine, it does not inhibit acetylcholinesterase, and cholinergic effects are not seen; therefore, an antimuscarinic agent (atropine or glycopyrrolate) is not needed. It will reverse deep induced paralysis in 2.9 minutes versus neostigmine at 48.8 minutes. Reversal of moderate block (appearance of second twitch in train-of-four stimulation) with rocuronium is 2 mg/kg. For deep block (no twitches in train-of-four stimulation), a dose of 4 mg/kg is used. For immediate reversal, use 16 mg/kg. Sugammadex may make hormonal contraception less effective for up to 7 days.[21]

Anticonvulsant

Most seizures are transient and managed by protection of the patient's head with cushioning and removing sharp objects from around the patient's area. Status epilepticus and prolonged or recurrent seizure require anticonvulsant therapy, such as benzodiazepines. They act on the inhibitory neurotransmitter GABA, the limbic system, the hypothalamus, and the thalamus to produce sedation, an antianxiety effect, and skeletal muscle relaxation. Diazepam at a dosage of 10 mg is acceptable if the IV line is intact. However, if a line is lost during a tonic-clonic convulsion, lorazepam 4 mg is the drug of choice, as it is long acting and allows IM administration. Lorazepam also can be used for management of acute withdrawal symptoms. Midazolam 5 mg may also be used, as it allows for IM administration.[25–27]

REVERSAL AGENTS
Naloxone

Naloxone is used for the management of opioid overdose with unintended respiratory depression. It is an antagonist for all opioid receptor subtypes. It will reverse all effects of opioids, including analgesia, respiratory depression, and chest wall rigidity. Because of its onset of action of 1 to 2 minutes, it is unsuitable for management of desaturation secondary to opioid-induced chest wall rigidity. Succinylcholine is the first-line agent for this. After administration of Naloxone, patients should be monitored in office for 1 hour to rule out resedation. A typical dose is 0.1-mg increments titrated to effect with a maximum of 0.8 mg. Formulation is usually 0.4 mg/mL in a 1-mL vial, which can be diluted with normal saline in a 10-cc syringe for a 0.1-mg/mL solution. Caution should be used, as use may result in significant release of catecholamines resulting hypertension, seizures, ventricular tachycardia, ventricular fibrillation, or fluid shift triggering pulmonary edema.[28]

Flumazenil

Flumazenil is used for management of benzodiazepine overdose, resulting in unconsciousness in planned moderate sedation, postoperative drowsiness, central nervous system depression, respiratory depression, or emergence delirium. It reverses the sedation, anxiolysis, amnesia, muscle relaxation, and anticonvulsant effects of benzodiazepines by inhibiting GABA receptors. Patients should be monitored in office for at least 1 hour to rule out re-sedation. A typical dose is 0.1 to 0.2 mg titrated to effect. It should not be given to patients with a seizure disorder managed by benzodiazepines.[21]

Anticholinergics

Anticholinergics is used for management of hemodynamically significant bradycardia, dizziness or motion sickness-related symptoms, and increased salivation. The target of anticholinergic medications is muscarinic receptors. When activated, these receptors cause parasympathetic effects on specific organs. The primary anticholinergic medications are atropine, glycopyrrolate, and scopolamine. Atropine has the fastest onset and blocks vagal stimulation to the heart, allowing for unopposed sympathetic stimulation. This makes it the drug of choice for hemodynamically unstable bradycardia with a typical dose of 0.5 mg IV titrated to effect. It also can be used in smaller doses of 0.01 mg/kg to counteract the hypersalivation effect of ketamine during procedural sedation. It should not be given to patients with ischemic heart disease, acute narrow-angle glaucoma, prostatic hypertrophy, urinary retention, acute hemorrhage, or hyperthyroidism. Physostigmine, a cholinesterase inhibitor, can reverse anticholinergic syndrome (emergence delirium) encountered with use of scopolamine, benzodiazepines, or diphenhydramine.[21]

ANTIHYPERTENSIVE AGENTS
Esmolol

Esmolol is a beta-1 selective antagonist with a very short duration of action. It decreases the force and rate of heart contractions. A typical dose is 20 mg titrated to effect. The duration of action is under 20 minutes. It can be used for management of hypermetabolic state. Caution should be used with patients with asthma and chronic obstructive pulmonary disease.[21]

Labetalol

Labetalol is a selective alpha-1 blocker and nonselective beta-blocker. It has intrinsic sympathetic activity and will not decrease resting cardiac function as much as esmolol. It lowers blood pressure by blockade of alpha-1 receptors in vascular smooth muscle and beta-1 receptor in the heart. The dosage is 20 mg titrated to effect. Duration of action is 2 to 18 hours. Caution should be used in patients with asthma, bradycardia, and congestive heart failure. Any patient given antihypertensive should be assessed carefully before discharge for risk of orthostatic hypotension.[21]

Hydralazine

Hydralazine is a direct-acting smooth muscle relaxant used to treat hypertension. It acts as a vasodilator to decrease peripheral resistance and lowers the blood pressure and decreases afterload. It can cause reflex sympathetic stimulation, which increases the heart rate and cardiac output. A typical dose 5 mg IV titrated up to 25 mg. Onset is 5 minutes with a duration 2 hours. It can be used for patients with asthma and can cause flushing, hypotension, headache, and nausea/vomiting. It should not be given to patients with tachycardia, coronary artery disease, constrictive pericarditis, lupus, pulmonary hypertension, high-output heart failure (thyrotoxicosis), dissection aortic aneurysm, or porphyria.[29]

ANTIARRHYTHMIC
Amiodarone

Amiodarone is used for the treatment of ventricular fibrillation, pulseless ventricular tachycardia refractory to defibrillation and epinephrine administration, and stable ventricular tachycardia. It is also used for Wolff-Parkinson-White syndrome with reentry phenomenon. It works by blocking potassium channels by slowing down conduction in the atrioventricular (AV) node and increasing threshold for ventricular fibrillation. In cardiac arrest algorithm, it is given as a 300-mg bolus. It should not be given with other antiarrhythmics or beta-blockers, as it may cause sinus arrest.[30]

Adenosine

Adenosine is used for the treatment of paroxysmal supraventricular tachycardia. It works by slowing conduction in the AV node and interrupting the reentry pathways. A typical dose is 6 mg push. It has a very rapid onset and may cause transient sinus bradycardia or asystole with administration. It may also cause chest pain, hypotension, flushing, and bronchospasm. It should not be given to patients with asthma or those taking dipyridamole or theophylline.[31]

DIURETICS
Furosemide (Lasix)

Furosemide (Lasix) is used to treat fluid buildup due to congestive heart failure, acute pulmonary edema, acute decompensated heart failure, and resistant hypertension. It is also used to prevent kidney injury during malignant hyperthermia. It is a loop diuretic that works on the thick ascending limb of loop of Henle. A dose is typically 0.5 to 1 mg/kg IV over 1 to 2 minutes for acute pulmonary edema and hypertensive crisis. Onset of action is 5 minutes after IV administration, and duration is 2 hours. Oral administration of Lasix will "last 6 hours," hence the name. It should not be used in patients with lupus, liver disease, renal impairment, and sulfa allergies. It can cause electrolyte imbalance, hypotension, and ototoxicity.[21]

Antiemetics

Antiemetics are used for treatment of nausea and vomiting after procedural sedation. It is important to know the known risk factors, like younger age, female sex, nonsmoker, and history of postoperative nausea vomiting. Also, high risks are obesity, gastroesophageal reflux disease, gastroparesis, and diabetes. It is important to limit known triggers like N_2O, fentanyl, and etomidate.[21]

Ondansetron

Ondansetron is used to prevent nausea and vomiting after procedural sedation. It is a 5-HT3 receptor antagonist that acts on both peripheral vagal nerve terminals and central chemoreceptor trigger zone of the area postrema in the medulla. Dose is usually 4 mg IV. It is associated with prolonged QT interval, which may lead to torsades de pointes. It should not be given to patients with congenital long QT syndrome and congestive heart failure.[21]

Metoclopramide

Metoclopramide is used to prevent nausea and vomiting after procedural sedation. It is a dopamine D2 receptor antagonist that acts on the chemoreceptor trigger zone in the central nervous system. The dose is 10 mg. It can cause movement disorders like tardive dyskinesia. It should

not be used in patients with Parkinson disease. It can also trigger neuroleptic malignant syndrome (NMS), characterized by high fever, confusion, rigid muscles, and autonomic imbalance. The management for NMS is stopping the offending agent, rapid cooling, dantrolene, and benzodiazepines.[21] One may also consider supplementing with additional known antiemetics like Decadron, propofol, and scopolamine transdermal patch.

SUMMARY

Anxiety control and patient comfort are integral parts of the OMFS practice. Knowledge of emergency drugs is part of a safe anesthesia practice, which includes proper patient selection, anesthesia technique, drug regimen, monitoring, and emergency preparedness.

This article focuses on describing many of the characteristics and properties of drugs that are helpful in the treatment of anesthetic emergencies in the OMFS office. This list should not be considered mandatory or all-inclusive.

Any OMFS office should be prepared to deal with emergencies. The provider should be cognizant of the drugs discussed in this article. Knowledge of the indication and appropriate use of the drugs described provides a sound basis for the management of adversity that may arise during sedation or anesthesia in an outpatient OMFS office.

CLINICS CARE POINTS

- A list of core emergency drugs includes oxygen, nitroglycerin, aspirin, epinephrine, albuterol, aromatic ammonium, diphenhydramine, and glucose.
- American Association of Oral and Maxillofacial Surgeons Anesthesia committee recommends the oral surgery office maintain supplies of the following medications: vasopressors, corticosteroids, bronchodilators, muscle relaxants, narcotic antagonists, benzodiazepine antagonists, antihistamines, antiarrhythmics, anticholinergics, coronary artery vasodilators, antihypertensives, and drugs for treatment of malignant hyperthermia.
- Triggers for malignant hyperthermia include sevoflurane, isoflurane, desflurane, and succinylcholine.
- Malignant hyperthermia can be treated with dantrolene or Ryanodex.

- Sugammadex can reverse neuromuscular blockade of Rocuronium.
- Naloxone can reverse overdose of fentanyl.
- Flumazenil can reverse overdose of versed.
- Physostigmine can reverse anticholinergic syndrome (emergence delirium) from use of glycopyrrolate.
- Basic life support, advanced cardiovascular life support, and pediatric advanced life support algorithms and guidelines should be routinely reviewed and readily available.

DISCLOSURE

The authors have nothing to disclose.

REFERENCES

1. Perrott DH, Yuen JP, Andresen RV, et al. Office-based ambulatory anesthesia: outcomes of clinical practice of oral and maxillofacial surgeons. J Oral Maxillofac Surg 2003;61:983–95.
2. Coyle TT, Helfrick JF, Gonzalez ML, et al. Office-based ambulatory anesthesia: factors that influence patient satisfaction or dissatisfaction with deep sedation/general anesthesia. J Oral Maxillofac Surg 2005;63:163–72.
3. Rosenberg M. Preparing for medical emergencies: the essential drugs and equipment for the dental office. J Am Dent Assoc 2010;141(Suppl 1):14S–9S.
4. Dym H. Preparing the dental office for medical emergencies. Dent Clin North Am 2008;52:605–8.
5. Dym H. Emergency drugs for the dental office. Dent Clin North Am 2016;60:287–94.
6. Dym H. Oral sedation in the dental office. Dent Clin North Am 2016;60(2):295–307.
7. Anesthesia in outpatient facilities. In: Parameters of care: clinical practice guidelines for oral and maxillofacial surgery (AAOMS ParCare 2012). 5th edition. Rosemont, IL: American Association of Oral and Maxillofacial Surgeons; 2012. p. e31–49.
8. Malamed S. Introduction. In: Malamed S, editor. Medical emergencies in the dental office. 7th edition. St. Louis (MO): Elsevier Mosby; 2015. p. 70–102.
9. Malamed SF. Sedation: a guide to patient management. 6th edition. St. Louis: Mosby; 2010.
10. Haas D. Preparing dental office staff members for emergencies: developing a basic action plan. J Am Dent Assoc 2010;141(Suppl):8S–13S.
11. Kloner RA. Cardiovascular effects of tadalafil. Am J Cardiol 2003;92:37M–46M.
12. Wysowski DK, Farinas E, Swartz L. Comparison of reported and expected deaths in sildenafil (Viagra) users. Am J Cardiol 2002;89:1331–4.
13. Haas DA. Management of medical emergencies in the dental office. Anesth Prog 2006;53:20–4.
14. Malamed SF. Viewpoint: EpiPens: dental necessity or extravagance? Chicago: ADA News; 2016. p. 2.
15. AAAI Board of Directors. The use of epinephrine in the treatment of anaphylaxis. J Allergy Clin Immunol 1994;94:666–8.
16. Hall RE, Malamed SF. Drugs for medical emergencies in the dental office. In: ADA/PDR guide to dental therapeutic. 4th edition. Chicago: ADA Publishing; 2006.
17. Dym H. Stocking the oral surgery office emergency cart. Oral Maxillofac Clin North Am 2001;13:103–18.
18. Zeitler DI. Drugs for treating allergic reactions. Oral Maxillofacial Surg Clin N Am 2001;13:43.
19. Pallasch TJ. This emergency kit belongs in your office. Dent Mange 1976;16:43.
20. American Association of Oral and Maxillofacial Surgeons Committee on Anesthesia. Office anesthesia evaluation manual. 8th edition. Rosemont, IL: The Association; 2012.
21. ClinicalKey, Elsevier. Available at: www.ClinicalKey.com. Accessed October 6, 2020.
22. Becker DE, Haas DA. Management of complications during moderate and deep sedation: respiratory: respiratory and cardiovascular considerations. Anesth Prog 2007;54:59–69.
23. Streeten DH. Corticosteroid therapy. I. Pharmacological properties and principles of corticosteroid use. JAMA 1975;232:944–7.
24. Soliday RK, Conley YP, Henker R, et al. Pseudocholinesterase deficiency: a comprehensive review of genetic acquired and drug influences. AANA J 2010;78:313–20.
25. Silbergleit R, Durkalski V, Lowenstein D, et al. NETT Investigators: intramuscular versus intravenous therapy for prehospital status epilepticus. N Engl J Med 2012;366:591–600.
26. Anderson GD, Saneto RP. Current oral and non-oral routes of antiepileptic drug delivery. Adv Drug Deliv Rec 2012;64:911–8.
27. Wolf P. Acute drug administration in epilepsy: a review CNS. Neurosci Ther 2011;17:442–8.
28. Dahan A, Aarts L, Smith TW, et al. Incidence, reversal, and prevention of opioid-induced respiratory depression. Anesthesiology 2010;112:226–38.
29. Varon J. Treatment of acute severe hypertension: current and newer agents. Drugs 2008;68(3):283–97.
30. Berg RA, Hemphill R, Abella BS, et al. Part 5: adult basic life support: 2010 American Heart Association Guidelines for cardiopulmonary resuscitation and emergency cardiovascular care. Circulation 2010;122:S685–705.
31. Neumar RW, Otto CW, Link MS, et al. Part 8: adult advanced cardiovascular life support: 2010 American Heart Association Guidelines for Cardiopulmonary Resuscitation and Emergency Cardiovascular Care. Circulation 2010;122(suppl 3):S729–67.

Update on Medications for Oral Sedation in the Oral and Maxillofacial Surgery Office

Monica Hanna, DMD*, Peter Chen, DDS, MS, Earl Clarkson, DDS

KEYWORDS

• Anxiolysis • Moderate sedation • Clinical technique • Benzodiazepines

KEY POINTS

- Dental anxiety is a leading cause of postponing dental treatment and can be reduced using oral sedation.
- Effective sedation and pain control are integral components of dental care for the fearful and anxious patient.
- Oral medications used to achieve minimal sedation in adult patients have a wide margin of safety to prevent loss of consciousness.
- Pharmacology of medications commonly used for conscious sedation in dentistry as well as clinical guidelines for administration are highlighted in this article.

INTRODUCTION

Dental anxiety is a leading cause of postponing treatment and/or complete avoidance of professional oral care. A study conducted by the American Dental Association (ADA) in the United States has shown that only 52.3% of adults reported dental visits every 6 months and 15.4% once per year.[1] An estimated 18.2% of children aged 5 to 18 years,[2] 26.5% of adults aged 19 to 64 years, and 16.7% of seniors older than 65 years have untreated caries.[3] Dental anxiety has been cited as a main barrier for patients in seeking needed care: 22% of people forgo their dental care because of fear of the dentist.[4] Ultimately, dental anxiety leads to poor oral health, which leads to a reduced quality of life. Therefore, effective sedation and pain control are integral components of dental care for the fearful and anxious patient.

Anxiety and pain control can be defined as the application of various physical, chemical, and psychological modalities to the prevention and treatment of preoperative, operative, and postoperative patient anxiety and pain to allow dental treatment to occur in a safe and effective manner.[5] A survey conducted in the United States found that 18% of adults would visit the dentist more frequently if they were given a drug to make them less nervous.[6] All patients, regardless of the level of anxiety, ought to receive treatment in a safe and fearless environment.

Pain and anxiety has been managed with anesthesia since the 1840s. Dentistry has continued to build upon the foundation of anesthesia in dentistry and has been instrumental in developing safe and effective sedative and anesthetic techniques. The oral route remains the safest, most established, and most commonly used route of drug administration. The oral route offers the following advantages versus other routes of drug administration:

1. Lower incidence of adverse reactions
2. Decreased severity of adverse reactions

Oral & Maxillofacial Surgery, NYC Health + Hospitals/Woodhull, 760 Broadway, Brooklyn, NY 11206, USA
* Corresponding author.
E-mail address: Mhanna0113@gmail.com

Oral Maxillofacial Surg Clin N Am 34 (2022) 9–19
https://doi.org/10.1016/j.coms.2021.08.008
1042-3699/22/© 2021 Elsevier Inc. All rights reserved.

3. High degree of patient acceptance and compliance
4. Convenience of administration
5. Cost-effectiveness
6. Additional equipment or personnel not required

LEVELS OF SEDATION AND ANALGESIA

The 4 levels of sedation and analgesia describe a drug-induced state of consciousness that occurs along a dose-related continuum. The continuum of analgesia progresses from a high state of consciousness to unconsciousness (**Fig. 1**). **Table 1** summarizes the 4 levels of sedation.[7]

Level 1: Minimal Sedation (Anxiolysis)

Minimal sedation is a drug-induced state during which patients respond normally to verbal commands. Cognitive function and physical coordination may be impaired; however, airway reflexes and ventilatory and cardiovascular functions are unaffected. Patients receive anxiolytic or analgesic drugs for alleviating pain, anxiety, or insomnia.

Level 2: Moderate Sedation/Analgesia

The 2001 Joint Commission replaced the term "conscious sedation" with the new term "moderate sedation and analgesia"; this is a drug-induced depression of consciousness in which patients have purposeful responses to verbal commands with or without light tactile touch. A withdrawal reflex from painful stimuli is not considered a purposeful response. Spontaneous ventilation is adequate with no interventions required to maintain a patent airway, and cardiovascular function is usually maintained.

Level 3: Deep Sedation/Anesthesia

In a state of deep sedation, the patient cannot be easily aroused, but does respond purposefully following repeated or painful stimulation. The patient may lose the ability to independently maintain ventilatory function, so the patient may require assistance in maintaining a patent airway. Spontaneous ventilation also may be inadequate for the patient. Cardiovascular function is usually

maintained, and cardiac monitors should be placed. Deep sedation and analgesia may be delivered by an anesthesiologist or privileged practitioner (ie, oral surgeon, intensivist).

Level 4: General Anesthesia

In general anesthesia, the patient is unarousable even by painful stimulation. The patient often loses the ability to independently maintain ventilatory function and often requires assistance in maintaining a patent airway. Positive pressure ventilation is further required because of depressed spontaneous ventilation or drug-induced neuromuscular function depression. Cardiovascular function may also be impaired.

Anesthesia is delivered by an anesthesiologist and is not in the scope of discussion of this article.

Moderate sedation is the focus of this article, as we outline the drug-induced depression of consciousness. An understanding of the full continuum is necessary because patients may pass through minimal to moderate with oral sedatives and can deepen to deep sedation, requiring awareness and response by the practitioner to protect airway and provide ventilation. The classification of the levels of sedation and anesthesia also helps deliver a uniform level of care, with specific requirements and hospital policy for each level.

METHODS OF ANXIETY AND PAIN CONTROL

Oral medications are suitable for minimal and moderate (conscious) sedation in the dental office. When nitrous oxide/oxygen (N_2O-O_2) is used in combination with sedative agents, levels of anesthesia deeper than minimal sedation can be reached.

Oral medications used to achieve minimal sedation in adult patients have a wide margin of safety to prevent loss of consciousness. The ADA is very specific about the dose of drug used to produce minimal sedation. When the intent is minimal sedation for adults, the appropriate initial dosing of a single enteral drug is no more than the maximum recommended dose (MRD) of a drug that can be prescribed for unmonitored home use.[5] MRD is defined as the maximum US Food and Drug

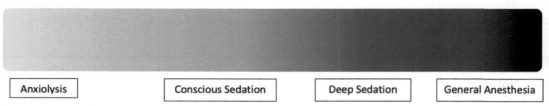

| Anxiolysis | | Conscious Sedation | | Deep Sedation | | General Anesthesia |

Fig. 1. Spectrum of sedation.

Table 1
Continuum of depth of sedation

	Responsiveness	Airway	Spontaneous Ventilation	Cardiovascular Function
Minimal sedation (anxiolysis)	Normal response to verbal stimulation	Unaffected	Unaffected	Unaffected
Moderate sedation/ analgesia	Purposeful response to verbal stimulation or tactile stimulation	No Intervention	Adequate	Usually maintained
Deep sedation	Purposeful response following repeated or painful stimulation	Intervention may be required	May be inadequate	Usually maintained
General anesthesia	Unarousable, even with painful stimulus	Intervention often required	Frequently inadequate	May be impaired

Administration (FDA)-recommended dose of a drug as printed in FDA-approved labeling for un-monitored home use.[8] Incremental and supplemental dosing also apply to minimal sedation. Incremental dosing is the administration of multiple doses of a drug until a desired effect is reached, but not to exceed the MRD. Supplemental dosing is a single additional dose of the initial dose of the initial drug that may be necessary for prolonged procedures, not to exceed one-half of the initial dose, and should not be administered until the dentist has determined the clinical half-life of the initial dosing has passed. The total aggregate dose must not exceed 1.5 times the MRD on the day of treatment.[5] If the administration of enteral drugs exceeds the MRD during a single appointment or if more than one enteral drug is administered to achieve the desired sedation effect, it is considered to be moderate sedation and the moderate sedation guidelines apply.[8]

It is important to emphasize that sedation and general anesthesia are a continuum, therefore, an individual's response may not always be predictable (see **Fig. 1**). Hence, practitioners intending to produce a given level of sedation must be able to rescue patients whose level of sedation becomes deeper than initially intended. Rescue of a patient is an intervention by a practitioner proficient in airway management and advanced life support, correcting adverse physiologic consequences of the deeper-than-intended level of sedation, and returning the patient to the originally intended level of sedation.[9]

EDUCATIONAL REQUIREMENTS

The ADA first developed clinical guidelines, including educational requirements, for the use of sedation in dentistry in 1996 and has been most recently updated in 2016. In the ADA's Policy Statement on the Use of Sedation and General Anesthesia by Dentists, it is stated that:

Dentists who wish to utilize minimal or moderate sedation are expected to successfully complete formal training which is structured in accordance with the Association's *Guidelines for Teaching Pain Control and Sedation to Dentists and Dental Students.* The knowledge and skills required for the administration of deep sedation and general anesthesia are beyond the scope of predoctoral and continuing education. Only dentists who have completed an advanced education program accredited by the Commission on Dental Accreditation (CODA) that provides training in deep sedation and general anesthesia are considered educationally qualified to use these modalities in practice.[10]

The 2016 ADA Clinical Guidelines for the Use of Sedation and General Anesthesia by Dentists state that to administer minimal sedation

1. The dentist must demonstrate competency by having successfully completed[8]:
   a. Training in minimal sedation consistent with that prescribed in the ADA *Guidelines for Teaching Pain Control and Sedation to Dentists and Dental Students*;
      Or
   b. Comprehensive training in moderate sedation that satisfies the requirements described in the Moderate Sedation section of the ADA *Guidelines for Teaching Pain control and Sedation to Dentists and Dental Students* at the time training was commenced;
      Or
   c. An advanced education program accredited by the CODA that affords comprehensive

and appropriate training necessary to administer and manage minimal sedation commensurate with these guidelines; And

d. A current certificate in Basic Life Support (BLS) for Healthcare Providers.

2. Administration of minimal sedation by another qualified dentist or independently practicing qualified anesthesia health care provider requires the operating dentist and his or her clinical staff to maintain current certification in BLS for Healthcare Providers.

The 2016 ADA Clinical Guidelines for the Use of Sedation and General Anesthesia by Dentists state that to administer moderate sedation

1. The dentist must demonstrate competency by having successfully completed[8]:

a. A comprehensive training program in moderate sedation that satisfies the requirements described in the Moderate Sedation section of the ADA *Guidelines for Teaching Pain Control and Sedation to Dentists and Dental Students* at the time training was commenced; Or

b. An advanced education program accredited by the CODA that affords comprehensive and appropriate training necessary to administer and manage moderate sedation commensurate with these guidelines; And

c. A current certificate in BLS for Healthcare Providers and either current certification in Advanced Cardiac Life Support (ACLS) or equivalent or completion of an appropriate dental sedation/anesthesia emergency management course on the same recertification cycle that is required for ACLS

2. Administration of moderate sedation by another qualified dentist or independently practicing qualified anesthesia health care provider requires the operating dentist and his or her clinical staff to maintain current certification in BLS for Healthcare Providers.

Individual state dental boards have the responsibility to ensure that only qualified dentists use sedation and general anesthesia.

PREPROCEDURAL PRACTICES

Before any level of sedation/analgesia administration, the practitioner must evaluate the following parameters.

Patient History and Evaluation

Thorough patient evaluation is critical in determining which patients to consider for any sedative procedure. Several factors need to be taken into consideration including the patient's chief complaint; comprehensive medical, social, and surgical history; complete list of medications, drug, and food allergies; review of systems; comprehensive examination of the maxillofacial region; a detailed physical examination; and appropriate laboratory results.

A focused medical history includes major organ systems, airway; allergies; medications; use of alcohol, tobacco, and recreational drugs; anesthesia and sedation history; and a risk assessment. After proper assessment, the dentist can consider the need for any further testing that may be required before proceeding with sedation.

Assign an American Society of Anesthesiologists Physical Status Score

When examination is complete, the dentist should have the knowledge to assign patients an American Society of Anesthesiologists (ASA) classification and determine the appropriate anesthesia modality (**Table 2**).[5] Patients with significant

Table 2 American Society of Anesthesiologists physical status class	
ASA Score	**Criteria**
ASA 1	Healthy patient without systemic disturbance
ASA 2	Patient with mild to moderate systemic disturbance that results in no functional limitations
ASA 3	Patient with severe systemic disturbance that results in functional limitations
ASA 4	Patient with severe systemic disturbance that is, life threatening with or without planned procedure
ASA 5	Moribund patient not expected to survive with or without the planned procedure
E	Any patient in whom the procedure is emergent

Data from American Dental Association (ADA). Guidelines for teaching pain control and sedation to dentists and dental students. ADA House of Delegates. Chicago: American Dental Association; 2016.

medical considerations (ASA III, IV) may require consultation with their primary care physician or consulting medical specialist before being sedated. In addition, patients with an elevated body mass index are at increased risk for airway-associated morbidity. Ultimately, the clinician must understand their limits based on training, experience, confidence, and ability when making the decision to treat.

Examination of Patient's Airway

Airway patency and spontaneous ventilation remain intact with moderate sedation and analgesia, but a patient receiving moderate sedation/analgesia may unexpectedly progress to deep sedation/analgesia, during which airway obstruction, respiratory depression, and apnea may occur. These adverse events may be predicted and potentially avoided with a focused presedation airway examination.

A simple technique, known as the Mallampati Classification System, predicts the degree of difficulty of endotracheal intubation and should be used in combination with the other elements of airway examination. As the class number increases, the difficulty of intubation increases. For patients to participate in the examination, a Mallampati airway class should be assigned, as described in the following discussion, and documented. Patients should be seated upright with their head in a neutral position. The tongue is protruded maximally without phonation, and the oral cavity is examined and classified as follows:

Class I: Tonsillar pillars easily visualized.
Class II: Entire uvula visualized.
Class III: Only the base of the uvula is visualized.
Class IV: Only the hard palate is visualized.

Verify Appropriate Preprocedural Fasting

Adherence to standards of preprocedure fasting established by the ASA[5] is essential for enhancing the quality and efficiency of patient care and reducing the severity of complications related to pulmonary aspiration of gastric contents should it occur (**Table 3**).

Obtain Informed Consent

The patient or patient's parent or legal representative must be informed of the risks, benefits, and alternatives to the proposed plan for any level of sedation and analgesia. Documentation of informed consent for sedation/analgesia must be in the medical record.

Table 3
American Society of Anesthesiologists fasting guidelines

Ingested Material	Minimum Fasting Period
Clear liquids	2 h
Breast milk	4 h
Infant formula	6 h
Nonhuman milk	6 h
Light meal	6 h
Fatty meal	8 h

Data from American Dental Association (ADA). Guidelines for teaching pain control and sedation to dentists and dental students. ADA House of Delegates. Chicago: American Dental Association; 2016.

Preoperative Evaluation and Preparation

As summarized by the ADA[8]

- The patient, parent, legal guardian, or caregiver must be advised regarding the procedure associated with the delivery of any sedative agents, and informed consent for the proposed sedation must be obtained.
- Determination of adequate oxygen supply and equipment necessary to deliver oxygen under positive pressure must be completed.
- An appropriate focused physical evaluation should be performed.
- Baseline vital signs including body weight, height, blood pressure (BP), pulse rate, and respiration rate must be obtained unless invalidated by the nature of the patient, procedure, or equipment. Body temperature should be measured when clinically indicated.
- Preoperative dietary restrictions must be considered based on the sedative technique prescribed.
- Preoperative verbal and written instructions must be given to the patient, parent, escort, legal guardian, or caregiver.

In addition to the aforementioned practices, the practitioner must have proper documentation of a plan for sedation and analgesia and must assure that the patient has an appropriate escort for outpatients.

CLINICAL GUIDELINES
Personnel and Equipment Requirements

- At least one other person trained in BLS for Healthcare Providers must be present in addition to the dentist.[8]
- A positive pressure oxygen delivery system suitable for the patient being treated must be immediately available.

- Documentation of compliance with manufacturers' recommended maintenance of monitors, anesthesia delivery systems, and other anesthesia-related equipment should be maintained. A preprocedural check of equipment for each administration of sedation must be performed.
- When inhalation equipment is used, it must have a fail-safe system that is appropriately checked and calibrated. The equipment must also have either a functioning device that prohibits the delivery of less than 30% oxygen or an appropriately calibrated and functioning in-line oxygen analyzer with audible alarm.
- An appropriate scavenging system must be available if gases other than oxygen or air are used.
- In addition, for moderate sedation
  - The equipment necessary for monitoring end-tidal CO_2 and auscultation of breath sounds must be immediately available
  - The equipment necessary to establish intravascular (IV) or intraosseous access should be available until the patient meets discharge criteria

Minimal Sedation Monitoring and Documentation

- A dentist, or at a dentist's direction, an appropriately trained individual, must remain in the operatory during active dental treatment to monitor the patient continuously until the patient meets discharge criteria.
- Monitoring must include
  - Consciousness: Level of sedation
  - Oxygenation: Oxygen saturation by pulse oximetry
  - Ventilation: Chest excursions must be observed and respirations must be verified
  - Circulation: BP and heart rate (HR) must be evaluated preoperatively, intraoperatively, and postoperatively
- An appropriate sedative record must be maintained including all drugs administered, time administered, and route of administration, including local anesthetics, dosages, and monitored physiologic parameters.

Moderate Sedation Monitoring and Documentation

- A qualified dentist administering moderate sedation must remain in the operatory room to monitor the patient continuously until the patient meets recovery criteria. When the patient recovers to a minimally sedated level, a qualified auxiliary may be directed by the dentist to remain with the patient and continue monitoring until the patient meets discharge criteria. Furthermore, the dentist must remain in the facility at all times until the patient is discharged.
- Monitoring must include consciousness, oxygenation, ventilation, and circulation as performed for minimal sedation with the following additions:
  - Ventilation: The dentist must monitor ventilation by monitoring end-tidal CO_2 as well as continual observation of qualitative signs, including auscultation of breath sounds with a precordial or pretracheal stethoscope.
  - Circulation: Continuous electrocardiographic monitoring of patients with cardiovascular disease should be considered.
- Documentation includes an appropriate time-oriented anesthetic record as with minimal sedation with additions of continual recording of pulse oximetry, BP, HR, respiratory rate, and level of consciousness.

Recovery and Discharge

- Oxygen and suction equipment must be immediately available if a separate recovery area is used.
- The qualified dentist or appropriately trained clinical staff must continually monitor the patient during recovery until the patient is ready for discharge by the dentist.
- The qualified dentist must determine and document that level of consciousness, oxygenation, ventilation, and circulation are satisfactory for discharge.
- Postoperative verbal and written instructions must be given to the patient, parent, escort, legal guardian, or caregiver.
- If a pharmacologic reversal agent is administered before discharge criteria have been met, the patient must be monitored for a longer period than usual before discharge, because resedation may occur once the effects of the reversal agent have waned.

Emergency Management

- If a patient enters a deeper level of sedation than the dentist is qualified to provide, the dentist must stop the procedure until the patient is returned to the intended level of sedation.
- The qualified dentist is responsible for the sedative management, adequacy of the faculty and staff, diagnosis and treatment of

emergencies related to the administration of minimal or moderate sedation, and providing the equipment, drugs, and protocol for patient rescue.

ADMINISTRATION OF ORAL ANXIOLYTICS

Oral anxiolytics are administered according to several factors, including level of patient anxiety, intended sedation level, type and length of procedure, and state regulations. If indicated, the cooperative adult can be prescribed oral medication to be taken at bedtime the night before a procedure to promote stress-free rest. A single dose is then taken typically 1 hour before the procedure, in which case a responsible adult must escort the patient to the dental office. To ensure proper dosage and time of administration, the dentist may choose to administer the dose in the dental office under constant supervision approximately 1 hour before the start of the procedure. About 45 minutes after administration, the dentist should evaluate the comfort level of the patient and efficacy of the medication and make a clinical decision on when to proceed with treatment.

If N_2O-O_2 is administered in conjunction with sedative agents, it must be carefully titrated to the desired level of sedation throughout the procedure. Vital signs are continuously monitored and recorded every 5 minutes on the anesthesia-sedation record. On termination of N_2O-O_2, 100% oxygen should be administered to the patient for a minimum of 5 minutes and recovery should be assessed. Postoperative vital signs must be documented. If the patient is deemed stable for discharge, postoperative instructions must be given as outlined earlier according to ADA guidelines.

CONSIDERATIONS FOR ORAL MODERATE SEDATION ADMINISTRATION

When planning for oral moderate sedation, all plans of drug delivery should always be individualized for the patient. Furthermore, the technique of titration in small increments should always be applied when possible. The dose of any sedative should also be reduced 25% to 50% when combined with other sedatives/narcotics, if the patient is elderly or disabled, or the patient has severe major organ disease (cardiac, pulmonary, cerebral, hepatic, or renal). The practitioner should be well versed in each drug's safe and effective use, along with all the possible complications (**Table 4**). When planning for only moderate sedation, medications that have a high risk of producing deep sedation (ie, propofol) should be avoided.

Analgesic (Fentanyl Citrate)

Fentanyl citrate (Sublimaze) is the choice analgesic for moderate sedation. Other opioids, like morphine, hydromorphone, and meperidine, are not recommended for moderate sedation. Fentanyl is a short-acting narcotic/opioid analgesic for management of perioperative pain with no amnesic effect. This is a choice analgesic in patients with allergy to morphine or other narcotic/opioid analgesics. Fentanyl comes in both IV and oral routes, and may not be the first choice oral sedation, but provides a pediatric oral moderate sedation alternative. Initial adult dose is 25 to 100 µg given slowly over 3 minutes into an infusing line, followed with 25-µg increments while monitoring effects until desired analgesia is achieved, with the total dose not exceeding 200 µg in most cases.[11] Initial pediatric IV initial dose is 0.25 to 1 µg/kg given slowly over 3 minutes IV infusion; additional doses in 0.25- to 0.5-µg/kg increments may be given accordingly with a total dose not exceeding 3 µg/kg. Pediatric oral dose is 10 to 15 µg/kg given orally as Fentanyl Oralet, with an onset time of 15 to 20 minutes. The following are the adverse effects that should be considered:

- Hypoventilation and apnea, which may be further potentiated with other central nervous system (CNS) depressants (ie, benzodiazepines) and are reversible with naloxone (Narcan)
- Muscle rigidity, especially at higher doses and rapid infusion
- Bradycardia and hypotension
- Nausea and vomiting

Sedative Benzodiazepines

Benzodiazepines are the choice drugs for oral sedation and have a high margin of safety allowing patients to maintain their airway. Benzodiazepines are sedatives, anxiolytic, induce sleep, and prevent seizures.[11] Benzodiazepines act by facilitating the physiologic inhibitory effects of γ-aminobutyric acid (GABA), the major inhibitory neurotransmitter in the brain,[12] and have a high therapeutic index (ratio of the toxic dose of a drug to its therapeutic dose). Their high margin of safety makes them advantageous to use when compared with other classes of sedatives. Common benzodiazepines include midazolam, triazolam, diazepam, lorazepam, and alprazolam.

The most widely used premedication oral sedative is diazepam, and the most common perioperative oral sedative for conscious sedation is midazolam. Chloral hydrate and pentobarbital are oral sedatives for conscious sedations, included

Table 4
Moderate sedation analgesics and sedatives for adult dosing

	Recommended Dose	Indication/Advantages	Contraindications/Caution
Benzodiazepines			
Diazepam (Valium)	Adult oral: 5–10 mg 1 h before	Choice premedication sedative/anxiolytic	Contraindicated in patients with narrow-angle glaucoma
Midazolam (Versed)	Adult IV: 0.5–3 mg over 3 min, with 0.5–1 mg increments, total 5 mg Pediatric IV: 0.05 mg/kg over 3 min, 0.05 mg/kg increments, total 0.2 mg/kg Adult and pediatric oral dose: 0.5–0.75 mg/kg with 10- to 20-min onset	Choice benzodiazepine for moderate sedation Reversal agent: Flumazenil	Hypoventilation and apnea Vertigo and dizziness
Lorazepam (Ativan)	Adult oral: 2–4 mg 1–2 h before	Seldom used over Valium	Contraindicated in patients with narrow-angle glaucoma Caution in patients with depressive disorder or psychosis
Aprazolam (Xanax)	Adult oral: 0.25–1 mg	Indicated for panic-type anxiety	Contraindicated in patients with narrow-angle glaucoma Caution in patients on CYP34A inhibitors
Triazolam (Halcion)	Adult oral: 0.25–0.5 mg 1 h before (30 min prior for sublingual)	Available in sublingual route	Contraindicated in pregnancy (class X)
Oxazepam (Serax)	Adult oral: 10–30 µg 1 h prior	Indicated for short-term anxiety Lower incidence of drowsiness	
Analgesics			
Fentanyl citrate (Sublimaze)	Adult IV: 25–100 µg over 3 min, then 25-µg increments, total 200 µg Pediatric IV: 0.25–1 µg/kg over 3 min, then 0.25- to 0.5-µg/kg increments, total 3 µg/kg Pediatric oral: 10–15 µg/kg (onset 15–20 min)	Choice analgesic, especially for patient with morphine or narcotic/opioid allergy	Hypoventilation Apnea Muscle rigidity (especially rapid infusion) Bradycardia Hypotension Nausea/vomiting
Nonbenzodiazepines			
Zolpidem (Ambien)	5 mg oral	Safe for pregnant	Caution respiratory depression
Zaleplon (Sonata)	5–10 mg oral	Similar to Zolpidem (except caution pregnant)	Caution hypersensitivity, impaired hepatic function, elderly, and pregnant

in the scope of the article, but more commonly reserved for diagnostic imaging.

Midazolam hydrochloride (Versed) is used in both adult and pediatric patients for sedation, anxiolysis, and amnesia. Chloral hydrate and pentobarbital are other alternatives for pediatric patients but are not recommended for moderate sedation, because they are not reversible. All 3 are sedative with no analgesic effect. Versed is a short-acting benzodiazepine that acts as a CNS depressant, anticonvulsant, and muscle relaxant. Versed comes in both IV and oral routes and is the choice oral sedative in moderate sedation. The adult IV dose is 0.5 to 3 mg given slowly over 3 minutes as IV infusion, with 0.5- to 1-mg increments, with total dose not to exceed 5 mg.

The pediatric IV dose is 0.05 mg/kg slowly over 3 minutes as IV infusion, with 0.05 mg/kg increments every 3 minutes, with total dose not exceeding 0.2 mg/kg. The oral dose is 0.5 to 0.75 mg/kg orally with 10 to 20 minutes onset.[12] Adverse effects include

- Hypoventilation and apnea, which may be potentiated by narcotic/opioids, alcohol, and other CNS depressants, especially with rapid injection, but are reversible with flumazenil
- Vertigo and dizziness

Diazepam (Valium) is an effective oral sedative and anxiolytic with a 1-hour onset time and is the most commonly prescribed before patient arrival. The recommended dose is 5 to 10 mg as an anxiolytic 1 hour before treatment, with availability as tablet (2 mg, 5 mg, and 10 mg) or suspension (10 mg/5 mL). Diazepam, Lorazepam, and Alprazolam are contraindicated in patients with narrowangle glaucoma.

Lorazepam (Ativan) is another oral benzodiazepine but has a longer onset of 1 to 2 hours. The recommended dose is 2 to 4 mg administered 1 to 2 hours before treatment.[12] Caution must be applied to not oversedate patients with a depressive disorder or psychosis. Adverse effects include sedation, dizziness, weakness, and ataxia.

Alprazolam (Xanax) is another oral anxiolytic benzodiazepine, with indication for patients with panic-type anxiety. Caution should be exercised for oversedation when patients are concurrently on cytochrome P (CYP) 34A inhibitors. The recommended oral dose is 0.25 to 1 mg.[12]

Triazolam (Halcion) is another benzodiazepine available in oral and sublingual forms, with a 1-hour and 30-minute onset, respectively. The initial dose is 0.25 to 0.5 mg.[12] Triazolam is contraindicated in the pregnant patient with a pregnancy classification of X.

Oxazepam (Serax) is a benzodiazepine for short-term anxiety given its rapid onset, short elimination half-life, no active metabolites, not affected by the CYP system, and lower incidence of drowsiness. The recommended initial dose of oxazepam is 10 to 30 mg 1 hour before treatment.[12]

Nonbenzodiazepines (Ambien and Zaleplon)

Nonbenzodiazepines have also been used as adjuncts to oral moderate sedation that provide similar but less profound pharmacologic effects of benzodiazepines. The most common are the sedative/hypnotics, Zolpidem (Ambien) and Zaleplon (Sonata), which are GABA receptor alpha-1 subunit agonists producing sedation and amnesia.

Zolpidem is the drug of choice for pregnant patients and has been proved to be effective in inducing and maintaining sleep in adults, with properties of gastrointestinal tract rapid absorption onset of 1 hour and peak effect in 1.6 hours.[13] Caution with Zolpidem includes risk of further respiratory depression especially in patients with compromised respiratory function. Recommended initial dose is 5 mg.

Zaleplon (Sonata) is similar pharmacologically and pharmacokinetically but has slightly higher caution in patients with imidazopyridine hypersensitivity and impaired hepatic function and the elderly and pregnant patient.[12] Initial adult oral dosing is 5 to 10 mg.

Antagonists (Naloxone and Flumazenil)

The moderate sedation plan that includes analgesics (fentanyl) and sedatives (midazolam) must always include the antagonist dosing as well (**Table 5**). Naloxone (Narcan) is a narcotic/opioid antagonist used for reversal of respiratory depression and hypotension. The adult initial dose is 0.05 to 0.2 mg by rapid IV push and repeated every minute until respiratory depression or apnea is reversed, with a maximal dose of 0.8 mg.[14] The pediatric initial dose is 0.01 to 0.1 mg/kg via rapid IV push, until reversal, with a maximal dose of 0.8 mg.[14] Special care must be considered with naloxone delivery to patients with cardiac disease or known opioid tolerance and hence should follow small incremental dosing. Naloxone also has a shorter duration of action than some narcotics/opioids and hence requires observation for up to 2 hours from the last dose and may require readministration after 30 to 60 minutes. Known adverse effects of naloxone include pain leading to tachycardia, myocardial ischemia, and pulmonary edema, especially in elderly patients if reversal is abrupt. Adverse effects also include

Table 5
Antagonist for reversal of sedative/analgesic agents

Naloxone (Narcan)	Adult initial dose: 0.05– 0.2 mg rapid IV push, repeat every minute PRN, maximum dose 0.8 mg	May require readministration after 30–60 min due to shorter duration of action	Tachycardia, MI, PE, especially in elderly patients if rapid reversal
Flumazenil (Romazicon)	Adult initial dose: 0.2 mg rapid IV push, repeat every minute PRN, maximum dose 1.0 mg	May require readministration after 20 min	Seizure, blurred vision, dizziness, dysrhythmias, excitement, agitation, anxiety confusion, incomplete reversal of amnesia, withdrawal symptoms

MI, Myocardial Infarction; PE, Pulmonary Edema; PRN, as needed.

withdrawal symptoms in patients chronically receiving narcotic/opioid analgesics, which may present as tremors, nausea, vomiting excitement, sweating, and hypertension.

Flumazenil (Romazicon) is a benzodiazepine antagonist used for reversal of the sedative and respiratory depressant effects. Adult initial dose is 0.2 mg given by rapid IV push, and repeated as needed every 1 minute, with a maximal dose of 1 mg. Pediatric initial dose is 0.1 mg as rapid IV push, and repeated every 1 minute as needed, with a maximal dose of 1 mg.[14] Flumazenil is contraindicated in patients who take benzodiazepines for seizure control, which may be life threatening. Further care for withdrawal symptoms should also be monitored while administering flumazenil. Flumazenil also has shorter duration of action than some benzodiazepines, so special care should be taken, including observation for up to 2 hours after last administered dose, and readministration of flumazenil might be necessary after 20 minutes. Adverse side effects of flumazenil include the following:

- Seizures, especially for patients with seizure disorders
- Blurred vision
- Dizziness
- Dysrhythmias
- Excitement, agitation anxiety, confusion
- Incomplete and inconsistent reversal of amnesia
- Withdrawal symptoms in patients on chronic benzodiazepines: tremors, sweating, hypertension, abdominal discomfort, seizures

SUMMARY

The application of oral sedation aids the trained practitioner to provide care to the anxious dental patient. Proper training and understanding of pharmacologic properties allow for safe and effective application of analgesics and sedatives for oral sedation. Midazolam and diazepam are well-established safe medications for oral sedation, with a predictable antagonist in emergency situations.

CLINICS CARE POINTS

- Sedation and general anesthesia are a continuum, therefore an individual's response may not always be predictable.
- Practitioners intending to produce a given level of sedation must be able to rescue patients whose level of sedation becomes deeper than initially intended.
- When planning for oral moderate sedation, all plans of drug delivery should always be individualized for the patient. The practitioner should also be well versed in each drug's safe and effective use, along with all the possible complications.
- Benzodiazepines are the choice drugs for oral sedation and have a high margin of safety allowing patients to maintain their airway.
- Midazolam and diazepam are well-established safe medications for oral sedation, with a predictable antagonist in emergency situations.

DISCLOSURE

The authors have nothing to disclose.

REFERENCES

1. Yarbrough C, Nasseh K, et al. Key differences in dental care seeking behavior between medicaid and non-medicaid adults and children 2014. Available at: https://www.ada.org/~/media/ADA/Science%20and%20Research/HPI/Files/HPIBrief_0814_4.pdf?la=en.
2. American Dental Association (ADA). Untreated caries rates falling among low-income children. Available at: https://www.ada.org/~/media/ADA/Science%20and%20Research/HPI/Files/HPIgraphic_0617_2.pdf?la=en.
3. American Dental Association (ADA). Racial disparities in untreated caries narrowing for children. Available at: https://www.ada.org/~/media/ADA/Science%20and%20Research/HPI/Files/HPIGraphic_0617_1.pdf?la=en.
4. American Dental Association (ADA). Oral health and well-being in the United States (Rep.). Available at: https://www.ada.org/en/science-research/health-policy-institute/oral-health-and-well-being.
5. American Dental Association (ADA). Guidelines for teaching pain control and sedation to dentists and dental students. ADA House of Delegates. Chicago: American Dental Association; 2016.
6. Smith TA, Thomas M. *The relation between mood and reported dental fear and attendance* (abstract 2044). J Dent Res 1998;77:887.
7. American Society of Anesthesiologists (ASA). Continuum of depth of sedation: definition of general anesthesia and levels of sedation/analgesia 2019. Available at: https://www.asahq.org/standards-and-guidelines/continuum-of-depth-of-sedation-definition-of-general-anesthesia-and-levels-of-sedationanalgesia.
8. American Dental Association (ADA). Guidelines for the use of sedation and general anesthesia by dentists. ADA House of Delegates. Chicago: American Dental Association; 2016.
9. American Association of Oral and Maxillofacial Surgeons (AAOMS). Parameters and pathways: clinical practice guidelines for oral and maxillofacial surgery (AAOMS ParPath o1) anesthesia in outpatient facilities. Available at: https://www.aaoms.org/images/uploads/pdfs/parcare_anesthesia.pdf.
10. American Dental Association (ADA). Policy statement: the use of sedation and general anesthesia by dentists. ADA House of Delegates. Chicago: American Dental Association; 2007.
11. Donaldson M, Gizzarelli G, Chanpong B. Oral Sedation: A Primer on Anxiolysis for the Adult Patient. Anesth Prog 2007;54(3):118–29.
12. Malamed SF. Sedation: a guide to patient management. 5th edition. St Louis (MO): Mosby; 2009.
13. Giovannitti JA, Trapp LD. Adult sedation: oral, rectal, IM, IV. Anesth Prog 1991;38(4–5):154–71.
14. Goodchild JH, Feck AS, Silverman MD. Anxiolysis in general dental practice. Dent Today 2003;22(3):106–11.

A Review of Sedation Agents

Hillel Ephros, DMD, MD[a],*, Sneha Shah, DMD[a], Robert J. Herrod, DMD[a,b]

KEYWORDS

- Sedation • Anxiolysis • Benzodiazepine • Opioid • Dissociative anesthesia • Titration

KEY POINTS

- Each of the agents used to produce sedation and/or general anesthesia has a pharmacologic profile that must be understood by the clinician.
- Initial dosing, titration, maintaining a desirable level of sedation, termination of the anesthetic event, and recovery vary by agent.
- A balanced anesthesia technique involves using more than one of these agents to lower doses, reduce drug-specific toxicity, and to meet the needs of the procedure.
- Patient safety and successful sedation are achieved by thorough preanesthetic evaluation, proper patient selection, and appropriate use of these agents.

MIDAZOLAM

Midazolam (Versed) is among the most widely used hypnotic sedatives for procedural sedation. It is a short-acting benzodiazepine with a structural formula of $C_{18}H_{13}ClFN_3$ (**Fig 1**). It consists of a benzene ring and an imidazole ring that closes at physiologic pH, increasing its lipid solubility.[1] Midazolam is a white crystalline compound that is insoluble in water. HCl is added to midazolam to create the acidic environment required to solubilize midazolam in aqueous solutions for storage.[2] Midazolam is most commonly titrated intravenously in the oral and maxillofacial surgeon's office, but it can also be administered orally, nasally, and intramuscularly.

Clinical Pharmacology

Benzodiazepines are gamma aminobutyric acid (GABA) receptor agonists that increase the affinity of these receptors for the GABA ligand. This in turn results in an increase in the frequency with which the chloride channels open, allowing intracellular influx of chloride ions. The influx of chloride ions hyperpolarizes postsynaptic neurons, inhibiting their ability to produce an action potential.[3] Similar to fentanyl, midazolam is metabolized by the CYP3A4 enzyme in the liver and intestines into water-soluble, glucuronidated end products and is excreted principally in urine.[1]

Indications and Usage

Outside of the operating room, labeled indications include sedation, anxiolysis, and amnesia. Midazolam is indicated for the initiation of general anesthesia before the administration of any other medications, as well as maintenance of anesthesia as a component of a balanced anesthesia technique.[2]

Dosage and Administration

When used in conjunction with other medications in a balanced anesthetic technique, midazolam is typically administered up to a 0.05 to 0.10 mg/kg dose, which is divided up into smaller boluses titrated to effect. Additional 0.5 mg to 1 mg boluses can be given intermittently to ensure adequate sedation for the duration of the procedure.[2]

[a] Department of Oral & Maxillofacial Surgery, St. Joseph's University Medical Center, 703 Main Street, Paterson, NJ 07503, USA; [b] Private Practice, 50 E. Main Street, Little Falls, NJ 07424, USA
* Corresponding author.
E-mail address: ephrosh@sjhmc.org

Oral Maxillofacial Surg Clin N Am 34 (2022) 21–34
https://doi.org/10.1016/j.coms.2021.09.001
1042-3699/22/

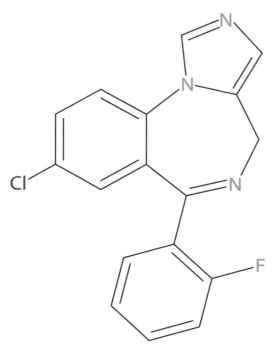

Fig. 1. Midazolam.

Contraindications

Fortunately, the contraindications for the use of midazolam are limited to patients with known hypersensitivities, acute narrow-angle glaucoma, hypotension, and shock.[2,4]

Warnings and Precautions

As other sedatives, midazolam, classified as a controlled substance IV, can cause central nervous system (CNS) depression, cardiovascular and respiratory depression, and obstructive and central apnea. Individualized anesthetic plans should be devised for each patient. Clinical vigilance is required along with the application of all indicated monitoring devices so that the patient can be monitored throughout the procedure and until full recovery. An oxygen source, resuscitative medications, appropriate bag-valve-mask, and advanced airway equipment should be easily accessible in case an airway or cardiovascular event occurs.[2]

Adverse Reactions

The most common adverse reactions to midazolam include hiccups, coughing, nausea, vomiting, thrombophlebitis, thrombosis, disinhibition, respiratory depression, hypotension, tachycardia, and pain on injection.[4]

Drug Interactions

Midazolam should be avoided or subject to dose modification for patients taking other CNS depressants. Midazolam is metabolized by CYP3A4 enzymes, so concurrent use of CYP3A4 inhibitors such as diltiazem, verapamil, erythromycin, and cimetidine can lead to prolonged sedation. Although these agents and others that have gained attention, such as grapefruit juice, may lead to increased blood levels of midazolam, the clinical significance is likely minimized when the drug is used intravenously with careful titration to the desired level of sedation.[2]

Use in Specific Populations

Midazolam carries a Food and Drug Administration (FDA) risk factor "D" for pregnant patients. Chronic benzodiazepine use should be avoided in pregnant patients, as a correlation with increased incidence of cleft palate, CNS defects, and dysmorphism exists in the current literature.[3] Although studies suggest that a single dose is unlikely to produce harm, benzodiazepine administration during the second and third trimesters has been shown to be associated with neonatal withdrawal syndrome and floppy infant syndrome.[2]

Nursing mothers have historically been advised to stop breast feeding for 24 hours following administration of benzodiazepines. However, more recent data have shown that this is not necessary.[5,6] In 2019, the American Society of Anesthesiologist's Committee on Obstetric Anesthesia published a recommendation for nursing patients to resume breastfeeding following administration of anesthesia, because the anesthetic agents used are excreted in breast milk at only very low levels.[7]

As with other sedation medications, consideration for decreased dosing should be made for geriatric patients, as they tend to have higher peak plasma concentrations of benzodiazepines than nongeriatric patients.[2]

Accumulation of midazolam and its active metabolites can occur in patients with renal and hepatic impairment, leading to excessive sedation and toxic accumulation. An assessment of kidney and liver function must be performed in patients with a history that warrants such investigation. A dose reduction of 50% is required for patients whose glomerular filtration rate has dropped less than 10 mL/min or if the patient is on dialysis.[3]

How Supplied/Storage and Handling

Intravenous (IV) midazolam comes in 2 dosage forms: 1 mg/mL and 5 mg/mL. The investigators strongly suggest limiting the oral and maxillofacial surgery office stock to one dosage or the other to avoid medication errors. Most will choose the 1 mg/mL formulation that requires no dilution and facilitates ease of titration by the IV route. The oral form of midazolam comes in a 2 mg/mL concentration. Alternatively, the IV form can be mixed with juice to the appropriate dose and administered orally. These ampules are stored at room temperature.[2]

Utility, Risks, and Benefits in Oral and Maxillofacial Surgical Practice

Midazolam has numerous benefits with minimal risks, making it an ideal medication for ambulatory anesthesia. These benefits include its sedative, amnestic, anxiolytic, central muscle relaxant, and anticonvulsant properties. Midazolam has modest dose-dependent hemodynamic and respiratory effects.[3] Its innovative structure allows it to be packaged and administered as an aqueous solution that attains lipid solubility on entering the bloodstream. As such, the incidence of phlebitis/thrombophlebitis at the IV site is significantly lower than with diazepam, the benzodiazepine that was widely used in oral and maxillofacial surgery before the release of midazolam in the early 1980s.

Midazolam is an excellent agent for use in combination with an opioid such as fentanyl. A balanced anesthesia approach using these two drugs may reduce the dose requirement for each and may allow overlapping effects such as sedation to be enhanced synergistically while limiting drug-specific toxicities. In addition, the specific benefits of each of the agents, midazolam's anxiolysis and amnesia and the analgesia and euphoria associated with fentanyl, are likely to combine well, producing a balanced and successful procedural sedation.

Among the significant benefits offered by midazolam is the availability of a specific reversal agent. Although the need for reversal is mitigated by the appropriate use of midazolam, particularly when carefully titrated via the IV route as described, the existence of flumazenil adds to the safety of midazolam and the clinician's comfort with its use in the ambulatory setting.

FENTANYL

Fentanyl was invented in Belgium in the 1950s by Dr Paul Janssen out of an interest in developing an opioid that was more effective than those that were in use at that time. Janssen surmised that he might be able to increase the lipid solubility of meperidine to create a more effective opioid analgesic. Over the next couple of years, he developed fentanyl.[8] Today, fentanyl (Sublimaze) is the opioid of choice in many oral and maxillofacial surgery offices, playing an important role in balanced ambulatory anesthesia. Fentanyl is an opioid receptor agonist that has a potency approximately 100 times that of morphine for its analgesic and sedative properties.[9] Fentanyl's molecular formula is $C_{22}H_{28}N_2O$ (**Fig. 2**).[10] Routes of fentanyl administration include IV, intramuscular, intrathecal, epidural, transmucosal, and transdermal.

Clinical Pharmacology

Fentanyl is a μ-opioid receptor agonist that inhibits the presynaptic release and postsynaptic response to excitatory neurotransmitters such as substance P and acetylcholine.[1] IV fentanyl has roughly a 20- to 30-second onset of action with a duration of 20 to 30 minutes. It is rapidly metabolized to inactive end products in the liver by CYP3A4 through dealkylation and hydroxylation.[3] Fentanyl is primarily eliminated in the urine, and approximately 10% undergoes biliary excretion.[1]

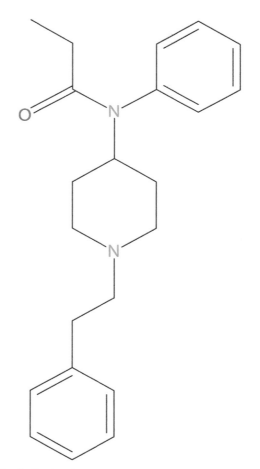

Fig. 2. Fentanyl.

Indications and Usage

Fentanyl is currently FDA approved for perioperative analgesia, as an adjunct to general or regional anesthetics, and for pain management.[10]

Dosage and Administration

There are many different algorithms for which oral and maxillofacial surgeons can use fentanyl in a balanced anesthetic technique. At the author's institution, an initial loading dose of fentanyl of 0.5 to 1 mcg/kg is given followed by incremental 25 mcg to 50 mcg boluses titrated to effect.

Contraindications

Contraindications for the use of fentanyl are generally only limited to patients with hypersensitivity.[10]

Warnings and Precautions

Fentanyl, classified as a controlled substance II/IIN, can cause CNS depression, dose-dependent respiratory depression, cardiovascular depression, and serotonin syndrome. Individualized anesthetic plans should be devised for each patient. Clinical vigilance is required along with the application of all indicated monitoring devices so that the patient can be monitored throughout the procedure and until full recovery. An oxygen source, resuscitative medications, appropriate bag-valve-mask, and advanced airway equipment should be easily accessible in case an airway or cardiovascular event occurs.[10]

Adverse Reactions

The most common adverse reactions include hypertension, hypotension, dizziness, blurred vision, nausea, emesis, diaphoresis, pruritus, urticaria, laryngospasm, anaphylaxis, respiratory depression, apnea, rigidity, and bradycardia.[10] Chest wall rigidity is a feared complication of administration of fentanyl and is related to the dose and speed of administration. Cases of chest wall rigidity have even been reported with doses as little as 50 mcg intravenously.[9]

Drug Interactions

Fentanyl should be avoided in patients who are taking medications that elevate serotonin levels, such as monoamine oxidase inhibitors, serotonin reuptake inhibitors, and linezolid. Dose reduction should be considered in those taking CYP3A4 inhibitors.[10] Use of fentanyl in patients who are taking serotonergic agents can lead to serotonin syndrome, with a range of symptoms including agitation, confusion, tachycardia, muscular twitching or rigidity, shivering, hyperpyrexia, dysrhythmias, and seizures.[3,11]

Use in Specific Populations

Fentanyl is a pregnancy category C drug; however, it is generally advisable to avoid elective procedures under anesthesia for pregnant patients. Historically, it has been recommended that breastfeeding patients pump and discard for 24 hours following anesthesia. However, several studies have shown clinically insignificant amounts of fentanyl in breast milk following its administration, suggesting that cessation of breastfeeding may be unwarranted.[6] Nursing patients may resume breastfeeding in the postoperative period once they are awake and alert, as long as the administered dose of fentanyl is within recommended dosing parameters.[5] The American Society of Anesthesiologists currently recommends lowering the dosage of or avoiding fentanyl in lactating patients; however, the American Society of Anesthesiologists does not recommend counseling patients to "pump and dump," following administration of anesthesia.

When using in geriatric patients, doses of fentanyl should be decreased and titrated slowly while closely monitoring for respiratory and CNS depression.

For patients with renal impairment, dose adjustments are not needed until the glomerular filtration rate becomes less than 50 mL/min. For patients whose glomerular filtration rate (GFR) is 10 to 50 mL/min, doses should be decreased to approximately 75% of the typical dose. If the GFR drops to less than 10 mL/min, the dose should be decreased to 50% the usual dose.[3]

The metabolism of a single dose of fentanyl is believed to be relatively unchanged in patients with liver failure. However, elimination is likely prolonged in patients with severe liver disease. As such, typical initial doses can be given, but caution should be exercised in administering repeat doses to prevent toxic accumulation.[12]

How Supplied/Storage and Handling

Fentanyl is currently available only as a 50 mcg/mL solution in various ampule volumes including 2 mL, 5 mL, 10 mL, and 20 mL. These ampules are stored away from light and at room temperature.[10]

Utility, Risks, and Benefits in Oral and Maxillofacial Surgical Practice

In addition to its anesthetic and analgesic properties, fentanyl offers a variety of advantages when used in the office-based ambulatory setting. When providing open airway anesthesia, as is commonly done in the practice of oral and maxillo-facial surgery, fentanyl's ability to blunt the cough reflex and attenuate a hyperactive airway may be of substantial value. Fentanyl also has the added benefit of being relatively inexpensive compared with other available opioids. Undesirable effects of fentanyl include an increase in incidence of postoperative nausea and vomiting (PONV).[3] Liberal use of opioids should be avoided for patients with a reported history of prior postanesthetic nausea, motion sickness, and other known risk factors for PONV. Prophylactic measures to prevent this unpleasant complication such as fluid boluses and administration of IV dexamethasone or other antiemetic medications should be considered when planning to use fentanyl for at-risk patients. Risk assessment for PONV should be part of the preanesthetic workup for all patients being evaluated for ambulatory anesthesia.

As with midazolam, fentanyl has an effective and readily available reversal agent, naloxone. Naloxone should be used only when indicated, and in such cases, the patient should be monitored carefully for signs of renarcotization. When reversal becomes necessary during a balanced anesthesia technique with both midazolam and fentanyl, a quick but careful evaluation of the patient's condition should lead to the correct choice of reversal agent. Both flumazenil and naloxone must be in the emergency kits of oral and maxillo-facial surgeons who are using midazolam and fentanyl, and reversal protocols should be well known or readily accessible.

PROPOFOL

Propofol (Diprivan) is a general anesthetic inductive agent that is speculated to allosterically increase binding affinity of GABA for $GABA_A$; this promotes hyperpolarization of nerve membranes and exerts neuroinhibitory effects within the reticular activating system of the brainstem. It structurally consists of a phenol ring substituted with two isopropyl groups with chemical formula $C_{12}H_{18}O$ (**Fig. 3**). Propofol is available for IV injection in a 10 mg/mL oil-in-water nonpyrogenic emulsion, which often causes pain during injection.[1]

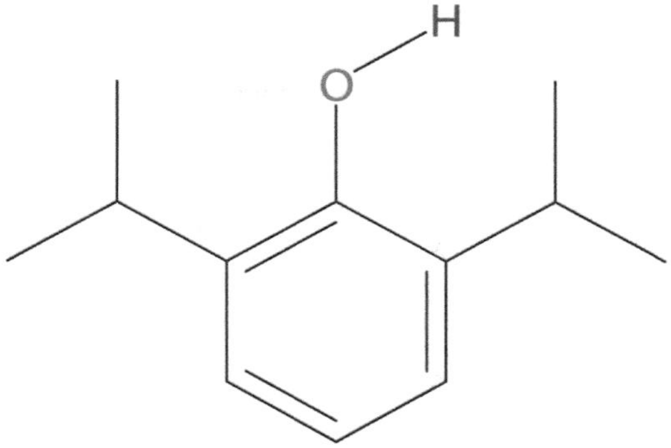

Clinical Pharmacology

Propofol is a rapidly acting IV medication commonly used for induction and maintenance of general anesthesia and sedation. Its onset from time of injection is approximately 40 seconds, due to rapid equilibration between the plasma and the brain. The half-time of blood brain equilibration is 1 to 3 minutes. Cardiorespiratory depression is likely to occur from bolus dosing or from a rapid

Fig. 3. Propofol.

increase in the rate of infusion of propofol. Generally, 3 to 5 minutes should be allowed between doses of propofol to adequately assess clinical effects. When propofol is dosed such that spontaneous ventilation is maintained, arterial hypotension may occur with little or no change in heart rate and no decrease in cardiac output. When propofol is dosed such that assisted or controlled ventilation is required, a decrease in cardiac output may occur. The reflex tachycardia seen with older induction agents such as methohexital is not a prominent feature of propofol and may not be seen at all.[1,13]

Propofol induction is frequently associated with apnea in all patient populations, which is exacerbated by the concurrent administration of opioid medications. Propofol is rarely associated with release of histamine and, on the contrary, may be associated with bronchodilation. It also does not reduce adrenal response to adrenocorticotropic hormone and is not a triggering agent for malignant hyperthermia. Following redistribution, propofol is cleared via hepatic conjugation into inactive metabolites and renally excreted. Rapid awakening within 10 to 15 minutes usually occurs when propofol has been used for a few hours or longer or even for extended periods at the minimum effective therapeutic concentration, as in an intensive care setting. When used at higher levels, propofol redistribution from fat and muscle to plasma may prolong recovery. Mild euphoria on awakening is common after propofol administration, and even at subhypnotic doses, propofol is associated with decreased postoperative nausea and vomiting.[1,13]

Indications and Usage

Propofol may be used as an induction and maintenance agent for general anesthesia in a variety of settings, including monitored anesthesia care, combined sedation and regional anesthesia such as for outpatient oral and maxillofacial surgery procedures, and for intensive care unit sedation of mechanically ventilated patients.

Dosage and Administration

The dosage and method of administration of propofol varies with the desired level of sedation and clinical purpose. Before drawing up the medication, the bottle should be shaken to achieve a uniform consistency. Notable phase separation indicates that the product is no longer stable. In adults, a 2 to 2.5 mg/kg bolus will induce general anesthesia within 30 seconds. Depending on the desired depth of anesthesia, periodic propofol bolus dosing may be used to maintain satisfactory anesthesia without overdosing. Changes in vital signs in response to surgical stimuli or a patient response indicating light anesthesia may be managed using propofol boluses of roughly 10 to 30 mg for sedation or 20 to 50 mg for general anesthesia. Concurrent inhalation of nitrous oxide and oxygen with propofol titration may achieve satisfactory anesthesia for minor procedures. A propofol infusion pump is also a useful tool for achieving and maintaining a desired anesthetic plane. FDA labeling recommends a rate of 50 to 100 mcg/kg/min for adults to optimize recovery time. This range may be expanded and broken down to 25 to 100 mcg/kg/min for moderate sedation, 75 to 150 mcg/kg/min for deep sedation, and 100 to 300 mcg/kg/min for general anesthesia. Infusion rates should be titrated down in the absence of clinical signs of light anesthesia.[1,13]

Contraindications

Propofol is contraindicated in patients with a known hypersensitivity to the drug itself or any of the preparation constituents. The FDA recommends that propofol be avoided in patients with true soy or egg allergies. However, most egg allergies are to the albumin in egg white and thus do not preclude the use of propofol emulsion, which specifically contains lecithin extracted from egg yolk. Several investigators have published reports indicating that concerns about the use of propofol in patients with the food allergies noted previously are unfounded.[13,14]

Warnings and Precautions

Propofol injection causes significant pain, which may be attenuated by pretreatment of the vessel with 1% lidocaine or by administering an opioid medication before propofol. If using lidocaine, the recommendation is no more than 20 mg per 200 mg propofol so that 1 or 2 mL of 1% plain lidocaine should suffice in advance of the first propofol

bolus. Long-term sedation of critically ill children or young adult neurosurgical patients may result in propofol infusion syndrome, which is characterized by lipemia, rhabdomyolysis, hyperkalemia, metabolic acidosis, hepatomegaly, renal failure, electrocardiogram changes and/or cardiac failure, and death. This unusual syndrome is generally associated with high-dose infusion of propofol; decreased oxygen delivery to tissues; serious neurologic injury and/or sepsis; or the concurrent administration of high doses of steroids, vasoconstrictors, or inotropes.[1,15]

Adverse Reactions

Anaphylaxis, although rare, has been reported in patients with a history of allergic reaction to other medications, especially neuromuscular blocking agents.[13]

Drug Interactions

Premedication with midazolam can reduce the propofol requirement by 10%. The respiratory effects of propofol, including reduced respiratory drive and its impact on cardiac output, are enhanced by opioid administration.[13,15]

Use in Specific Populations

Elderly, debilitated, and medically fragile patients are more susceptible to undesirable cardiorespiratory depression, so bolus dosing should be avoided or performed with great care in these populations. A reduced induction dose of 1 to 1.5 mg/kg is recommended for these patients, due to reduced clearance and higher blood concentrations. On the contrary, healthy pediatric patients aged 3 to 16 years require a higher induction dose of 2.5 to 3.5 mg/kg. Pediatric patients also require a correspondingly higher infusion rate for maintenance of general anesthesia, with younger pediatric patients requiring even higher rates than older pediatric patients. There are no adequate and well-controlled studies of propofol administration in pregnant women, and a pregnancy category has not been assigned, but animal studies have suggested adverse effects on the mother and/or the fetus when propofol is administered during pregnancy.

Pharmacokinetics of propofol in adult patients with chronic renal or hepatic impairment is no different from that of normal healthy adults.[13]

How Supplied/Storage and Handling

Propofol is packaged as a 1% (10 mg/mL) aqueous solution consisting of soybean oil, glycerol, and egg lecithin that is opaque white. This formulation may support bacterial growth, so the vial is handled using sterile technique and must be used within 6 hours of opening. Although current preparations contain 0.005% disodium edetate or 0.025% metabisulfite as preservatives to slow the growth of microorganisms, this does not qualify as an antimicrobial preparation by US pharmacopeia standards. It is a schedule IV controlled substance.[13,16]

Utility, Risks, and Benefits in Oral and Maxillofacial Surgery/Ambulatory Anesthesia Practice

Propofol is usually titrated to effect to achieve, maintain, or deepen sedation during outpatient oral and maxillofacial surgery procedures. Typically, a benzodiazepine and an opioid medication will be given to achieve a baseline moderate sedation. Propofol is then administered in 10 to 30 mg bolus doses, usually during administration of local anesthesia or other stimulating portions of the surgical procedure. The oral and maxillofacial surgeon must be prepared to manage the respiratory consequences of propofol use including apnea during open airway sedation. For older clinicians who have experience with methohexital, the benefits of propofol are clear. Deep sedation with propofol is generally smoother, untoward reactions are fewer, recovery is quicker, and postoperative nausea is less likely than with methohexital.[16]

KETAMINE

Ketamine (Ketalar) is a phencyclidine derivative (**Fig. 4**) that acts as an N-methyl-ᴅ-aspartate (NMDA) receptor antagonist to induce a state of "dissociative anesthesia" (**Fig. 4**). It does this by functionally dissociating the thalamus from the limbic cortex, the area of the brain involved with awareness of sensation, thereby preventing transmission of sensory impulses from the reticular activating system to the cerebral cortex.

Clinical Pharmacology

Ketamine's mechanism of action is via nonselective and noncompetitive antagonism of supraspinal NMDA inotropic glutamate receptors. It is known to have a rapid onset and short duration of action, due to high lipid solubility and fast redistribution. Its metabolite, norketamine, acts at the same receptor with about one-third the affinity of ketamine. It produces an atypical state of general anesthesia in which the patient may seem awake but does not respond to commands, does not react to painful stimuli, and usually has

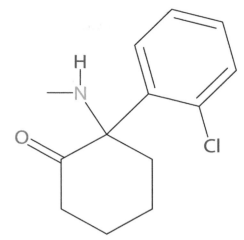

Fig. 4. Ketamine.

nystagmus. The analgesic effect of ketamine is explained, in part, by decreased neuronal signaling due to its action on NMDA receptors in the CNS and also by a speculated interaction with pain receptors in the spinal cord and with opioid receptors. Its unique ability to produce analgesia, anterograde amnesia, and unconsciousness makes this a very effective agent for procedural sedation.[17]

Ketamine induction preserves normal laryngeal-pharyngeal reflexes, normal or slightly enhanced skeletal muscle tone, and normal cardiovascular stimulation and respiratory drive. Ventilatory drive is minimally affected by an induction dose of ketamine, although a slight transient decrease in drive may be noticed, particularly in the context of opioid coadministration. Ketamine acts as a direct myocardial depressant when administered in large doses, likely due to inhibition of calcium transport; this is usually masked by its indirect cardiovascular stimulatory effect mediated by central stimulation of the sympathetic nervous system and inhibition of norepinephrine reuptake at nerve terminals. However, in patients with sympathetic blockade or catecholamine depletion, the direct myocardial depressant effects may be unveiled. The predominant indirect cardiovascular effects of ketamine are elevated blood pressure, increased heart rate, and enhanced cardiac output, which usually occur within a few minutes of administration and may be used strategically in a trauma setting in patients experiencing acute shock. Blood pressure increases may be quite significant but readings generally return to baseline within 15 minutes of administration. Large boluses should therefore be delivered with caution in patients with coronary artery disease, uncontrolled hypertension, congestive heart failure, or arterial aneurysms. Like propofol, ketamine does not cause histamine release and is also a potent bronchodilator (via sympathetic activation as well as direct smooth muscle relaxation), making it an ideal agent for patients at risk for developing bronchospasm.[16]

The distribution half-life after IV administration is 10 to 15 minutes, but its anesthetic effect can last 45 minutes. Emergence delirium is common but is attenuated by premedication with benzodiazepines. Ketamine undergoes hepatic metabolism by CYP enzymes to an active metabolite, norketamine, which is metabolized further in the liver. The elimination half-life is only 2 hours due to a relatively high hepatic extraction ratio of 0.9. The end products of ketamine metabolism are renally excreted.[17]

Indications and Usage

Ketamine may be used as the sole anesthetic agent for diagnostic and surgical procedures that do not require skeletal muscle relaxation. It may also be used as an induction agent for general anesthesia or a supplement to other drugs in the maintenance of general anesthesia or sedation. It is particularly useful as an intramuscular agent for uncooperative patients who are unable to tolerate IV placement.[1,17]

Dosage and Administration

Ketamine may be given via oral, nasal, subcutaneous, rectal, or epidural routes. However, for procedural sedation, it is best administered intramuscularly or intravenously. For traditional IV induction of anesthesia, a 1 to 4.5 mg/kg initial dose is recommended, administered slowly over 60 seconds to avoid respiratory depression and enhanced vasopressor response. On average, 2 mg/kg will produce surgical anesthesia within 30 seconds, which will last for 5 to 10 minutes. FDA labeling recommends 6.5 to 13 mg/kg intramuscular (IM) ketamine to induce 12 to 25 minutes of general anesthesia within 3 to 4 minutes. However, 3 to 7 mg/kg is typically an adequate induction dose, and 2 to 3 mg/kg is sufficient to gain control to obtain IV access or to provide local anesthesia for a very brief procedure. Maintenance with IV ketamine is titrated based on clinical observation of the patient. Approximately one-half to a full induction dose can be administered to redose ketamine, or 0.1 to 0.5 mg/min can be infused to maintain general anesthesia in adults. When administered as a supplement to other anesthetic medications, ketamine is administered at a lower dose and titrated based on the patient response. Ketamine

administration is associated with increased salivation, which may be preempted and treated by administration of an anticholinergic agent such as glycopyrrolate. Glycopyrrolate is preferred over scopolamine or atropine due to superior antisialagogue effects, milder cardiac effects, and poor CNS penetration.[15,17]

Contraindications

Ketamine is contraindicated in patients who are unable to tolerate a significant elevation in blood pressure, which may include patients with a variety of cardiovascular disease states. It is also contraindicated in patients with any known hypersensitivity to ketamine.[17]

Warnings and Precautions

Ketamine is known to have significant abuse potential and is a schedule III controlled substance. Physical dependance and withdrawal have been reported with long-term use. Memory or attention may become impaired, and tolerance may also develop in these patients. Vital signs and cardiac function must be closely monitored during administration of ketamine, as significant myocardial depressant or indirect stimulant effects may occur in susceptible patients. Postoperative confusion and agitation (emergence delirium) has been reported to occur in approximately 12% of patients. The likelihood and intensity of this phenomenon are reduced by premedication with a benzodiazepine before ketamine administration. Although respiratory depression is mild and transient, it may occur if ketamine is administered in too large a dose or too rapidly. Ketamine has been reported to elevate intracranial pressure, which should be monitored.[17]

Adverse Reactions

Hemodynamic instability, emergence delirium, respiratory depression, pediatric neurotoxicity, and drug-induced liver injury are all known adverse reactions associated with ketamine. All of these can be avoided or mitigated by prudent use and appropriate patient selection. Vomiting and aspiration may also occur with ketamine, so it is not recommended for patients who have not followed proper *nil per os* guidelines. Other adverse reactions that are not mentioned elsewhere but have been reported subjectively include diplopia, elevated intraocular pressure, hepatobiliary dysfunction, pain and rash localized to the site of injection, anaphylaxis, unpleasant dreams and emotional effects days to weeks after administration, and renal and urinary disorders.[17]

Drug Interactions

Sympathomimetics and vasopressin may enhance the sympathomimetic effect of ketamine, so dosing should be adjusted accordingly based on patient response. As with other sedative medications, coadministration of ketamine with benzodiazepines, opioids, and other CNS depressants may produce profound sedation, respiratory depression, coma, and death. Careful titration of ketamine should be performed when these other agents are concurrently used. Ketamine may lower seizure threshold by its interaction with theophylline and aminophylline, and another anesthetic agent should be considered instead in patients who are taking these medications.[17]

Use in Specific Populations

As propofol, ketamine has not been studied in an adequate or well-controlled manner in pregnant women and has not been assigned a pregnancy classification. However, animal studies have suggested developmental delay in the fetus when the mother received high doses of ketamine. Despite a track record of use for pediatric sedation, safety and efficacy in pediatric patients younger than 16 years have not technically been established. Negative effects on the developing brain are estimated to be possible between the third trimester of gestation and the first several months of life. Regardless, benefit of administration must be weighed against this potential risk in pediatric patients who require appropriate anesthesia. Ketamine administration is also not well studied in patients older than 65 years. However, dosing should be cautious, keeping in mind possible comorbidities and concurrent home medications.[17]

How Supplied/Storage and Handling

Ketamine is prepared as a clear solution as the hydrochloride salt. It is prepared in the following multidose vial concentrations: 200 mg in 20 mL, 500 mg in 10 mL, or 500 mg in 5 mL. It should be stored at 20 to 25°C (68–77°F) with an acceptable range from 15 to 30°C (59–86°F), and it should be protected from light.[17]

Utility, Risks, and Benefits in Oral and Maxillofacial Surgery/Ambulatory Anesthesia Practice

The principal uses of ketamine in oral and maxillofacial surgical practice include IM injection for uncooperative adult patients and for children who will not tolerate IV placement. A 2 mL maximum fluid volume of ketamine combined with midazolam and glycopyrrolate may be drawn up for this purpose using the 100 mg/mL formulation of ketamine to allow adequate initial dosing of all 3 agents in this small volume. The IM combination may be adequate to complete a very short procedure but should be used to achieve cooperation for IV placement so that any necessary additional titration can then be done IV. Ketamine is a useful drug to attain deep IV sedation in OMS/ambulatory anesthesia and is particularly applicable for patients who have been administered a benzodiazepine with or without an opioid and still require apnea-inducing doses of propofol to attain surgical anesthesia. Because of its analgesic property, ketamine may also be used in lieu of opioid administration during sedation. Ketamine may be preferred for patients who are susceptible to bronchospasm, such as asthmatics, or in children, who are less tolerant of the cardiovascular depressive effect of other anesthetic agents than are adult patients.[15,16]

Other Agents

Two additional sedative/hypnotics are of interest to the oral and maxillofacial surgeon. Methohexital was the general anesthetic/deep sedation agent of choice for many years in oral surgery practice and, although largely displaced by propofol, is still available and effective. No discussion of ambulatory anesthesia in oral and maxillofacial surgery would be complete without mention of methohexital, at least for historical perspective and to provide context for current practice. Dexmedetomidine has also been available for quite some time but has not become part of standard anesthesia practice in the oral and maxillofacial surgery community as have the other agents discussed previously.

METHOHEXITAL

Methohexital (Brevital) is an ultrashort-acting barbiturate with the structural formula $C14H17N2NaO3$ (**Fig 5**). It is supplied as a white freeze-dried plug that is water soluble and prepared for parenteral administration. Methohexital is typically given by IV push and/or by continuous IV drip to induce anesthesia and maintain a desired level of sedation.

Clinical Pharmacology

Methohexital is more potent than other traditional barbiturate induction agents with a much shorter clinical duration of action; this is thought to be related to less fat storage than is seen with other barbiturates. Unlike these agents, it contains no sulfur, but its failure to produce analgesia is a property shared among the barbiturates.

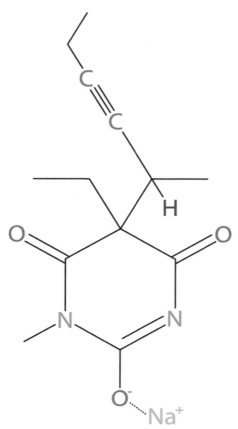

Fig. 5. Methohexital.

Methohexital and other members of this class of sedative/hypnotics interact with alpha and beta subunits of the GABA-A receptor and increase chloride ion influx, potentiating the inhibitory effect of GABA (ref Barb article refs 13–15). Induction of sleep is very rapid, generally 1 to 2 arm-brain circulations when given intravenously with slower onset expected with IM or rectal administration, routes that have little utility in the ambulatory anesthesia setting. After a single IV dose, duration of action is determined primarily by the redistribution rate. The drug is metabolized in the liver and excreted by the kidneys.[18]

Indications and Usage

Official indications include as an IV induction agent when followed by other anesthetics or as an IV induction agent and adjunct to nitrous oxide and oxygen for short procedures. It is also indicated for use as part of a balanced anesthetic technique that may include benzodiazepines and opioids as well as N2O/O2. As a solo agent, it may be used for very brief, minimally stimulating or nonpainful procedures and is also capable of producing a hypnotic state.[18]

Dosage and Administration

Product labeling provides a very specific dilutional regimen, and the diluent must be a bacteriostatic vehicle with a 1% solution in sterile water or saline acceptable for IV induction and intermittent bolus use. Sterile water is not recommended for continuous infusions, which are generally 0.2% solutions and require an isotonic diluent. An initial rate of administration for a 1% solution is about 1 mL/5 seconds with a total induction dose usually in the 50 to 100 mg range. Although the duration of a single dose is likely to be only 5 minutes, methohexital in oral and maxillofacial surgery practice is generally part of a balanced anesthesia technique, and with other agents and local anesthesia on board, a workable state of sedation may continue for significantly longer.

For induction of anesthesia, a 1% solution is administered at a rate of about 1 mL/5 seconds. Gaseous anesthetics and/or skeletal muscle relaxants may be administered concomitantly. The dose required for induction may range from 50 to 120 mg or more but averages about 70 mg. The usual dosage in adults ranges from 1 to 1.5 mg/kg. The induction dose usually provides anesthesia for 5 to 7 minutes. Use of methohexital to maintain a desired sate of sedation is accomplished by continuous infusion of a 0.2% solution, titrating the rate to effect. A starting rate of 3 mL/min, which is one drop per second, is a reasonable guideline. Intermittent bolusing of the 1% solution is also effective, particularly when a rhythm is found that keeps the patient comfortably sedated and tolerating the surgical procedure while still exchanging well. Boluses of 20 to 40 mg every 4 to 7 minutes are suggested in FDA product information; however, anticipatory titration is often difficult. For many patients there is a narrow pathway between inadequate sedation and the adverse effects seen with higher doses.[18]

Contraindications

Methohexital is contraindicated for use by clinicians inadequately prepared to assist ventilation and manage the expected and unusual consequences of it administration. It should not be used in facilities that lack the equipment and supplies to ensure that adverse effects can be managed properly. Methohexital is also contraindicated in patients who are not candidates for ambulatory general anesthesia, in those with porphyria, and in patients with known barbiturate hypersensitivities.[18,19]

Warnings and Precautions

As with other anesthetic agents, the principal concern is adequacy of ventilation with apnea more likely on induction with methohexital than with other barbiturates. Laryngospasm is not uncommon, particularly during induction. The use of methohexital demands careful consideration in patients with hepatic dysfunction, cardiovascular disease, or other underlying conditions that might be destabilized and in patients with a history of convulsive activity in whom seizures might be elicited. Appropriate care must be taken to avoid intraarterial injection and to manage this potentially catastrophic occurrence in the unlikely event that the drug is inadvertently administered intraarterially. Longer procedures may be associated with cumulative effects of methohexital including prolonged somnolence and respiratory and/or cardiovascular depression.[18,20]

Adverse Reactions

Beyond the major issues noted earlier, numerous adverse effects have been noted including bronchospasm, hypotension, tachycardia, hiccups, muscle hyperactivity, restlessness, emergence delirium, nausea, vomiting, allergic reactions, and pain at the injection site.[18]

Drug Interactions

Most of the significant drug interactions are additive effects of combining methohexital with other CNS depressants.

Use in Specific Populations

Although it is unlikely to be selected as an agent of choice for pediatric patients, it may be administered IV, IM, or rectally to induce anesthesia in children.

How Supplied/Storage and Handling

It is currently available in 500 mg and 2.5 g vials that are stored at room temperature. Solutions with appropriate diluents as described earlier are stable and may be used for up to 24 hours. These solutions are basic and therefore incompatible with acidic agents such as succinylcholine and atropine and should not be administered simultaneously or mixed in the same syringe as methohexital.[18]

Utility, Risks, and Benefits in Oral and Maxillofacial Surgical Practice

Although methohexital was the preferred agent for deep sedation and general anesthesia in oral and maxillofacial surgery practice before the release of propofol, its use has declined dramatically. One study comparing adverse effects of the 2 agents in oral and maxillofacial surgery facilities

concluded that propofol was associated with fewer. In general, propofol is more readily available and the current generation of oral and maxillofacial surgeons uses propofol as they did during training.[21]

DEXMEDETOMIDINE

Dexmedetomidine (Precedex) is a specific and selective alpha-2 adrenoceptor agonist with the structural formula C13H16N2 (**Fig. 6**). It binds to presynaptic alpha-2 adrenoceptors inhibiting the release of norepinephrine. It is reported to provide sedation that parallels natural sleep as well as anxiolysis, analgesia, and sympatholysis, all while producing minimal respiratory depression. Dexmedetomidine hydrochloride is a white powder that is freely soluble in water and when mixed in isotonic saline, is a sterile, nonpyrogenic ready-to-use solution for IV infusion. Unlike most sedation agents, it is not a controlled substance, and there are no data from human studies regarding dependence[22].

Clinical Pharmacology

The sedation produced by dexmedetomidine via alpha$_2$-adrenergic stimulation is associated with little or no respiratory depression at recommended sedative doses in healthy subjects. When administered intravenously, it redistributes quickly with a distribution half-life of 6 minutes and a terminal elimination half-life of 2 hours. Metabolism is in the liver through glucuronidation and cytochrome P450 biotransformation, primarily involving CYP2A6. No active or toxic metabolites have been identified. Products of dexmedetomidine metabolism are excreted almost entirely in the urine with no unchanged drug detected.[22,23]

Indications and Usage

The primary indication for dexmedetomidine is the initial sedation of intubated and mechanically ventilated patients in intensive care environments. In these settings, administration by continuous IV

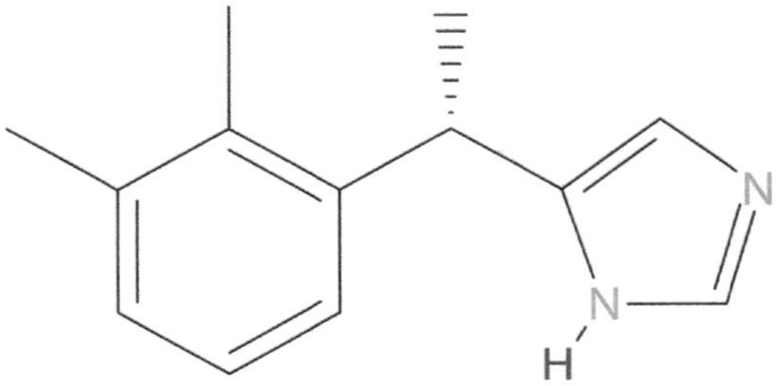

Fig. 6. Dexmedetomidine.

infusion is recommended for no more than 24 hours. The indication for use that is relevant to oral and maxillofacial surgeons is sedation of nonintubated patients for procedures including surgery. Although not listed in the FDA prescribing information, a variety of anxiety-provoking, uncomfortable, or painful procedures may be managed using dexmedetomidine, which may also offer benefits in the preoperative and postoperative periods.[24]

Dosage and Administration

Although dosing suggestions follow later, dexmedetomidine dosing is adjusted by titrating to the desired effect. The use of a controlled infusion device is recommended. The starting rate of 1 µg/kg over 10 minutes for awake fiberoptic intubation and surgical procedures should be adjusted down for less invasive manipulations and/or when treating patients for whom dose reductions are advisable. The range of maintenance infusion rates is likely to be from 0.2 to 1 µg/kg/h, with 0.6 µg/kg/h suggested at the onset of the maintenance phase. This rate should be adjusted based on appropriate clinical parameters. Dexmedetomidine is diluted with 0.9% sodium chloride injection to achieve the 4 µg/mL concentration that is used for either the loading dose or for a maintenance infusion.[22]

Contraindications

There are no contraindications to dexmedetomidine listed by the FDA.[22]

Warnings and Precautions

As with other sedation agents, clinicians are warned to use this agent only when the facility and personnel are appropriate for managing the expected and potential adverse effects of the drug. Significant reduction in heart rate should be anticipated and may be mitigated by the concurrent administration of glycopyrrolate or atropine, when indicated. Hypotension may occur and generally responds to slowing the infusion rate and fluid administration; although other measure may be required, isolated cases have been reported in which resuscitation was inadequate resulting in fatality. Hypertension has also been noted, particularly with the loading dose, as peripheral vasoconstriction may occur initially. Other reports suggest a biphasic blood pressure response, with higher blood levels associated with blood pressure elevation from baseline. Tolerance and tachyphylaxis are noted when dexmedetomidine is used for more than 24 hours and prolonged use increases the risk for adverse effects and withdrawal when the drug is stopped.[22–24]

Adverse Reactions

The principal adverse effects of dexmedetomidine are hypotension, bradycardia, and hypertension as described earlier. Others are noted but are less frequent and less severe, including nausea, atrial fibrillation, pyrexia, and xerostomia. Others occur in less than 4% of adults on continuous infusions in intensive care units and are presumably far less likely when dexmedetomidine is used for procedural sedation. As with most sedation agents, respiratory depression is a significant adverse effect of dexmedetomidine during procedural sedation.[22]

Drug Interactions

There are likely to be additive effects when dexmedetomidine is used concurrently with other CNS depressants, and dose adjustments must be considered. No other specific drug interactions are listed.[22]

Use in Specific Populations

As of 2020, the FDA's position on pediatric use of dexmedetomidine is that safety and efficacy have not been adequately evaluated. The available pediatric anesthesia literature on dexmedetomidine suggests that it may be a viable agent for procedural sedation in children and may actually possess benefits over more commonly used drugs. One publication did note that the use of glycopyrrolate to manage dexmedetomidine-associated bradycardia in children has resultant in significant hypertension.[25] Based on available data, dose reduction for patients older than 65 years is recommended as hypotension, and bradycardia occur more frequently in this population, even with short exposures to the drug for procedural sedation. Dose reduction is also advocated when using this agent in the management of individuals with hepatic impairment.[22]

How Supplied/Storage and Handling

Dexmedetomidine hydrochloride injection is clear and colorless and supplied in single-use glass vials. It is administered as a 4 µg/mL solution, and the unused portion must be discarded.[22]

Utility, Risks, and Benefits in Oral and Maxillofacial Surgical Practice

Although dexmedetomidine possesses qualities that make it an attractive alternative for appropriately selected patients, its use has not become widespread in the United States among oral and maxillofacial surgeons. Its ability to produce sedation with anxiolysis, analgesia, sympatholysis, and minimal respiratory depression suggests that it might be considered for ambulatory, open airway sedation in the oral and maxillofacial surgery office. In comparison with midazolam, dexmedetomidine is associated with less respiratory depressions and reduced analgesic requirements, but bradycardia is more likely, and a controlled infusion device is recommended.[23]

SUMMARY

The safety and success of the oral and maxillofacial surgery practice model for procedural sedation is well established. At the core of this is great attention to patient selection, prudent and appropriate use of the available agents, excellent monitoring using clinical parameters as well as the most current and effective technology, and a strong commitment to patient safety. The agents reviewed in this chapter must be well understood and respected by all clinicians who use them to facilitate the care of patients.

CLINICS CARE POINTS

- When using sedation agents, safety and efficacy are optimized by slow and careful titration coupled with appropriate patient and medication selection.
- Balanced anesthesia is likely to produce sedation with the benefits of each agent maximized and drug-specific toxicities minimized.
- When using propofol, rapid administration is appropriate, whereas fentanyl should be given slowly.
- When considering reversal for a patient who is oversedated after administration of both fentanyl and midazolam, the choice of initial reversal agent should be based on clinical findings.
- When using ketamine, the co-administration of glycopyrrolate may limit hypersecretion and make laryngospasm less likely.

DISCLOSURE

The authors have nothing to disclose.

REFERENCES

1. Butterworth JF, Mackey DC, Wasnick JD, et al. Morgan and mikhail's clinical anesthesiology. New York: McGraw-Hill; 2013.
2. Federal Drug Administration. Versed® (midazolam). Drugs@FDA: FDA-approved drugs; 2017. Available at: https://www.accessdata.fda.gov/drugsatfda_docs/label/2017/208878%20orig1s000lbl.pdf.
3. Mizukawa M, McKenna SJ, Vega LG. Anesthesia considerations for the oral and maxillofacial surgeon. 1st edition. Berlin: Quintessence Publishing; 2017.
4. Lingamchetty TN, Hosseini SA, Saadabadi A. Midazolam. In: StatPearls [Internet]. Treasure Island (FL): StatPearls Publishing; 2021. Available at: https://www.ncbi.nlm.nih.gov/books/NBK537321/.
5. Cobb B, Liu R, Valentine E, et al. Breastfeeding after anesthesia: a review for anesthesia providers regarding the transfer of medications into breast milk. Transl Perioper Pain Med 2015;1(2):1–7.
6. Nitsun M, Szokol JW, Saleh HJ, et al. Pharmacokinetics of midazolam, propofol, and fentanyl transfer to human breast milk. Clin Pharmacol Ther 2006; 79(6):549–57.
7. Statement on resuming breastfeeding after anesthesia. In: Statement on resuming breastfeeding after anesthesia. American Society of Anesthesiologists (ASA); 2019. Available at: https://www.asahq.org/standards-and-guidelines/statement-on-resuming-breastfeeding-after-anesthesia. Accessed June 19, 2021.
8. Stanley TH. Fentanyl. J Pain Symptom Manage 2005;29(5 Suppl):S67–71.
9. Stanley TH. The fentanyl story. J Pain 2014;15(12): 1215–26.
10. Federal Drug Administration. Sublimaze® (fentanyl citrate) USP. Drugs@FDA: FDA-Approved Drugs; 2017. Available at: https://www.accessdata.fda.gov/drugsatfda_docs/label/2016/016619s038lbl.pdf.
11. Volpi-Abadie J, Kaye AM, Kaye AD. Serotonin syndrome. Ochsner J 2013;13:533–40.
12. Lewis JH, Stine JG. Review article: prescribing medications in patients with cirrhosis—A practical guide. Aliment Pharmacol Ther 2013;37:1132–56.
13. Federal Drug Administration. Diprivan® (propofol) injectable emulsion, USP. Drugs@FDA: FDA-Approved Drugs; 2017. Available at: https://www.accessdata.fda.gov/drugsatfda_docs/label/2017/019627s066lbl.pdf.
14. Asserhoj LL, Mosbech H, Kroigaard M. No evidence for contraindications to the use of propofol in adults allergic to egg, soy or peanut. Br J Anaesth 2016; 116:77–82.
15. Miloro M, Peterson LJ. Pharmacology of Outpatient Anesthesia Medications. 3rd edition. In: Miloro M, Ghali GE, Larsen PE, et al, editors. Peterson's principles of oral and maxillofacial surgery, vol. 1. Shelton: Essay, People's Medical Pub. House-USA; 2011. p. 73–5.
16. Lam D, Laskin DM. Anesthesia. In: Lam D, Laskin DM, editors. Oral & maxillofacial surgery review: a study guide. Hanover Park: Essay, Quintessence Publishing Co, Inc; 2015. p. 56–7.

17. Federal Drug Administration. Highlights of pre-scribing information: Ketalar® (ketamine). Drugs@ FDA: FDA-Approved Drugs; 2020. Available at: https://www.accessdata.fda.gov/drugsatfda_docs/label/2020/016812Orig1s046lbl.pdf.

18. Federal Drug Administration. Highlights of prescrib-ing information: Brevital®(methohexital). Drugs@ FDA: FDA-Approved Drugs; 2020. Available at: https://www.accessdata.fda.gov/drugsatfda_docs/label/2008/011559s041lbl.pdf.

19. Skibiski J, Abdijadid S. Barbiturates. In: Stat pearls. Treasure Island (FL): StatPearls Publishing; 2021.

20. Martone CH, Naglehout J, Wolf SM. Mehgtohexital: a practical review for outpatient dental anesthesia. Anesth Prog 1991;38:195–9.

21. Lee JS, Gonzalez ML, Chuang SK, et al. Compari-son of methohexital and propofol use in ambulatory procedures in oral and maxillofacial surgery. J Oral Maxillofac Surg 2008;66:1996–2003.

22. Federal Drug Administration. Highlights of prescribing information: Precedex® (dexmedetomidine). Drugs@ FDA: FDA-Approved Drugs; 2020. Available at: https://www.accessdata.fda.gov/drugsatfda_docs/label/2013/021038s021lbl.pdf2.

23. Wang L, Zhang T, Huang L, et al. Comparison be-tween dexmedetomidine and midazolam for seda-tion in patients with intubation after oral and maxillofacial surgery. Clin Study Open Access 2020;2020. 7082597.

24. Mahmoud M, Mason KP. Dexmedetomidine: review, update and future considerations of paediatric peri-operative and periprocedural applications and limi-tations. Br J Anaesth 2015;115(2):171–82.

25. Mason KP, Zgleszewski S, Forman RE, et al. An exaggerated response to glycopyrrolate therapy for bradycardia associated with high-dose dexme-detomidine. Anesth Analg 2009;108:906–8.

Acute Pain Management

Nabil Moussa, DDS[a,b,*], Orrett E. Ogle, DDS[a,b]

KEYWORDS

- Acute • Pain • Medical management • Pathophysiology

KEY POINTS

- Notably, current public attention and perception have been directed to the widespread misuse and abuse of opioid medications. Dentists were found to be the most common prescriber of opioid analgesics to patients between 10 and 19 years old for postoperative pain management.
- Acute pain is a physiologic response to insult or injury. The pain may be secondary to surgical intervention or part of an infectious or pathologic process. Acute pain stimulation can be divided into 2 main mechanisms: peripheral and central stimulatory responses.
- The concept of multimodal or balanced analgesia in acute pain management recommends that combined analgesic regimens are much more effective in achieving postoperative pain control and avoiding untoward side effects. The method takes advantage of synergistic and additive effects of medications at a lower dose.
- Pharmacologic treatment modalities of pain control include acetaminophen, ibuprofen, anticonvulsants, opioids, gamma-aminobutyric acid agonists, and local anesthetics. Nonpharmacologic pain control includes application of ice, which is effective by reducing local inflammation.

INTRODUCTION

Acute pain is usually associated with tissue injury, inflammation, a surgical procedure, trauma, or a short-term disease process. In oral and maxillofacial surgery, acute pain can arise directly from a surgical procedure or from problems such as dental caries, infection, perforation of maxillary sinus, pericoronitis, and jaw fractures. Acute pain is of short duration and gradually improves as the injured tissues heal. Acute pain is always present following any surgical procedure.

The major factor in acute pain management is deciding on an appropriate intervention and/or analgesic that will provide the best pain relief to the patient. Although this article addresses acute pain management in general terms, it must be clear that treatment that is effective for one acute pain condition and patient may not be effective in others and the surgeon should therefore be disease and patient specific. In oral and maxillofacial surgery, acute pain often requires a procedure to relieve the pain (eg, treating of dry socket) in addition to pharmaceutical management. In this article, postoperative pain is presented as the exemplar for acute pain management. Postoperative pain should be addressed as soon as possible after the procedure.

Providing appropriate postoperative pain control can have significant impacts on both the patient and the surgeon. Patient perception and tolerance can differ dramatically from patient to patient. Titrating the appropriate analgesic requirement requires careful consideration of the invasive nature of the procedure and the expected patient response and tolerance of pain. Patient response and experience of pain are often subjective, making assessment difficult. In addition to past experiences, other patient factors that may also play a crucial role in the acute pain management include age, sex, race/ethnicity, and the severity of the pain.

a Department of Oral and Maxillofacial Surgery, The Brooklyn Hospital Center, New York, NY, USA;
b Department of Dentistry, Division of Oral and Maxillofacial Surgery, 121 Dekalb Avenue, Brooklyn, NY 11201, USA
* Corresponding author. Department of Dentistry, Division of Oral and Maxillofacial Surgery, 121 Dekalb Avenue, Brooklyn, NY 11201.
E-mail address: moussanabil@gmail.com

Oral Maxillofacial Surg Clin N Am 34 (2022) 35–47
https://doi.org/10.1016/j.coms.2021.08.014
1042-3699/22/© 2021 Elsevier Inc. All rights reserved.

Providing appropriate analgesia requires a depth of experience and knowledge of pain management. Providing the patient with the appropriate level of analgesia following a surgical procedure can have dramatic effects on the provider-patient relationship. The patient's quality of life can be heavily affected, including psychological effects. Uncontrolled postoperative pain has been documented to lead to the development of depression.[1] There is evidence in the literature to show that mismanagement of acute pain may even lead to central sensitization and the development of chronic pain.[1,2] A variety of analgesic options are available to clinicians when considering pain control. It is important to have a depth of understanding with regard to analgesic properties, adverse effects, duration of action, and pharmacology to appropriately control and provide appropriate postoperative acute pain relief. This article presents options for acute pain control and provides guidance and strategies for acute postoperative pain control.

IMPORTANCE AND SIGNIFICANCE

Appropriate use of analgesic is important in the postoperative care of patients after oral and maxillofacial surgery. Pain can have detrimental effects on the quality of life and postoperative experience of patients. Current standards of practice often involve acute pain management with the use of nonsteroidal antiinflammatory medications used in combination with acetaminophen.

All postsurgical pain is associated with inflammation, and to a great extent the control of acute pain is the control of inflammation. For this reason, nonsteroidal antiinflammatory drugs (NSAIDs) are the first-line analgesics for the control of postoperative dental pain. Opioids are never the first choice for management of acute postsurgical pain in dentistry. Acute pain normally resolves as healing from the surgical procedure occurs and can be managed without the use of opioids. In 2019, the Centers for Disease Control and Prevention (CDC) published a guideline for the use of opioids and advised against the use of opioids for acute pain (available at https://www.cdc.gov/acute-pain/postsurgical-pain/index.html and https://www.cdc.gov/drugoverdose/pdf/patients/Opioids-for-Acute-Pain-a.pdf).[3,4]

Notably, current public attention and perception have been directed to the widespread misuse and abuse of opioid medications. Controlled substance prescriptions have nearly doubled in the time period between 1994 and 2007.[5] Opioids are associated with high rates of abuse. In a study conducted by Volkow and colleagues,[6] the investigators analyzed the prescription practices of health care professionals in the United States. The investigators reviewed data acquired through the national database and focused the study primarily on the youth population. There were 201.9 million prescriptions for opioid analgesics in 2009, with 79.5 million to adolescents (39%). Most prescriptions were for products containing hydrocodone and oxycodone. Of the 201 million prescriptions, 11% (9.3 million) were for patients aged 10 to 29 years. Dentists were found to be the most common prescribers of opioid analgesics to patients between the ages of 10 and 19 years for postoperative pain management.[6] In 2015, the Department of Health and Human Services reported that 12.5 million people misused opioid prescription medication. Two million of those people were in the diagnostic category of prescription opioid use disorder, defined as a condition where psychotropic medications are used without a prescription for a use other than as directed by a physician or more often/longer than normally prescribed.[7,8] In addition, dentists were found to be the most likely source of unused prescriptions among high school seniors for nonmedical purposes obtained from previous medications (27% of prescriptions).[9]

BIOLOGY OF ACUTE PAIN

Acute pain is a physiologic response to insult or injury. The pain may be secondary to surgical intervention or part of an infectious or pathologic process. Acute pain stimulation can be divided into 2 main mechanisms: peripheral and central stimulatory responses. Sensory information is transmitted to the brain using a complex network of neurons within the spinothalamic tract (**Figs. 1** and **2**).[10,11] Understanding the chemical mediators and neurophysiologic pathways allows clinicians to have a better understanding and administer targeted therapies to control pain.[12]

Acute insult (eg, surgery or trauma) results in the activation of neurons commonly referred to as nociceptors. These afferent neurons, which project from the tissues to the central nervous system tissues, include but are not limited to skin, muscle, joints, and viscera (see **Fig. 1**). These nociceptors have direct contact with the central nervous system and their cell bodies located in the dorsal rood ganglion.[10,13] Also termed the first-order or primary afferent neuron, these neurons are divided into 3 classes based on their diameter and myelination. The 3 peripheral somatosensory classes are termed Aβ, Aδ, and C fibers (**Table 1**). The A class fibers Aβ and Aδ are rapidly conducting fibers with large diameter and are myelinated. The

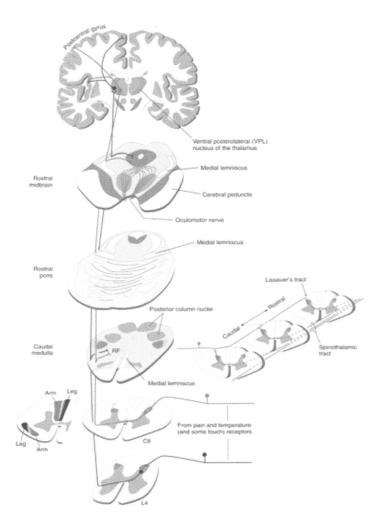

Fig. 1. The spinothalamic tract. First-order and second-order neurons are shown. Pain, temperature, and touch are transmitted through the afferents located in the posterior horn. The fibers are transmitted to the brain via medulla, pons, and midbrain to the thalamus and finally the sensory cortex or postcentral gyrus. Second-order neurons cross the midline. (*From* Vanderah TW, Gould DJ. Chapter 10: Spinal Cord. In: Vanderah, TW, Gould DJ. Nolte's The Human Brain. 7th ed. Elsevier. 2015.)

Aβ is a large myelinated fiber that is primarily responsible for touch but has modulatory effects on the function of the remaining Aδ and C fibers. The Aδ fibers, which are smaller and slower conducting, are responsible for pain stimulation along with the unmyelinated C fibers. Sharp sensation and pain perception are transmitted by Aδ fibers. The unmyelinated C fibers are thought to be the major players in pain perception and respond in a multimodal fashion. The nerve class responds to noxious mechanical, thermal, and chemical stimuli.

Insult and injury result in nociception through the release of inflammatory mediators. Excitatory neurotransmitters transfer information from the peripheral nervous system to the central nervous system through the actions of glutamate, an inflammatory neurotransmitter. Local modulation is achieved by the actions of chemical mediators, which include bradykinin (peptides), nerve growth factor (neurotrophins), and prostaglandins (lipids). The combined actions of local modulation sensitizes peripheral nociceptors by lowering their activation thresholds. The action of local nociception is further compounded by the release of neurotransmitter substance P. Substance P contributes to local injury via vasodilation, which results in leakage of proteins and fluids into the extracellular space. The combined action of the multimodal stimulants makes up the bases for nociceptive transmission of pain and activation of the peripheral nervous system.[10] Of particular importance in acute pain control is the release of arachidonic acid metabolites. Prostaglandin, which is a metabolite of arachidonic acid produced by the cyclooxygenase (COX) enzyme, acts to block potassium efflux from nociceptors and lowers the activation threshold.[10] Prostaglandin synthesis depends on

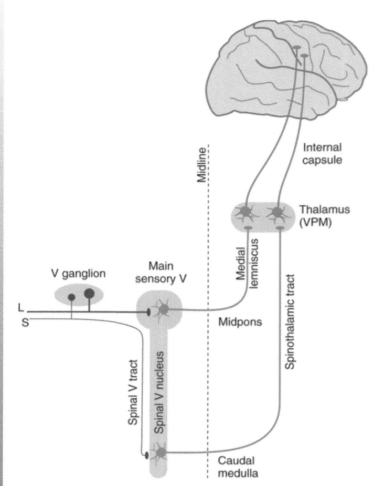

Fig. 2. Sensory afferents of the trigeminal nerve. First-order neurons travel to the main spinal trigeminal nucleus, cross the midline, and are transferred to the thalamus. Signals subsequently are transferred to the somatosensory cortex. (*From* Vanderah TW, Gould DJ. Chapter 12: Cranial Nerves and Their Nuclei. In: Vanderah, TW, Gould DJ. Nolte's Essentials of the Human Brain. 7th ed. Elsevier. 2015.)

the activities of COX-1 and COX-2. COX-1 has a primary activity in the peripheral tissues, whereas COX-2 acts within the gut and promotes mucus production. Prostaglandin additionally reserves the ability to modulate vasodilation of peripheral tissues as well as viscera such as the glomerular apparatus of the kidney.[14] This action further contributes to local inflammation and pain. Another important player in nerve sensitization is histamine. Histamine is released through stimulation of mast cells. Similarly to prostaglandin, histamine has stimulatory effects on nociceptors that cause pain with additional effects on vasodilation and local lymphocyte stimulation.[10] Multimodal analgesic strategies target these local inflammatory mediators to modulate pain.

Table 1
Classification of nociceptors based on diameter and myelination

Classification	Diameter (μm)	Myelin	Conduction Velocity (m/s)	Sensory Function
Aβ	Large (6–12)	Yes	>35	Touch
Aδ	Medium (1–5)	Thin	5–35	Fast pain
C	Small (0.2–1.5)	No	<2.0	Slow pain

From Bell A. The neurobiology of acute pain. Vet J. 2018 Jul;237:55-62.

Stimulation and afferent sensory input are transferred from the peripheral to the central nervous system and ultimately to the somatosensory cortex. Transfer of neurosensory signals from the periphery to the central nervous system involves the synapsis and transfer of information from the first-order neurons to the second-order neurons within the spinal cord or brain stem. Activation of the secondary somatosensory neurons is completed via the release of neurochemical agents such as glutamate, vasoactive peptide, somatostatin, calcitonin gene–related peptide, and substance P. Activated second-order neurons project to the somatosensory cortex via the thalamus and the brain stem using third-order neurons. The information is transferred up the spinal cord via the contralateral and ipsilateral spinothalamic tracts. Of these sensory highways, the anterior spinothalamic tract carries sensory information of pain, temperature, and touch (see **Fig. 1**).[10]

Pain from the maxillofacial region is transmitted to the central nervous system by the trigeminal nerve. The trigeminal nerve system is a complex arrangement of nerve transmission fibers and its transmission pathway is slightly different from what was described earlier. Sensory information from the dental and maxillofacial regions first travels to the subnucleus caudalis within the spinal trigeminal nuclear complex. The subnucleus caudalis is located in the medulla, and is the principal brain relay site of nociceptive information arising from the orofacial region. The subnucleus caudalis exhibits considerable similarity with the spinal dorsal horn and thus it is termed the medullary dorsal horn (MDH). Its similar laminar organization to the spinal dorsal horn is what has led to this alternative name. However, despite apparent homology in nociceptive processing, features of trigeminal pain processing in the MDH are distinctly different from that of the spinal dorsal horn.[15] The continuity of the spinal dorsal horn and MDH is collectively termed the trigeminocervical complex. Following injury and noxious stimulation of the dental and maxillofacial region, there is increased excitability and sensitization of trigeminal pain pathways in nonlaminar regions of the spinal trigeminal nuclear complex. The spinal trigeminal nucleus projects to the ventral posteromedial (VPM) nucleus in the contralateral thalamus via the ventral trigeminal tract. This sensory information is relayed from the thalamus to the primary motor cortex via the primary sensory cortex, allowing response to stimuli of the face. Both incoming nociceptive signals to the subnucleus caudalis and projecting nociceptive signals on their way to the thalamus can be modified (modulated) by descending nerve fibers from higher levels of the central nervous system or by drugs.[16]

PSYCHOLOGICAL EFFECTS OF PAIN

Mental distress and anxiety has a significant impact on the outcome of patient pain perception and experience in operative and postoperative pain control. Psychological preparation before surgery can help reduce acute postoperative pain by a variety of mechanisms. Negative emotions, cognitive preparation, behavior, and stress have been found to have a significant impact on postoperative pain experience.[17,18] Negative emotions compound postoperative pain by enhancing pain sensations. Cognitive emotions influence behavior when experiencing acute pain by affecting medication dosing and compliance with postoperative instructions.

In a prospective observational study conducted by Maple and colleagues,[18] patients undergoing a hand-assisted laparoscopic donor nephrectomy were asked to complete a perceived stress scale survey before surgery. The study used a high-resolution ultrasonography scan of surgical wounds on the first 3 postoperative days and once following discharge. The wound size and median intensity, which is a marker of tissue fluid that is edema, were measured. Improved median intensity reflected faster wound healing and resolution of tissue edema. The study found that increased emotional stability was associated with faster wound healing. Fifty-eight patients were involved in the study. The investigators concluded that stress had a negative impact on wound healing and that optimism and emotional stability had a positive impact on postoperative outcomes.[18] In 1993, Johnston and Vögele[20] conducted a meta-analysis investigating the benefits of psychological preparation before surgery. The study concluded that psychological preparation was beneficial in reducing use of pain medication, length of hospital stay, behavior recovery, and clinical recovery, and improving patient satisfaction.[19,20] A Cochrane Review conducted by Powell and colleagues[19] examined the benefits of psychological preparation before surgery. The investigators highlight the following preoperative interventions as beneficial in reducing postoperative pain: procedural information, sensory information, behavioral instruction, cognitive intervention, relaxation techniques, hypnosis, and emotion-focused interventions.[19] The anxiety of having to see the dentist and the fear of dentistry can activate the pituitary-adrenal axis, leading to an increased experience of pain.

The management of acute pain in the average oral surgical patient is not often affected by central neurophysiologic plasticity from chronic pain but it is important for dentists to screen patients for chronic pain elsewhere in the body; for example, arthritis, back pain, and migraine. Patients with chronic pain problems who have developed central neurophysiologic plasticity do not respond to the treatment of acute pain as would pain-free patients, and they may require adjustments to routine analgesics.

MULTIMODAL ANALGESIA

In 1993, Kehlet and Dahl[21] published an article that introduced the concept of multimodal or balanced analgesia in acute pain management. The investigators argued that appropriate pain control cannot be achieved by a single drug or method without significant side effects. The investigators recommended that combined analgesic regimens are much more effective in achieving postoperative pain control and avoiding untoward side effects. The method takes advantage of synergistic and additive effects of medications at a lower doses. This approach offsets side effect profiles.[21] Multimodal analgesic takes advantage of targeting therapy at the peripheral nervous system and central nervous system (**Fig. 3**).

Appropriate acute pain control following surgery must be tailored to the surgery that was completed in addition to the patient and the patient's specific tolerance. Dosing of medications involved in multimodal pain control are listed in **Table 2**.[22] In attempts to provide guidelines and recommendations for postsurgical pain control, the Enhanced Recovery After Surgery (ERAS) society guidelines were established. The ERAS society guidelines are available through the Web site www.erassociety.org/ and comprise a series of recommendations for multimodal anesthesia. These recommendations are published following careful consideration of the available research in the literature. Evidence-based recommendations are presented for a multitude of specialties.

CURRENTLY AVAILABLE ANALGESICS
Nonsteroidal Antiinflammatory Drugs

Nonsteroidal antiinflammatory medications include all medications that act on the enzymatic actions of COX-1 and COX-2. As previously discussed, through the production of arachidonic acid and subsequently prostaglandin synthesis, by COX-1 and COX-2, peripheral nerve sensitization is achieved by lowering the activation threshold. The NSAID class of drugs act to inhibit the actions of prostaglandin. The reduction in prostaglandin synthesis acts to diminish peripheral nociception and swelling associated with tissue damage and edema.[14] Variations in their targeted mechanisms have been formulated, and

selective COX-2 inhibitors aim to reduce adverse effects of reduced gastric mucus production. Inhibiting prostaglandin synthesis in the gastric mucosal tissues results in reduced protection of the lumen against the local environment, resulting in deepithelization and ultimately gastric ulceration. NSAIDs are particularly useful in inflammatory disorders, such as acute pain associated with arthropathies and trauma. By reducing tissue edema and prostaglandin synthesis, reductions in inflammatory mediators result in reduced tissue edema and pain.

NSAIDs come in several forms, including oral, intravenous, topical, and rectal routs of administration. Typical oral agents include aspirin, ibuprofen, ketorolac, and diclofenac. As previously mentioned, selective COX-2 inhibitors are available, such as Celecoxib and Parecoxib.[6] Ketorolac is an example of a commonly available intravenous agent. New topical agents, such as diclofenac, come in 5% to 16% concentration gels, which have gained increasing popularity in applications to the temporomandibular joints.

Acetaminophen

A well-known and familiar medication that is available over the counter for pain control is acetaminophen. Patients are often familiar with its use and are comfortable with administration. Acetaminophen and NSAIDs make up the mainstay of multimodal anesthesia. The medication is available in either intravenous or oral forms. With appropriate use and dosing, the medication has minimal side effects and can be used effectively in management of centrally mediated pain. Acetaminophen acts through modulation of the endogenous cannabinoid and serotonin systems. Early investigations of acetaminophen revealed that acetaminophen is metabolized into p-aminophenol, which crosses the blood-brain barrier. The metabolite N-acylphenolamine is produced by the actions of amide hydrolase, where it acts on vanilloid 1 and cannabinoid 1 receptors in the midbrain and medulla to modulate pain.[23–25] When used in combination with NSAIDs, it provided synergistic effects of anesthesia by modulation of the central nervous system by acetaminophen and the peripheral nervous system by NSAIDs.

Hepatotoxicity is of particular concern with the use of acetaminophen. Emergency physicians become particularly concerned with hepatotoxicity when acetaminophen doses exceed 12 g or 200 mg per kilogram of body weight in the pediatric population. N-acetylcysteine administration following acute ingestion has been shown to reduce acute hepatotoxicity following acute

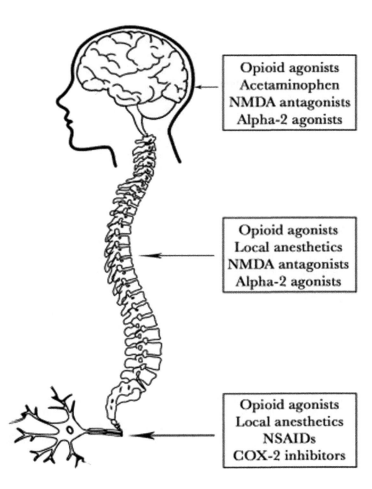

Fig. 3. Multimodal analgesic sites of action in the central and peripheral nervous system. NMDA, *N*-methyl-D-aspartate. (*From* Pitchon DN, Dayan AC, Schwenk ES, Baratta JL, Viscusi ER. Updates on Multimodal Analgesia for Orthopedic Surgery. Anesthesiol Clin. 2018 Sep;36(3):361-373.)

Table 2
Commonly used multimodal analgesic agents

Drug	Route	Dosing (mg)	Interval (h)
Acetaminophen	Oral	325–625	Q 4–6
Celecoxib	Oral	Loading 400 Maintenance 200	Q 12
Ibuprofen	Oral	400–800	Q 6–8
Naprosyn	Oral	250–500	Q 12
Ketorolac	Intravenous	30–60	Q 6
Pregabalin	Oral	Initial 75 Max 150 Increase as needed	Q 12 Q 12
Gabapentin	Oral	Initial 300 Max 600 Increase as needed	Q 24 Q 8

Abbreviation: Q, every.
Adapted from Pitchon DN, Dayan AC, Schwenk ES, Baratta JL, Viscusi ER. Updates on Multimodal Analgesia for Orthopedic Surgery. Anesthesiol Clin. 2018 Sep;36(3):361-373.

overdose of acetaminophen. Peak hepatotoxicity in stage III disease can result in hepatic failure, encephalopathy, hyperbilirubinemia, shock, increased prothrombin time, thrombocytopenia, and bleeding.[26]

Local Anesthetics

The efficacy of local anesthesia is well established. Clinicians have used local anesthesia via local infiltration and regional anesthesia to conduct surgery to provide comfort for patients during awake or general anesthetic procedures. Although not available for administration in the head and neck, regional anesthesia via the administration of regional anesthesia (eg, a Bier limb block) additionally provides an alternative method of pain control. Local anesthesia exerts its effects by controlling sodium channel conduction and depolarization of nerves. Several local anesthetics are available with different durations of action (**Table 3**). Local anesthetic duration of action depends on the degree of protein binding. Local anesthetics such as bupivacaine that have a high degree of protein binding are useful in the immediate postoperative period in controlling pain. By administering a nerve block after a procedure, postoperative pain can be controlled until oral medications can be obtained by the patient and allow for the manifestation of appropriate pain control before the local anesthesia wears off. New medications have been developed with a superior profile for long-lasting anesthetic effects. A liposomal form of bupivacaine (Exparel; Pacira Pharmaceuticals, Parsippany, NJ) has recently been gaining popularity for long-term control of postoperative pain. The duration of action of Exparel ranges from 72 to 96 hours. Local administration into the peripheral soft tissues in the surgical site allows long-term control of pain.[27]

Current literature has shown that systemic administration of local anesthesia in conjunction with general anesthesia may reduce postoperative pain. In a meta-analysis conducted by Marret and colleagues,[28] the investigators reviewed 8 clinical trials where 161 total patients received intravenous lidocaine during abdominal surgery. The trials were selected because of consistent use of a visual analog scale (VAS) for postoperative pain evaluation. In addition, the study recorded incidence of postoperative nausea and vomiting in patients. There was a statistically significant reduction in patient pain scores when receiving intraoperative lidocaine versus the control. The incidence of nausea and vomiting was 32% when receiving intravenous lidocaine and 52% in the control.[28]

Anticonvulsants

Gabapentinoid medications, which include gabapentin and the more recently developed pregabalin, have been traditionally used as anticonvulsants. Gabapentin and pregabalin act by inhibiting $\alpha2\delta$ voltage-gated Ca^{2+} channels.[29] Reduced activity of calcium channels suppresses the excitability of the dorsal horn neurons after tissue damage.[30] The use of gabapentin in perioperative acute pain control has been incorporated into ERAS protocols in attempts to prevent central and peripheral sensitization to pain.[29,31] Anticonvulsants act to aid in acute pain control to reduce opioid consumption in the form of opioid-sparing effects. This approach allows reduced dosing of opioids, reduced consumption, and reduced opioid-associated side effects such as respiratory depression, nausea, and vomiting.[32] Recommended dosing of pregabalin is a starting dose of 150 mg/d in 2 or 3 doses increasing to 300 mg/d and a maximum dose of 600 mg/d.

Although promising data are reported, some investigators argue that the evidence to support its routine use is weak, and some studies are reported to have a significant risk of bias. Kumar and Habib[31] published a meta-analysis of the most recent literature, arguing that the beneficial effects of gabapentinoids are inflated. In a retrospective review, Wright and colleagues[33] reported no statistically significant difference in morphine-equivalent dosing of patients who underwent abdominal surgery with the use of perioperative

---

Table 3
Properties of local anesthetics

Agent	Lipid Solubility	Protein Binding	Duration	PKa	Onset Time
Mepivacaine	1	75	Medium	7.6	Fast
Lidocaine	4	65	Medium	7.7	Fast
Bupivacaine	28	95	Long	8.1	Moderate
Tetracaine	80	85	Long	8.6	Slow

From Agarwal R, Obeid G, Abubaker AO, Benson KJ. Chapter 6: Local Anesthetics. In: Abubaker AO, Lam D, Benson, K, eds. Oral and Maxillofacial Surgery Secrets. 3rd ed. Elsevier; 2016: 77-86.

pregabalin dosing. The patients received perioperative multimodal pain control as per American Pain Society guidelines of acetaminophen 500 mg 3 times per day, celecoxib 400 mg and 900 mg of gabapentin daily.[33] In comparison, Mishriky and colleagues[32] performed a systematic review investigating the analgesic efficacy of perioperative pregabalin. The meta-analysis included studies observing postoperative pain in patients undergoing a variety of surgeries, including abdominal surgery, spine surgery, knee and hip arthroplasties, and plastic surgery. The investigators found a statistically significant reduction in opioid consumption with administration of pregabalin. Additional effects, including reduced hospital stay and reduced duration of postanesthesia care unit stay, were reported.[32] There is still debate with regard to routine use of gabapentinoids for perioperative acute pain control. However, there seems to be some benefit to its use in the hospital setting.

Gamma-aminobutyric Acid

Medications that act on gamma-aminobutyric acid (GABA) channels such as benzodiazepines are primarily used for sedation and anesthesia. The properties of benzodiazepines are well known and include sedation, hypnosis, anxiolysis, and amnesia. There are no known anesthetic properties to midazolam. In the acute pain setting, benzodiazepines are used to help manage acute pain by controlling anxiety.

There is evidence to suggest that the GABA channel modulates the complex array of descending pain pathways by augmenting the inhibitory pathways that originate in the rostroventral medulla, brain stem, nucleus tractus solitarius, paratracheal nucleus, hypothalamus, and the somatosensory cortex. Interactions depend on their activities on the afferent fibers and interneurons projected from the dorsal horn first-order afferent neurons. The GABA-mediated inhibitory pathways act by suppression of nociceptive stimulation of the central nervous system. Suppression results in reduced activity and sensory activation of the periaqueductal gray matter, thalamus, hypothalamus, parabrachial nuclei, nucleus tractus solitarius, and amygdala.

The evidence to support the efficacy of midazolam in aiding modulation of postoperative pain is weak at best. A prospective randomized, double-blinded, placebo-controlled trial investigating the effects of coadministration of midazolam with morphine was conducted by Auffret and collogues.[34] The study compared administration of 0.10 mg/kg of intravenous midazolam with a placebo to observe the effects on reducing morphine equivalents needed to control postoperative pain. Pain assessment was completed using a numeric rating scale. Ninety-one patients were involved and no significant difference in the pain score was observed between the control and test groups. The investigators concluded that midazolam does not enhance pain control as an adjunct to morphine when administered for acute pain control in the trauma setting. For routine patients, coadministration does not seem to have much impact on reducing acute pain. However, if clinically patients appear agitated and anxious, administration of midazolam provides comfort and anxiolysis. This decision should be based on clinical judgment of the physician.[34]

Opioids

Opioid receptors modulate pain in both the central and peripheral nervous systems. Receptors act to modulate between the complicated interplay of the descending and ascending neurosensory pathways. Opioids act through several types of receptors that have a variety of activities, which include κ, μ, δ, and σ (**Table 4**). Of particular note is the δ opioid receptor, which is responsible for analgesia. When stimulated, the peripheral and central nervous systems trigger an inhibitory response of pain processing and analgesia. This mechanism depends on the activities of exogenous opioids or endogenous opiates such as endorphin, encephalin, or dynorphin.[14]

CANNABINOIDS

Cannabinoids are gaining momentum and increasing popularity in the control of acute and

Table 4	
Outline of opioid receptors and their respective activities	
Receptor	**Effect**
Δ	Analgesia
M	Supraspinal analgesia μ1 Respiratory depression μ2 Physical dependance Muscle rigidity
Σ	Dysphoria Hallucinations
κ	Sedation Spinal analgesia

Adapted from Egan TD, Newberry C. Chapter 10: Opioids. In: Pardo, MC, Miller, RD. Basics of Anesthesia. 6th ed. Elsevier. 2012; 117.

chronic pain. Changes in public opinion and legislation have opened options for use in the medical field, opening access to the greater public. The 2 main active components of cannabinoid medications are Δ^9-tetrahydrocannabinol (THC) and cannabidiol (CBD), which act through the endocannabinoid system.[35] Cannabidiol in particular is useful in acute pain management because of its effects in modulating central and peripheral neuron activity and alteration in release of proinflammatory mediators. At present, 2 receptors have been identified: CB_1 and CB_2. Activation of the receptor CB_1 regulates central and peripheral neurons through retrograde synaptic messaging, which suppresses the nociceptive sensitization. The remaining CB_2 receptor affects the release of proinflammatory cytokines from immune cells and modulates cell inflammatory responses.[35,36] The main psychoactive component THC is thought to act through the antiinflammatory and analgesic mechanisms. THC is thought the suppress mast

cell activations, leukocyte trafficking and adhesion, neurogenic inflammation, oxidative stress, and endothelial activation.[37] Although the mechanism of pain modulation has been identified through animal models, the evidence to support its efficacy is weak. In a double-blinded crossover study, 18 heathy individual volunteers were administered capsules containing THC extract versus a placebo. A circular sunburn spot was induced on the skin surface of the upper leg and pain thresholds were measured. The investigators did not find that THC did not affect acute pain thresholds using this sunburn model.[38] In comparison, in a randomized clinical trial investigating the effect of inhaled cannabis for chronic pain in adults with sickle cell disease, the investigators did not find any statistically significant reduction in pain-associated symptoms compared with a placebo. The clinical trial compared chronic pain using a visual analog scare where participants inhaled vaporized cannabis and compared the pain ratings

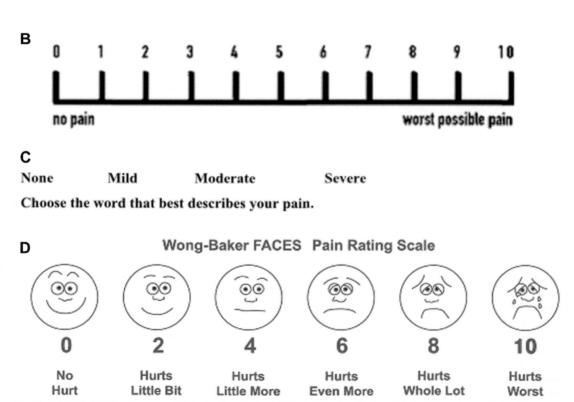

Fig. 4. (A) VAS. (B) The Numerical Pain Rating Scale. (C) Verbal Rating Scale of Verbal Descriptor Scale. (D) Wong-Baker FACES Pain Rating Scale. (*From* Karcioglu O, Topacoglu H, Dikme O, Dikme O. A systematic review of the pain scales in adults: Which to use? Am J Emerg Med. 2018 Apr;36(4):707-714.)

with a vaporized placebo. The study involved 23 participants who completed the study.[37] There is low-quality evidence indicating that cannabinoids may be a safe alternative for a small but significant reduction in subjective pain score when treating acute pain.[39]

NONPHARMACOLOGIC TREATMENT

Treating pain with hot and cold can be effective. After oral surgery, ice can be used for the acute pain and inflammation. The cold reduces blood flow to the surgical site, which tends to reduce the inflammation that causes pain. It may also temporarily reduce nerve activity, which can also relieve pain. Salt water rinses can help reduce inflammation by reverse osmosis. Edema fluid comes out of the cells because the salt concentration in the saline solution is greater than that in the cell.[40]

SUMMARY

The importance of clinical judgment in multimodal analgesia cannot be stressed enough. Appropriate acute pain control starts with administration of excellent local anesthesia. Properly conducted local nerve blocks and infiltration reduces the sensitization and anxiety of the patient for control of postoperative pain. First-line treatment should involve a combination of ibuprofen and Tylenol, weight based for children, in a staggered manner. The literature has provided evidence that this technique is equally effective in pain management as administering opioid analgesia. With the current public attention directed toward misuse of opioids, clinicians have become wary of their use. However, when used in the appropriate setting, administration of opioids is appropriate. For example, following major surgery, joint replacement, or orthognathic surgery, administration of multimodal anesthesia that includes the use of morphine or hydromorphone is appropriate and should be considered for patient comfort and pain control. Administration of oxycodone doses following invasive outpatient oral surgery is another indication for use of opioid analgesics. Examples where opioids should be considered include invasive wisdom teeth removal that involves removal of bone, full-mouth extractions with alveoloplasty, and local bone harvesting (symphysis and ramus). In adults in whom multimodal anesthesia is inadequate and opioid use is being avoided, as previously discussed, administration of gabapentin and pregabalin in combination with the use of ibuprofen and Tylenol provides superior postoperative acute pain control. The use of Exparel (liposomal bupivacaine) should be considered for invasive procedures when available. Although costly, postoperative analgesia by administering the medication provided superior acute pain control and drastically reduced oral and intravenous medication use. Appropriate clinical assessment of pain and the ability to evaluate effective pain control are important. Tailoring analgesia is both a science and a product of experience. A systematic approach for pain control has been developed. The VAS has been developed for evaluation of pain, which is easy to use and is additionally suitable for use in the pediatric population. The numeric rating scale (NRS) is an 11-point scale similar to the VAS that has been validated for pain evaluation in the literature. Tools such as the VAS and NRS allow evaluation of pain without the need for language translation and allow clinicians to better quantify patients' pain experience (**Fig. 4**).[41]

SUMMARY

Pain is a complicated and subjective entity that is difficult to quantify and treat. Clinicians must use all the knowledge and experience at their disposal to properly evaluate the degree of pain that each patient is experiencing. Having a solid foundation and deep understanding of pain and its mechanism is critical in administering appropriate acute pain control. Moreover, appropriate administration of opioid analgesics when indicated is important to avoid further contributing to the opioid epidemic. With the use of multimodal anesthesia, opioid administration can be minimized. Using visual scales that quantify pain, such as the FACES pain rating scale, gives clinicians another tool to tailor medications to achieve appropriate postoperative acute pain control. The key to controlling acute pain is to use all the tools at clinicians' disposal and to provide the patients with empathy and understanding of their situations. Achieving good acute pain control improves patient experience, quality of life, and operative experience.

CLINICS CARE POINTS

- Patient perception and tolerance can differ dramatically from patient to patient. Titrating the appropriate analgesic requirement requires careful consideration of the invasive nature of the procedure and the expected patient response and tolerance of pain.

- There is evidence in the literature to show that mismanagement of acute may even lead to central sensitization and the development of chronic pain.
- Opioids are associated with high rates of abuse. There were 201.9 million prescriptions for opioid analgesics in 2009, with 79.5 million to adolescents (39%). In 2015, the Department of Health and Human Services reported that 12.5 million people misused opioid prescription medication.
- Psychological preparation before surgery can help reduce acute postoperative pain by a variety of mechanisms. Stress had a negative impact on wound healing and optimism and emotional stability had a positive impact on postoperative outcomes.
- In 1993, Kehlet and Dahl[21] published an article that introduced the concept of multimodal or balanced analgesia in acute pain management. The investigators argued that appropriate pain control cannot be achieved by a single drug or method without significant side effects. The method takes advantage of synergistic and additive effects of medications at a lower dose, which offsets the side effect profiles.
- Through production of arachidonic acid, and subsequently prostaglandin synthesis, by COX-1 and COX-2, peripheral nerve sensitization is achieved by lowering the activation threshold.
- Acetaminophen acts through modulation of the endogenous cannabinoid and serotonin systems. The metabolite N-acylphenolamine is produced by the actions of amide hydrolase where it acts on vanilloid 1 and cannabinoid 1 receptors in the midbrain and medulla to modulate pain.
- The administration of regional anesthesia (eg, a Bier limb block) provides a method of pain control. Local anesthesia exerts its effects by controlling sodium channel conduction and depolarization of nerves. By administering a nerve block after a procedure, postoperative pain can be controlled until oral medications can be obtained by the patient and this allows for manifestation of appropriate pain control before the local anesthesia wears off.
- Gabapentin and pregabalin act by inhibiting $\alpha 2\delta$ voltage-gated Ca^{2+} channels.[29] Reduced activity of calcium channels suppresses the excitability of the dorsal horn neurons after tissue damage.
- Medications that act on GABA channels, such as benzodiazepines, are primarily used for sedation and anesthesia. In the acute pain setting, benzodiazepines are used to help manage acute pain by controlling anxiety.
- Opioid receptors modulate pain through the δ opioid receptor, which is responsible for analgesia. When stimulated, the peripheral and central nervous systems trigger an inhibitory response of pain processing and analgesia.
- The 2 main active components of cannabinoid medications are THC and CBD, which act through the endocannabinoid system. At present, 2 receptors have been identified: CB1 and CB2. Activation of the receptor CB1 regulates central and peripheral neurons through retrograde synaptic messaging. This process suppresses nociceptive sensitization.

DISCLOSURE

The authors have nothing to disclose.

REFERENCES

1. Cogan J. Pain management after cardiac surgery. Semin Cardiothorac Vasc Anesth 2010;14(3):201–4.
2. Ziehm S, Rosendahl J, Barth J, et al. Psychological interventions for acute pain after open heart surgery. Cochrane Database Syst Rev 2017;7(7):Cd009984.
3. Centers for Disease Control and Prevention NCfIPaC. Acute pain 2019. Available at: https://www.cdc.gov/acute-pain/postsurgical-pain/index.html. Accessed April 14, 2021.
4. Centers for Disease Control and Prevention NCfIPaC. Opioids for acute pain. What you need to know 2019. Available at: https://www.cdc.gov/drugoverdose/pdf/patients/Opioids-for-Acute-Pain-a.pdf. Accessed April 04, 2021.
5. Fortuna RJ, Robbins BW, Caiola E, et al. Prescribing of controlled medications to adolescents and young adults in the United States. Pediatrics 2010;126(6):1108–16.
6. Volkow ND, McLellan TA, Cotto JH, et al. Characteristics of opioid prescriptions in 2009. JAMA 2011;305(13):1299–301.
7. The Opioid Epidemic in the U.S.. 2018. Available at: https://www.hhs.gov/sites/default/files/2017-opioids-infographic.pdf. Accessed January 22, 2021.
8. Han B, Compton WM, Blanco C, et al. Prescription opioid use, misuse, and use disorders in U.S. adults: 2015 national survey on drug use and health. Ann Intern Med 2017;167(5):293–301.
9. McCabe SE, West BT, Boyd CJ. Leftover prescription opioids and nonmedical use among high school seniors: a multi-cohort national study. J Adolesc Health 2013;52(4):480–5.

10. Dinakar P, Stillman AM. Pathogenesis of pain. Semin Pediatr Neurol 2016;23(3):201–8.
11. Todd Vanderah DG. Nolte's the human brain. 7th edition. Elsevier; 2015.
12. Pasero CM. Pain assessment and pharmacologic management. Elsevier/Mosby; 2011.
13. Bell A. The neurobiology of acute pain. Vet J 2018; 237:55–62.
14. Beverly A, Kaye AD, Ljungqvist O, et al. Essential elements of multimodal analgesia in enhanced recovery after surgery (ERAS) guidelines. Anesthesiol Clin 2017;35(2):e115–43.
15. Ren K, Dubner R. The role of trigeminal interpolaris-caudalis transition zone in persistent orofacial pain. Int Rev Neurobiol 2011;97:207–25.
16. Conti PC, Pertes RA, Heir GM, et al. Orofacial pain: basic mechanisms and implication for successful management. J Appl Oral Sci 2003;11(1):1–7.
17. Rainville P, Bao QVH, Chrétien P. Pain-related emotions modulate experimental pain perception and autonomic responses. Pain 2005;118(3):306–18.
18. Maple H, Chilcot J, Lee V, et al. Stress predicts the trajectory of wound healing in living kidney donors as measured by high-resolution ultrasound. Brain Behav Immun 2015;43:19–26.
19. Powell R, Scott NW, Manyande A, et al. Psychological preparation and postoperative outcomes for adults undergoing surgery under general anaesthesia. Cochrane Database Syst Rev 2016;(5):Cd008646.
20. Johnston M, Vögele C. Benefits of psychological preparation for surgery: a meta-analysis. Ann Behav Med 1993;15(4):245–56.
21. Kehlet H, Dahl JB. The value of "multimodal" or "balanced analgesia" in postoperative pain treatment. Anesth Analg 1993;77(5):1048–56.
22. Pitchon DN, Dayan AC, Schwenk ES, et al. Updates on multimodal analgesia for orthopedic surgery. Anesthesiol Clin 2018;36(3):361–73.
23. Ohashi N, Kohno T. Analgesic effect of acetaminophen: a review of known and novel mechanisms of action. Front Pharmacol 2020;11:580289.
24. De Petrocellis L, Bisogno T, Davis JB, et al. Overlap between the ligand recognition properties of the anandamide transporter and the VR1 vanilloid receptor: inhibitors of anandamide uptake with negligible capsaicin-like activity. FEBS Lett 2000;483(1):52–6.
25. Palazzo E, de Novellis V, Marabese I, et al. Interaction between vanilloid and glutamate receptors in the central modulation of nociception. Eur J Pharmacol 2002;439(1–3):69–75.
26. Fisher ES, Curry SC. Evaluation and treatment of acetaminophen toxicity. Adv Pharmacol 2019;85:263–72.
27. Vyas KS, Rajendran S, Morrison SD, et al. Systematic review of liposomal bupivacaine (Exparel) for postoperative analgesia. Plast Reconstr Surg 2016; 138(4):748e–56e.
28. Marret E, Rolin M, Beaussier M, et al. Meta-analysis of intravenous lidocaine and postoperative recovery after abdominal surgery. Br J Surg 2008;95(11): 1331–8.
29. Gross JL, Perate AR, Elkassabany NM. Pain management in trauma in the age of the opioid crisis. Anesthesiol Clin 2019;37(1):79–91.
30. Dahl JB, Mathiesen O, Møiniche S. Protective premedication': an option with gabapentin and related drugs? A review of gabapentin and pregabalin in in the treatment of post-operative pain. Acta Anaesthesiol Scand 2004;48(9):1130–6.
31. Kumar AH, Habib AS. The role of gabapentinoids in acute and chronic pain after surgery. Curr Opin Anaesthesiol 2019;32(5):629–34.
32. Mishriky BM, Waldron NH, Habib AS. Impact of pregabalin on acute and persistent postoperative pain: a systematic review and meta-analysis. Br J Anaesth 2015;114(1):10–31.
33. Wright R, Wright J, Perry K, et al. Preoperative pain measures ineffective in outpatient abdominal surgeries. Am J Surg 2018;215(5):958–62.
34. Auffret Y, Gouillou M, Jacob GR, et al. Does midazolam enhance pain control in prehospital management of traumatic severe pain? Am J Emerg Med 2014;32(6):655–9.
35. Maurer GE, Mathews NM, Schleich KT, et al. Understanding cannabis-based therapeutics in sports medicine. Sports Health 2020;12(6):540–6.
36. Pertwee RG. The diverse CB1 and CB2 receptor pharmacology of three plant cannabinoids: delta9-tetrahydrocannabinol, cannabidiol and delta9-tetrahydrocannabivarin. Br J Pharmacol 2008;153(2): 199–215.
37. Abrams DI, Couey P, Dixit N, et al. Effect of inhaled cannabis for pain in adults with sickle cell disease: a randomized clinical trial. JAMA Netw Open 2020; 3(7):e2010874.
38. Kraft B, Frickey NA, Kaufmann RM, et al. Lack of analgesia by oral standardized cannabis extract on acute inflammatory pain and hyperalgesia in volunteers. Anesthesiology 2008;109(1):101–10.
39. Gazendam A, Nucci N, Gouveia K, et al. Cannabinoids in the management of acute pain: a systematic review and meta-analysis. Cannabis Cannabinoid Res 2020;5(4):290–7.
40. Ogle OE. New approaches to pain management. Dent Clin North Am 2020;64(2):315–24.
41. Karcioglu O, Topacoglu H, Dikme O, et al. A systematic review of the pain scales in adults: which to use? Am J Emerg Med 2018;36(4):707–14.

Pharmacologic Treatment for Temporomandibular and Temporomandibular Joint Disorders

Amanda Andre, DDS*, Joseph Kang, DDS, Harry Dym, DDS

KEYWORDS

• TMD • Pharmacotherapy • Intra-articular injections • Botox • Prolotherapy

KEY POINTS

• Drug therapy for the treatment of temporomandibular joint disorder is often prescribed as an adjunct for noninvasive or minimally invasive treatments.
• Nonsteroidal anti-inflammatory drugs (with proton pump inhibitors) and muscle relaxants are first-line therapies shown to improve symptoms of temporomandibular joint disorder.
• Oral benzodiazepines, tricyclic antidepressants, and anticonvulsants are alternative therapies that may be considered in resistant or refractory temporomandibular joint disorder, in consultation with the patient's physician.
• Botox injections have shown to be safe and effective for treatment for myofascial temporomandibular joint disorder as intramuscular injections. Intra-articular injections have shown marked improvement in symptoms. Evidence suggests they share similar effectiveness.
• Prolotherapy with hypertonic glucose is effective for treating hypermobility and subluxation of the temporomandibular joint.

INTRODUCTION

Temporomandibular joint (TMJ) disorders refers to multietiological conditions defined by pain and/or loss of function of the TMJ, the muscles of mastication, and other associated structures.[1,2] When symptoms are limited to the muscles of mastication, the term myofascial pain dysfunction is often used. The goals of therapy for patients with temporomandibular joint disorder (TMD) focus on the reduction of pain and the improvement or restoration of function. The current thinking on the etiology of TMD places a greater emphasis on the biochemical processes involved within the joint and therefore emerging therapies focus on

halting the disease process.[3] Management strategies included noninvasive, minimally invasive, invasive, or surgical interventions and salvage modalities. Noninvasive modalities are oftentimes preferred as the first line of treatment. Drug therapy is often prescribed as an adjunct for noninvasive or minimally invasive treatments. Although most patients respond well to conservative measures,[2] those who cannot find relief for their symptoms through noninvasive therapies can suffer from debilitating functional limitations and pain that can negatively affect their overall quality of life.[4] Increasing severity of symptoms, impediments to daily activities, and failure of conservative measures may be an indication for more invasive

The authors of this article have received no external funding or grants or any remuneration regarding any commercial items mentioned within the article.

The Brooklyn Hospital Center, 121 Dekalb Avenue, Brooklyn, NY 11201, USA

* Corresponding author.

E-mail address: aafernandez@tbh.org

Oral Maxillofacial Surg Clin N Am 34 (2022) 49–59

https://doi.org/10.1016/j.coms.2021.08.001

1042-3699/22/Published by Elsevier Inc.

treatments, including surgical intervention. This article aims to review some of the most commonly used pharmacologic agents available to oral and maxillofacial surgeons for the treatment of mild to moderate TMD (**Box 1**).

MEDICINE THERAPIES
Nonsteroidal Anti-Inflammatory Drugs

Nonsteroidal anti-inflammatory drugs (NSAIDs) decrease inflammation in the TMJ and associated muscles of mastication to provide relief of pain, promoting its use as a first-line treatment for TMD.[5] The primary mechanism of action of NSAIDs is through the inhibition of cyclo-oxygenase (COX) enzymes. COX-1 functions as a protective agent in the gastrointestinal (GI) tract. COX-2 is responsible for the synthesis of key biological mediators, such as prostaglandins (namely prostaglandin E_2) and leukotrienes from arachidonic acid, which are essential for the inflammation cascade. Inhibition of COX-2, and therefore prostaglandin E_2, cause a decrease in the classical signs of inflammation, namely, redness, swelling, and pain.[6] For anti-inflammatory effects in TMD, NSAIDs should be taken around the clock for at least 2 weeks, even in the absence of pain.[7]

Commonly prescribed NSAIDs for TMD include ibuprofen, naproxen, diclofenac, and piroxicam.

To study the efficacy of NSAIDs, investigators conducted a double-blind, placebo-controlled study comparing naproxen (nonselective, 500 mg twice a day), celecoxib (COX-2 selective, 500 mg twice a day), and placebo (twice a day) for 6 weeks. Naproxen was shown to significantly decrease symptoms of painful TMJ disc displacement at week 3 to week 6 on a visual analog scale (VAS) pain scale compared with celecoxib and placebo, although celecoxib also showed minor improvements in symptoms.[8] Kurita Varoli and colleagues[5] demonstrated that, in combination with an occlusal splint, NSAID (sodium diclofenac, 50 mg twice a day) was more effective than placebo (only occlusal splint), promoting significant pain relief after the third day, and the occlusal splint provided relief after the eighth day. These results indicate the additive effects of multiple treatment modalities to treat TMD.

NSAIDs are widely used and considered safe for prolonged use in healthy patients, up to 2 months in consultation with the patient's primary care physician.[1] The most common and serious adverse effect of NSAIDs is the risk for GI bleeding. Owing to its inhibitory effects on COX-1, NSAIDs can cause ulcers and bleeding of the GI tract and, therefore, they are contraindicated in patients with active GI disease, especially the elderly.[9] In patients with a high GI risk, COX-2 selective (eg, celecoxib) or a nonselective NSAID with a proton pump inhibitor (eg, omeprazole) may offer protection from upper GI events.[10] Other considerations with NSAIDs include cardiovascular disease, likely owing to the inhibition of COX-2 and its decreased prostaglandin I2 production, predisposing to endothelial injury.[11] In patients with low GI risk and high cardiovascular risk, naproxen may be preferred owing to its lower cardiovascular risk.[10] Furthermore, NSAIDs are metabolized by the renal system, causing alterations to renal blood flow, electrolyte balance, and platelet function.[12] Consequentially, NSAIDs should be avoided in patients with kidney disease.

Muscle Relaxants

Muscle relaxants inhibit overactive muscles of mastication and associated muscles to decrease myofascial pain and decrease the load on the TMJ. These spasmolytics have shown to decrease skeletal muscle tone and are beneficial for patients with chronic orofacial pain associated with increased muscle activity and TMD.[13] They act at the level of the cortex, brain, or spinal cord, causing inhibition of polysynaptic pathways at

---

Box 1
Drugs used in the treatment of temporomandibular dysfunction/TMJ disorders by route of administration

Medicine therapies (by mouth)

- Nonsteroidal anti-inflammatory drugs
- Opioids
- Corticosteroids
- Antidepressants
- Anticonvulsants
- Antiepileptics
- Muscle relaxants
- Sedatives, hypnotics

Injections

  Intramuscular

  - Botulinum toxin

  Intra-articular

  - Corticosteroids
  - Local anesthetics
  - Hypertonic dextrose (prolotherapy)
  - Platelet-rich plasma
  - Hyaluronic acid

the central nervous system (CNS). Commonly prescribed medications in this class of drugs include cyclobenzaprine, baclofen, tizanidine, carisoprodol, and methocarbamol.

A recent meta-analysis concluded that cyclobenzaprine improved TMD muscle pain in the short term through its effects over local spasms and associated acute musculoskeletal pain.[14] A review of 8 studies supports that cyclobenzaprine can significantly decrease pain intensity on a VAS pain scale from myofascial TMD versus placebo at 3-weeks follow-up. Further evidence is necessary to evaluate the effectiveness of prolonged use beyond 3 weeks and associated side effects of cyclobenzaprine.

The most prominent short-term side effect of centrally acting muscle relaxants is sedation, owing to its inhibitory effects against the CNS. Other potential side effects include malaise, tachycardia, dysrhythmia, and additive effects with other CNS depressants, such as alcohol, benzodiazepine, opioids, and barbiturates.[15] Cyclobenzaprine has a similar structure to tricyclic antidepressants (TCAs) and, therefore, can cause additional side effects familiar with this class of drugs, such as xerostomia, owing to its anticholinergic activity.[16] Furthermore, it is contraindicated for patients with congestive heart failure, arrhythmias, hyperthyroidism and may have serious adverse drug interactions with monoamine oxidase inhibitors and tramadol (increased risk of seizure).[1]

To decrease its sedative side effects, cyclobenzaprine is commonly prescribed at lower doses (10 mg) when treating TMD and is started as 1 dose per day at bedtime.[1] As mentioned, it can be prescribed for up to 3 weeks safely; long-term therapy should be managed in consultation with the patient's physician. Follow-up is critical to reassess the patient's tolerance to adverse effects.

Benzodiazepines

Benzodiazepines are used primarily as an anxiolytic medication, but have shown benefit to patients with acute muscle spasms and sleep disorders. Benzodiazepines enhance the effect of the neurotransmitter gamma-aminobutyric acid at its receptor, which mediates inhibitory synaptic transmission throughout the CNS. It does this by facilitating the opening of chloride channels, therefore causing hyperpolarization of the neurons in the CNS.[17] As a treatment modality for myofascial TMD, benzodiazepines promote muscle relaxation, sedation, and induce sleep.[18,19] Benzodiazepines commonly prescribed include diazepam, lorazepam, and alprazolam.

The effectiveness of benzodiazepines for TMD has been well-supported, specifically longer acting formulations with anticonvulsant activity, such as diazepam. In 1 double-blind placebo-controlled study of patients with myofascial jaw pain, investigators compared diazepam (5 mg 4 times a day for 4 weeks), ibuprofen (600 mg 4 times a day for 4 weeks), diazepam and ibuprofen combined, and placebo.[20] They demonstrate that diazepam has a significantly greater decrease in myofascial and TMD pain than placebo. Ibuprofen alone was less effective at pain relief than diazepam, but diazepam and ibuprofen combined proved better than ibuprofen alone. This finding may indicate that the use of benzodiazepines as a secondary therapy should the patient fail first-line NSAID therapy for TMD.

Benzodiazepines present adverse effects such as drowsiness, confusion, amnesia, and impaired coordination. Side effects are dose dependent and may prove useful to the clinician to titrate dosages.[20] Psychomotor deficits, such as memory impairment, are magnified in the geriatric population, owing to decreased biotransformation, decreased clearance, and increased receptor sensitivity.[21] As a CNS depressant, benzodiazepines should be avoided with other depressants, such as opioids, alcohol, or centrally acting muscle relaxants. Other contraindications include myasthenia gravis, acute narrow-angle glaucoma, or any medications of CYP 4503A4 substrates (eg, grapefruit juice, azole antifungals, erythromycin, calcium channel blockers).[22] Another concern with benzodiazepines is the development of tolerance and physical dependence with prolonged use. Withdrawal symptoms include anxiety, agitation, restlessness, insomnia, and seizures.[1] Clinicians can minimize the negative effects of physical and psychological dependence by limiting the course of therapy to no more than 4 weeks.[23] In light of these adverse effects, benzodiazepines are not the first-line pharmaceutical treatment of choice for TMD, but are an alternative for refractory TMD symptoms.

Antidepressants

Antidepressants have been well-supported to show the effectiveness in the management of pain arising from TMD. The major classes of antidepressants are TCAs, selective serotonin reuptake inhibitors monoamine oxidase inhibitors, and dual selective norepinephrine and serotonin reuptake inhibitors. The mechanism of action of antidepressants for analgesia is not clear, but some investigators suggest that their action on the neuronal circuits that regulate emotion show improvements in pain symptoms, even in the absence of concomitant depression.[24] Although selective serotonin reuptake inhibitors are shown to have improved side effects, TCAs and selective norepinephrine and serotonin reuptake inhibitors display superior pain relief compared with the others.[24] Commonly prescribed TCAs and selective norepinephrine and serotonin reuptake inhibitors include amitriptyline, nortriptyline, duloxetine, and venlafaxine.

To study the analgesic efficacy for TMD, a double-blind study of chronic patients with TMD pain concluded that low-dose amitriptyline (25 mg once per day for 14 days) significantly improved VAS pain scores during treatment and up to 1 week after treatment compared with placebo.[19] Although higher doses of amitriptyline are commonly prescribed to control depression, increased dosage of amitriptyline to 50 to 75 mg/d did not increase analgesic effects.[19]

TCAs, such as amitriptyline, can produce unwanted anticholinergic side effects, including sedation, dizziness, blurred vision, constipation, and dry mouth.[22] Exogenous epinephrine may cause adverse cardiovascular effects, and therefore dental anesthetics with epinephrine should be limited to 0.04 mg (2 carpules containing 1:100,000 epinephrine) per appointment for patients taking TCAs.[22] Furthermore, TCAs are absolutely contraindicated in patient's taking monoamine oxidase inhibitors owing to potential lethal serotonin syndrome causing confusion, fever, ataxia, myoclonus, and severe hypertension.[23] Although antidepressants are effective and safe as therapy for TMD, it is recommended for prescribing clinicians to comanage antidepressants with the patient's physician for long-term use and supervision of side effects.[1] Last, antidepressants require strict follow-up to not only assess efficacy and side effects, but also patient compliance because it may take up to a few weeks before therapeutic effects are seen clinically.[1] However, not all patients respond to TCAs or other antidepressants; alternatives, such as anticonvulsants (eg, gabapentin), may prove useful for these resistant patients.[25]

Anticonvulsants

Anticonvulsant medications are frequently prescribed for neuropathic pain, including orofacial pain and TMD. Medications in this class commonly prescribed for TMD include gabapentin and pregabalin. As structurally similar medications, gabapentin and pregabalin act in the CNS by inhibiting specific voltage-gated calcium channels causing a decrease in the release of excitatory neurotransmitters, such as glutamate and substance P.[25] The decrease in these excitatory neurotransmitters diminishes neuronal hyperexcitability and abnormal synchronization, promoting antiseizure activity, analgesia, and anxiolysis.[25]

In a double-blind, 12-week randomized controlled clinical trial, investigators demonstrated that gabapentin showed significant pain decrease on a VAS pain score versus placebo for myogenous TMD.[26] After the initial dose of 300 mg/d, patients' dose was increased by 300 mg every 3 days until pain was controlled with no adverse effects, with a maximum dose of 4200 mg. There were significant decreases in spontaneous pain by week 8 (mean dose, 3315 mg/d) and in the number of tender sites by week 12 (mean dose, 3426 mg/d).

Notable side effects of gabapentin include dizziness and drowsiness. Other adverse effects are memory impairment, xerostomia, peripheral edema, and hypoventilation.[27] Contraindications for gabapentin are patients with depression, myasthenia gravis, severe chronic kidney disease, and pulmonary disease.[27] Although anticonvulsants are not a first-line treatment for TMD, they may be useful as adjuvant analgesics in patients who have a history of failed TMJ surgeries or patients with longstanding unremitting pain.[23]

Opioids

Although there are recent and emerging studies on the efficacy of arthrocentesis and intra-articular injections of morphine to manage TMD, there is a gap in the literature supporting oral or subcutaneous opioids in the use of chronic orofacial pain.[23] Nonetheless, opioids may be considered acceptable therapy in a small subset of patients who have persistent TMD pain after failure of relief of symptoms after surgery or implants.[13] Common opioids prescribed for chronic pain include oral morphine, oxycodone, hydromorphone, and transdermal fentanyl patches.

Opioids can cause patients to have physical dependence and tolerance, along with other side effects, including sedation, dizziness, nausea, vomiting, constipation, and respiratory depression. Patients may exhibit drug-seeking behavior by reporting TMD pain.[23] Clinicians should perform an assessment of patients' previous drug use and past and current psychiatric status, often in consultation with a behavioral medicine specialist.[23] Additionally, clinicians should establish treatment goals with patients, including realistic goals for pain and function, and consider how therapy will be discontinued if benefits do not outweigh the risks.[28] Contraindications for opioids include patients taking other CNS depressants, such as spasmolytics, benzodiazepines, antidepressants, and antipsychotics, owing to the additive sedative effects.[1]

With the lack of data on the efficacy of opiate analgesics and its adverse effects of dependence, tolerance, and others mentioned elsewhere in this article, nonopioid pharmacologic therapy should be considered, if not exhausted, before initiating opioid therapy (**Table 1**). More information on prescribing opioids for chronic pain can be found in the 2016 guidelines from the Centers for Disease Control and Prevention.[28]

INJECTIONS
Botulinum Toxin

The botulinum toxin (BTX) is produced by the gram-positive anaerobic bacterium *Clostridium botulinum* and it derives its effect from the toxin's ability to inhibit the release of acetylcholine at the neuromuscular junction leading to dose-dependent paresis of the muscle. In addition, the neurotoxin has been shown to act in the CNS via interaction with the central endogenous opioid system and to play a role in reducing the inflammatory response via suppression of mediators such as calcitonin gene-related peptide, substance P, and glutamate.[29–31] The most commonly used products in North America are BOTOX (Allergan, Inc, Irvine, CA), XEOMIN (Merz Pharmaceuticals GmbH, Frankfurt, Germany), and Dysport (Ipsen Ltd, Maidenhead, Berkshire, UK). BTX serologic type A products come in the form of a white powder that requires reconstitution with saline to achieve the desired concentration. Because the effectiveness of each product varies, the dosages required for optimal effect also vary. As an example, BOTOX is known to be 50 to 100 times more effective than Dysport. Therefore, the clinician must practice caution when choosing the dose based on the product.[32,33]

BTX injections target the muscles of mastication to improve myofascial TMD. Injection of the masseter and temporalis muscles has been shown to lessen pain levels on a VAS pain score for patients with TMD when chewing and at rest.[34] BOTOX recommended doses are 10 to 25 units for the temporal muscle, 25 to 50 units for the masseter muscle, and 7.5 to 10.0 units for the lateral pterygoid muscle.[32] BTX injections effects begin to appear 3 to 4 days after injections, the peak effect is achieved in 3 to 4 weeks, and redosing is typically required after 3 to 4 months. This is sometimes referred to as the rule of 3–4s. Various protocols have been suggested and BTX therapy should be tailored to the needs of each patient. The authors recommend starting with a low

dose, keeping meticulous records of the sites of injection and scheduling follow-ups at 1 week, 3 weeks, and 3 months for optimal titration of the patient's dose.

It is important to understand that, although BTX injections offer temporary relief of symptoms, it has not been directly linked to treating the underlying etiology of TMD. Although this therapy modality has shown its value in alleviating pain, it may be better used as an adjunct. There is still no consensus on the therapeutic benefits of BTX injections for the management of TMD and/or myofascial TMD and further high evidence studies are needed.[35]

Corticosteroids

Corticosteroid injections are highly cost effective and readily available. The effectiveness of corticosteroid injections into the TMJ for the treatment of acute symptoms of osteoarthritis has been shown in the literature. Improvements in pain, symptoms, and function have been described for the treatment of TMJ osteoarthritis, rheumatoid arthritis, and juvenile idiopathic arthritis.[36] Intra-articular injections for the treatment of juvenile idiopathic arthritis TMD have shown to be the most promising modality because it has the potential of preventing mandibular growth alterations by reaching complete resolution in a majority of cases and potentially increasing the maximal incisional opening of this patient population. The best results are seen in patients under the age of 6 years and computed tomography-guided injections are recommended.

Some studies have reported that steroids can exacerbate degenerative changes in the joint with repeated use. Intracutaneous or subcutaneous injections can also cause local skin atrophy, local calcifications and hypopigmentation. It is advised that the frequency of injections does not exceed every 3 to 4 months to prevent these unwanted side effects. Special care should be taken to localize the joint components accurately and avoid spillage of the steroids during penetration and withdrawal. In some cases, sodium hyaluronate injections may be used as an alternative; when compared with corticosteroid injections, it has shown to have equally effective results.[2,37]

Hyaluronic Acid

Hyaluronic acid (HA) is a linear glycosaminoglycan present in synovial fluid that aids in joint lubrication. Degradation of HA is often present in cases of TMJ degeneration. Intra-articular joint injections with HA have shown positive results for increasing mouth opening and decrease in pain associated

Table 1
Pharmacologic therapy for TMD

Drug Class	Prescription	Indications	Contraindications	Phase of Treatment
NSAIDs[a]	Naproxen 500 mg PO q12 h × 14 d Ibuprofen 400 mg PO q6h × 14 d	Early disc displacement Myofascial TMD Synovitis Arthritis	Active GI disease Prior history of GI ulcers or bleeding Impaired kidney function	Initial, first line
Proton pump inhibitors[a]	Omeprazole 40 mg PO q24 h × 4–8 wk	High GI risk	Penicillin Warfarin Diazepam Clopidogrel	Initial, first line
Muscle relaxants	Cyclobenzaprine 10 mg PO q24 h at bedtime × 14 d	Myofascial TMD Clinical evidence of muscle spasm	CNS depressants (alcohol, opioids, benzodiazepines) Tramadol TCAs, MAOIs Congestive heart failure, arrhythmias Hyperthyroidism	Initial, secondary
Benzodiazepines	Diazepam 5 mg PO q6 h × 14 d	Chronic TMD pain Comanage with physician	Geriatric population CNS depressants (alcohol, opioids, muscle relaxants) Myasthenia gravis Acute narrow-angle glaucoma CYP 4503A4 substrates (grapefruit, azoles, erythromycin, CCBs) Substance use disorder Prolonged use (>4 wk)	Alternative, secondary
Antidepressants (TCA)	Amitriptyline 25 mg PO q24 h × 14 d (increase dosage by 25 mg, up to 75 mg)	Chronic TMD pain Comanage with physician	Exogenous epinephrine, limit 0.04 mg (2 carpules) MAOIs Centrally acting muscle relaxants Opioids	Alternative, tertiary
Anticonvulsants	Gabapentin 300 mg PO q24 h (increase titration of dosage 300 mg every 3 d until adequate pain control with no adverse effects, maximum 4200 mg)	Chronic TMD pain Comanage with physician Failed TMJ surgery	Depression Myasthenia gravis Severe chronic kidney disease Chronic obstructive pulmonary disease Opioids	Alternative, tertiary

Commonly prescribed medications in specific drug class with indications, contraindications, and phase of treatment.
Abbreviations: CCB, calcium channel blocker; CNS, central nervous system; MAOI, monoamine oxidase inhibitor.
[a] Medications to be taken together if necessary.

with TMD.[38] However, intra-articular injections with sodium hyaluronate seem to be as effective as corticosteroid and sodium injections. The Bjørnland 2007 trial found that although intra-articular injections of HA and corticosteroids have similar effectiveness over several parameters, TMJ pain seems to be slightly less after 6 months after injections of sodium hyaluronate, and an immediate improvement of TMJ sounds after treatment can be seen.[39] The current US Food and Drug Administration labeling for sodium hyaluronate is limited to osteoarthritis of the knee, and although growing evidence of its efficacy for the treatment of TMD is emerging, the effects of HA intra-articular injections have not been found to be significantly superior to platelet-rich plasma (PRP) injections or corticosteroid injections. Consequently, insurance coverage in the United States is limited and the cost of treatment is greater than similar modalities.

Platelet-Rich Plasma

PRP is medium with a high concentration of platelets, rich with growth factors and regenerative properties derived from the patient's blood. Typically, there are 3 to 10 times the normal platelet concentration of whole blood. When injected into the joint, platelets secrete a large number of growth factors such as transforming growth factor β1, platelet-derived growth factor, and vascular endothelial growth factor, among others. As a result, PRP has been shown to stimulate proteoglycan and collagen II production, the synthetic capacity of chondrocytes, bone regeneration, and cartilage repair. This therapy has gained popularity owing to its ease of preparation, low cost, and association with few postoperative complications.

A systematic review by Bousnaki and colleagues[38] compared the effect of PRP with HA, Ringer's lactate, and saline. The review included 6 randomized controlled trials that showed significant improvements after PRP injections in pain intensity and maxillomandibular opening when compared with baseline in all studies. Although this provides strong evidence for the potential benefit of intra-articular injections of PRP in patients with TMD, a standardized protocol for the preparation of the PRP has yet to be established.

Prolotherapy Dextrose

Prolotherapy or regenerative injection therapy refers to a technique in which a nonpharmacologic irritant, such as hypertonic dextrose, is injected into the joint space. The objective is to strengthen and repair the TMJ ligaments by stimulating the proliferation of collagen and fibro-osseous junctions.[40] Dextrose is transported into human cells via GLUTs 1 to 4 and interacts with cytokines to

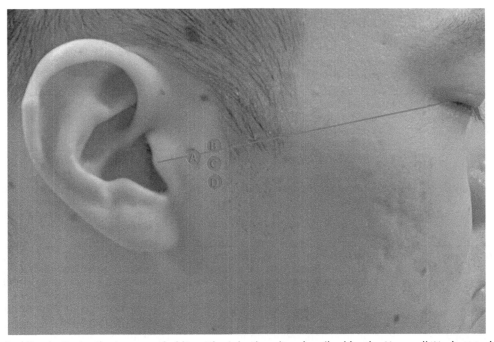

Fig. 1. Red line indicates the tragocanthal line. The injection sites described by the Hemwall–Hackett technique are illustrated as (A) posterior disk attachment, (B) superior capsular attachment, (C) superior joint space, and (D) inferior capsular attachment.

induce cell growth or repair.[41] Multiple clinical trials have shown prolotherapy to have favorable outcomes for the treatment of temporomandibular subluxation, hypermobility of the joint, and pain.[4,40–42]

A recent study by Dasukil and colleagues[4] assessed the effect of prolotherapy treatment on the quality of life of patients with TMD. In the study, patients were asked to answer a questionnaire before prolotherapy injections and 2 years after their treatment. Of the 25 patients who met the criteria, all patients reported a statistically significant improvement in all domains (functional limitation, physical pain, psychological discomfort, physical disability, psychological disability, social disability, and handicap). The authors concluded that the beneficial effects of prolotherapy can persist at least 2 years after treatment, deeming the technique promising for improving the quality of life of patients who suffer from TMD.

There is no general consensus on the concentration of dextrose indicated for the treatment of TMJ hypermobility. Dextrose concentrations between 10% and 50% have been reported in the literature. Similarly, various injection techniques have been suggested. It is important to document subjective and objective findings before treatment to better analyze the efficacy of the prolotherapy treatment. Local anesthetics can be injected into the site to increase patient comfort during and after the procedure.

One of the injection techniques was published by Hemwall-Hackett[43] (refer to **Fig. 1**). The injection sites are marked in the skin, which include the superior joint space, the posterior disc attachment and superior and inferior capsular attachments. The posterior disc attachment can be located by asking the patient to open their mouth by approximately 10 mm, then palpating the depression that forms anterior to the tragus of the ear. Before injection, the site should be decontaminated with alcohol wipes. A needle is inserted in an anteromedial direction to avoid penetration into the ear and 1 mL of dextrose is deposited at

Table 2
Potential complications and contraindications of pharmacologic management of TMD

Treatment	Complications	Contraindications
BTX injections	Local: diffusion to neighboring tissues, transient numbness, ptosis, local edema, bruising, pain and/or muscle weakness on injection site, bruising Systemic: flu-like symptoms, production of neutralizing antibodies at high doses, mild nausea, development of tolerance[31,33,44]	Pregnancy, neuromuscular disorders (ie, myasthenia gravis)
Intra-articular corticosteroid Injections	Infection, exacerbation of degenerative joint changes, skin atrophy, local calcifications, hypopigmentation[2,36,37]	Infections, idiopathic thrombocytopenic purpura
PRP	Bleeding, bruising, pain on injection site	Anticoagulation therapy, coagulopathies, sepsis
HA injections	Pain, bruising, redness, itching, and swelling	Hypersensitivity to HA, bleeding disorder, hypersensitivity reaction to gram-positive bacterial proteins (for products derived from bacterial source), infection.
Iontophoresis	Local paresthesia, itching, irritation, erythema, edema, and galvanic urticaria, burning sensation	Cardiac arrhythmias, hypercoagulability, cardiac pacemakers, superficial blood vessels, orthopedic implants, and areas of skin with lesions and impaired sensation.
Prolotherapy dextrose injections	Pain on injection, reduction in maximum incisal opening[40]	Local abscess, acute infection, bleeding disorders, septic arthritis

a depth of 20 mm. To locate the superior joint space, the patient's mouth is widely opened, and the needle is directed anteromedially to contact with the medial wall of the glenoid fossa and another milliliter is injected—the site should be about 10 mm anterior to the tragus of the ear and 2 mm bellow the tragocanthal line. The last milliliter is split between the superior and inferior capsular attachments, 0.5 mL of the solution is injected into the lateral margin of the glenoid fossa, and 0.5 mL of the solution is applied to the condylar neck. Another technique advocates for injection into the lateral pterygoid muscle attachment, posterior disc attachment, and stylomandibular ligaments. Multiple sessions are necessary to achieve the desired effect and therefore injections are typically performed every 4 to 6 weeks. For postoperative pain control, it is contraindicated to use anti-inflammatory drugs, which may directly interfere with healing (**Table 2**).

Emerging Treatments

New therapies and modalities of treatment for TMD are currently being studied. Imotun is an avocado-soybean unsaponifiable extract that has shown anabolic, anticatabolic, and anti-inflammatory effects on chondrocytes, currently being studied in the orthopedic literature for osteoarthritis.[45] Avocado-soybean unsaponifiable extract inhibits the breakdown of cartilage, and promotes cartilage repair via the synthesis of collagen by inhibiting inflammatory cytokines (eg, IL-1, IL-6, IL-8, tumor necrosis factor) and metalloproteinases.[46] Furthermore, it stimulates chondrocytes and synoviocytes through proteoglycan and synovial fluid synthesis.[46] At the clinical level, avocado-soybean unsaponifiable extract decreases pain and stiffness while improving function in the joints.[46]

SUMMARY

Noninvasive and minimally invasive pharmacologic therapies are effective treatment strategies to approach mild to moderate TMD. Although it is beyond the scope of this article, the accurate diagnosis of TMD and its severity is critical to apply the appropriate therapy, because there are multiple etiologies of TMD (ie, myofascial, articular, hypermobility). Therefore, a thorough knowledge of each drug class, as well as their properties and indications, are necessary for oral and maxillofacial surgeons involved in the management of TMD. Finally, it is important to understand the limits of pharmacologic therapy and when to advance to surgical intervention, when indicated, to treat TMD. The beneficial effects of

pharmacologic and surgical treatments should be scrutinized against the potential harm and surgical risk, adverse drug effects, and the risk of dependency of these management modalities.

CLINICS CARE POINTS

- Accurate diagnoses between different temporomandibular disorders (ie, myofascial pain, articular, hypermobility) is necessary to appropriately manage symptoms.
- Conservative pharmacologic management of mild to moderate temporomandibular disorders has been shown effective as first-line treatment.
- Comanage medications with the primary care physician for alternative pharmacologic therapies including benzodiazepines, antidepressants, and anticonvulsants.
- Intramuscular and intra-articular injections are safe mildly invasive procedures that predictably treat moderate temporomandibular disorders refractory to conservative therapy.

DISCLOSURE

None.

REFERENCES

1. Ouanounou A, Goldberg M, Haas DA. Pharmacotherapy in temporomandibular disorders: a review. J Can Dent Assoc 2017;83:h7.
2. Karlis V, Glickman R. Nonsurgical management of temporomandibular disorders. In: Miloro M, editor. Peterson's principles of oral and maxillofacial surgery. Ontario: BC Decker Inc; 2004. p. 949–61.
3. Dym H, Israel H. Diagnosis and treatment of temporomandibular disorders. Dent Clin North Am 2012;56(1):149–61, ix.
4. Dasukil S, Arora G, Shetty S, et al. Impact of prolotherapy in temporomandibular joint disorder: a quality of life assessment. Br J Oral Maxillofac Surg 2020;59(5):599–604.
5. Kurita Varoli F, Sucena Pita M, Sato S, et al. Analgesia evaluation of 2 NSAID drugs as adjuvant in management of chronic temporomandibular disorders. Sci World J 2015;2015:359152.
6. Ricciotti E, FitzGerald GA. Prostaglandins and inflammation. Arteriosclerosis, Thromb Vasc Biol 2011;31(5):986–1000.
7. Wright EF, Klasser GD. Manual of temporomandibular disorders. Hoboken: John Wiley & Sons; 2019.

8. Ta LE, Dionne RA. Treatment of painful temporomandibular joints with a cyclooxygenase-2 inhibitor: a randomized placebo-controlled comparison of celecoxib to naproxen. Pain 2004;111(1–2):13–21.

9. Ouanounou A, Haas DA. Pharmacotherapy for the elderly dental patient. J Can Dent Assoc 2015;80(18):f18.

10. Scarpignato C, Lanas A, Blandizzi C, et al. Safe prescribing of non-steroidal anti-inflammatory drugs in patients with osteoarthritis–an expert consensus addressing benefits as well as gastrointestinal and cardiovascular risks. BMC Med 2015;13(1):1–22.

11. Solomon DH, Cannon CP, Saperia GM. NSAIDs: adverse cardiovascular effects. Waltham: UpToDate; 2020.

12. Radi ZA, Khan KN. Cardio-renal safety of non-steroidal anti-inflammatory drugs. J Toxicol Sci 2019;44(6):373–91.

13. Dionne RA. Pharmacologic treatments for temporomandibular disorders. Oral Surg Oral Med Oral Pathol Oral Radiol Endodontol 1997;83(1):134–42.

14. Häggman-Henrikson B, Alstergren P, Davidson T, et al. Pharmacological treatment of oro-facial pain–health technology assessment including a systematic review with network meta-analysis. J Oral Rehabil 2017;44(10):800–26.

15. Dym H, Bowler D, Zeidan J. Pharmacologic treatment for temporomandibular disorders. Dent Clin North Am 2016;60(2):367–79.

16. PA M. Sedative-hypnotics, antianxiety drugs, and centrally acting muscle relaxants.. In: Yagiela JADF, Neidle EA, editors. Pharmacology and therapeutics for dentistry. 5th edition. St Louis: Elsevier Mosby; 2004. p. 193–218.

17. Griffin CE, Kaye AM, Bueno FR, et al. Benzodiazepine pharmacology and central nervous system–mediated effects. Ochsner J 2013;13(2):214–23.

18. Rizzatti-Barbosa CM, Martinelli DA, Ambrosano GM, et al. Therapeutic response of benzodiazepine, orphenadrine citrate and occlusal splint association in TMD pain. Cranio 2003;21(2):116–20.

19. Rizzatti-Barbosa CM, Nogueira MT, De Andrade ED, et al. Clinical evaluation of amitriptyline for the control of chronic pain caused by temporomandibular joint disorders. Cranio 2003;21(3):221–5.

20. Singer E, Dionne R. A controlled evaluation of diazepam and ibuprofen for chronic orofacial pain. J Orofac Pain 1997;11:139–47.

21. Laroche ML, Charmes JP, Nouaille Y, et al. Is inappropriate medication use a major cause of adverse drug reactions in the elderly? Br J Clin Pharmacol 2007;63(2):177–86.

22. Haas D. Pharmacologic considerations in the management of temporomandibular disorders. J Can Dent Assoc 1995;61(2):105–9, 112.

23. Hersh EV, Balasubramaniam R, Pinto A. Pharmacologic management of temporomandibular disorders. Oral Maxill Surg Clin North America 2008;20(2):197–210.

24. Micó JA, Ardid D, Berrocoso E, et al. Antidepressants and pain. Trends Pharmacol Sci 2006;27(7):348–54.

25. Calandre EP, Rico-Villademoros F, Slim M. Alpha2-delta ligands, gabapentin, pregabalin and mirogabalin: a review of their clinical pharmacology and therapeutic use. Expert Rev Neurother 2016;16(11):1263–77.

26. Kimos P, Biggs C, Mah J, et al. Analgesic action of gabapentin on chronic pain in the masticatory muscles: a randomized controlled trial. Pain 2007;127(1–2):151–60.

27. Quintero GC. Review about gabapentin misuse, interactions, contraindications and side effects. J Exp Pharmacol 2017;9:13.

28. Control CfD, Prevention. CDC guideline for prescribing opioids for chronic pain—United States, 2016. MMWR Recomm Rep 2016;65(1):1–49.

29. Drinovac Vlah V, Filipović B, Bach-Rojecky L, et al. Role of central versus peripheral opioid system in antinociceptive and anti-inflammatory effect of botulinum toxin type A in trigeminal region. Eur J Pain 2018;22(3):583–91.

30. Matak I, Lacković Z. Botulinum toxin A, brain and pain. Prog Neurobiol 2014;119-120:39–59.

31. Hoque ABA, McAndrew M. Use of botulinum toxin in dentistry. N Y State Dental J 2009;75(6):52–5.

32. Sipahi Calis A, Colakoglu Z, Gunbay S. The use of botulinum toxin-a in the treatment of muscular temporomandibular joint disorders. J Stomatol Oral Maxillofac Surg 2019;120(4):322–5.

33. Park KS, Lee CH, Lee JW. Use of a botulinum toxin A in dentistry and oral and maxillofacial surgery. J Dent Anesth Pain Med 2016;16(3):151–7.

34. Patel J, Cardoso JA, Mehta S. A systematic review of botulinum toxin in the management of patients with temporomandibular disorders and bruxism. Br Dent J 2019;226(9):667–72.

35. Thambar S, Kulkarni S, Armstrong S, et al. Botulinum toxin in the management of temporomandibular disorders: a systematic review. Br J Oral Maxillofac Surg 2020;58(5):508–19.

36. Habib GS, Saliba W, Nashashibi M. Local effects of intra-articular corticosteroids. Clin Rheumatol 2010;29(4):347–56.

37. Heir GM. The efficacy of pharmacologic treatment of temporomandibular disorders. Oral Maxillofacial Surg Clin 2018;30(3):279–85.

38. Bousnaki M, Bakopoulou A, Koidis P. Platelet-rich plasma for the therapeutic management of temporomandibular joint disorders: a systematic review. Int J Oral Maxill Surg 2018;47(2):188–98.

39. Bjørnland T, Gjaerum A, Møystad A. Osteoarthritis of the temporomandibular joint: an evaluation of the

effects and complications of corticosteroid injection compared with injection with sodium hyaluronate. J Oral Rehabil 2007;34(8):583–9.

40. Zhou H, Hu K, Ding Y. Modified dextrose prolotherapy for recurrent temporomandibular joint dislocation. Br J Oral Maxillofac Surg 2014;52(1):63–6.

41. Reeves KD, Sit RW, Rabago DP. Dextrose prolotherapy: a narrative review of basic science, clinical research, and best treatment recommendations. Phys Med Rehabil Clin N Am 2016;27(4):783–823.

42. Dasukil S, Shetty SK, Arora G, et al. Efficacy of prolotherapy in temporomandibular joint disorders: an exploratory study. J Maxillofac Oral Surg 2021; 20(1):115–20.

43. Hauser RA, Hauser MA, Blakemore KA. Dextrose prolotherapy and pain of chronic TMJ dysfunction. Pract Pain Management 2007;7(9):49–57.

44. Niamtu J 3rd. Complications in fillers and Botox. Oral Maxillofac Surg Clin North Am 2009;21(1): 13–21, v.

45. Abouelhuda AM. Non-invasive different modalities of treatment for temporomandibular disorders: review of literature. J Korean Assoc Oral Maxillofac Surg 2018;44(2):43.

46. Christiansen BA, Bhatti S, Goudarzi R, et al. Management of osteoarthritis with avocado/soybean unsaponifiables. Cartilage 2015;6(1):30–44.

Pharmacologic Management of Neuropathic Pain

Yoav Nudell, DDS, MS[a],*, Harry Dym, DDS[b], Feiyi Sun, DDS[a],
Michael Benichou, DMD[a], Jonathan Malakan, DDS[b],
Leslie R. Halpern, DDS, MD, PHD, MPH[c]

KEYWORDS

- Orofacial pain • Temporomandibular joint disorder • Neuropathic pain disorder
- Traumatic neuropathic pain

KEY POINTS

- Chronic orofacial pain is multifactorial in origin, affecting lives in negative, even debilitating ways. There are many powerful therapeutic options to treat a broad spectrum of both acute and chronic orofacial pain conditions.
- The oral health care clinician must be diligent when diagnosing clinical presentations as odontogenic and other dental conditions as a primary versus secondary cause of orofacial pain. A careful deciphering of signs and symptoms for an accurate diagnosis will set the foundation for specific treatment to improve long-term prognosis and resolution of most of the orofacial pain conditions.
- Orofacial pain can be the result of a diverse set of pain disorders. When general dentists and especially oral and maxillofacial surgeons consult, many Orofacial pain patients will require treatment for a neuropathic pain disorder. Once a definitive diagnosis has been established for the patient's pain disorder, the primary approach of pain management is through astute pharmacotherapy and potentially invasive and noninvasive techniques.

INTRODUCTION

General dentists and especially oral and maxillofacial surgeons will oftentimes be asked to consult with patients who have had a history of ongoing acute and chronic facial and oral pain. Many of these patients will have had multiple root canal therapies, extractions, and other assorted treatments for possible temporomandibular joint (TMJ) disorder, before they visit surgeons' offices. After repeated visits to multiple practitioners, they will ultimately be diagnosed with a neuropathic pain (NP) disorder. NP conditions are a definitive entity that must be well understood by oral and maxillofacial surgeons along with possible treatment approaches. This article is primarily devoted to medication management once the diagnosis of NP, a true trigeminal neuralgia (TN), or a variant of TN often referred to as traumatic neuropathic pain (TNP) or traumatic TN. A more in-depth discussion regarding the physiologic factors involved in the etiology of TNP is addressed in many other textbooks on the treatment of chronic orofacial pain (OFP) patients.

The International Association for the Study of Pain defines pain as "an unpleasant sensory and emotional experience associated with actual or potential tissue damage, or described in terms of such damage."[1–3] Pain has significant effects on the physiology, psychology, and sociology of the population. The World Health Organization

---

[a] Oral and Maxillofacial Surgery, The Brooklyn Hospital Center, 155 Ashland Place, Brooklyn, NY 11201, USA;
[b] The Brooklyn Hospital Center, 155 Ashland Place, Brooklyn, NY 11201, USA; [c] The University of Utah, School of Dentistry, 530 South Wakara Way, Salt Lake City, UT 84108, USA
* Corresponding author.
E-mail address: ynudell@gmail.com

Oral Maxillofacial Surg Clin N Am 34 (2022) 61–81
https://doi.org/10.1016/j.coms.2021.09.002
1042-3699/22/

(WHO) estimated that more than 1 in every 3 people suffers from acute or chronic pain.[1,2]

OFP refers to pain associated within the head and neck regions, soft and hard tissues, as well as both extraorally and intraorally. Jeffrey P Okeson, an international authority on OFP, divides OFP into physical (axis 1) and psychological (axis 2) conditions.[3] Chronic OFP includes such phenomena as atypical odontalgia, burning mouth syndrome (BMS), and idiopathic facial pain. These entities are often considered diagnoses of exclusion, thus definitive diagnosis and therapeutic solution is a challenge. Physical conditions include disorders of the TMJ and the local musculoskeletal structures (eg, masticatory muscles, tendons, cervical spine); intraoral dental and pulpal pain of somatic origin; NPs, which include episodic (eg, TN) and continuous (eg, peripheral and centralized mediated) characteristics; and neurovascular disorders/headaches (eg, migraine and temporal arteritis). In addition, OFP can often be a presenting symptom for systemic illnesses such as chronic pain seen in fibromyalgia, gastroesophageal reflux disease (GERD)/irritable bowel disease, posttraumatic stress disorder or other psychological disorders, myocardial ischemia and cancerous lesions locally or elsewhere in the body.[4]

The oral health care clinician must be diligent when diagnosing clinical presentations as odontogenic and other dental conditions as a primary versus secondary cause of OFP.[4–6] A careful deciphering of signs and symptoms for an accurate diagnosis will set the foundation for specific treatment to improve long-term prognosis and resolution of most of the OFP syndromes.

The aim of this chapter is to provide the practitioner with therapeutic options to treat a broad spectrum of both acute and chronic OFP syndromes. The focus will be nonsurgical (pharmacologic management) that the oral health care physician can implement to treat this population of patients.

PRINCIPLES OF PHARMACOLOGIC TREATMENT FOR NP

Chronic NP is multifactorial in origin, affecting lives in negative, even debilitating, ways that oftentimes require pharmacologic modality of treatment for management. The International Association for the Study of Pain (IASP) defines NP as *pain caused by a lesion or disease of the somatosensory system.*[7] NP is therefore a clinical descriptor rather than the diagnosis, differentiated by positive or negative symptoms.[8] Positive NPs would be separated among stimulus-dependent, stimulus-

independent, or paresthesias. The trigger for such positive NP could be perioral touch or cold on patients with orofacial NP. Negative NPs are described as numbness, loss of reflexes, and weakness in the involved nerve area. On the face, orofacial NP typically follows the dermatome of the trigeminal nerve. There are 5 well-studied mechanisms contributing to NP conditions identified, including ectopic activity, peripheral sensitization, central sensitization, impaired inhibitory modulation, and activation of microglia. Duration of pain will indicate different disease processes. Episodic NP, characterized by shooting pains lasting seconds to minutes, is typical of TN or glossopharyngeal neuralgia. Whereas, continuous NP arises because of neural structures and can vary in intensity without resolution, as in atypical odontalgia or nerve injury-neuromas. Treatment modalities are directed at the different etiologies including trauma, infection, chemotherapy, surgery, neurotoxins, inflammation, and tumor infiltration.

Local anesthesia may be helpful in discerning between peripheral or central origin of NP. Only once a nonpharmacologic, noninvasive trial of treatment for NP has failed, should pharmacologic modalities be used. When a single pharmacologic agent has failed to provide adequate pain relief, oftentimes a multimodal approach is taken because of the risk of side effects when increasing dosage. Through numerous review articles, different pharmacologic treatment algorithms are available.

With numerous pharmacologic agents available, special attention should be directed to the origin of the NP—such as, peripheral neuropathy secondary to diabetes, postherpetic neuralgia (PHN), central neuropathy secondary to multiple sclerosis, NP status after spinal cord injury, HIV, chemotherapy-induced peripheral neuropathy, and so forth—which would help identify best pharmacologic agent with the highest potential for reducing NP. Although different neuromodulators have been shown to provide transient relief, there is a lack of understanding regarding long-term usage of these drugs.[9]

Analgesic drugs are typically the primary choice for relief in patients suffering from NP.[10,11] Morphine, like the body's endogenous endorphins, acts on the central nervous system (CNS) to modify pain signaling. Tricyclic antidepressants (TCAs) can act to increase catecholaminergic analogs that travel systemically to targets for relief by both acting as membrane stabilizers and transsynaptic effects.[12,13] The salicylates can act as anti-inflammatory agents that inhibit cyclooxygenase pathways with inhibition of prostaglandins.

Anticonvulsant medications can act as membrane stabilizers because they suppress hyperexcitability.[11] It is important for the clinician to apply careful dosing because of the potential for side effects, allergic reactions, and risk of drug dependence. Pharmacotherapy options are broad and varied, based on a diversity of analgesics whose dosing and concentrations vary with the type of NP being treated.

ACUTE FACIAL PAIN VERSUS NP

Within OFP, it is important to differentiate acute facial pain from neuropathic pain.

Acute Facial Pain

Pain presenting acutely is often relatively easy to definitively diagnose and effectively manage. The underlying sources include odontogenic, periodontal oral mucosa, hard tissue, or a combination of multiple of these sources. Odontogenic pain is often short in duration and sharp, then progresses to a dull ache depending on whether there exists reversible or nonreversible pulpitis. Pain within the mucosa presents as raw (sore or tender), aching, and burning. Periodontal disease also presents as a continuous or intermittent ache.

Other etiologies include maxillary sinusitis and salivary gland disorders. Maxillary sinusitis may or may not have pain associated with etiologies such as oral antral communications and bacterial/viral disease. Salivary diseases are often due to obstruction of ducts with consequent infection. Pain pathways from the trigeminal system will not only innervate the site but refer to other areas of the head and neck. Imaging/ultrasound can aid in localization and evaluation for surgical intervention.

Neuropathic Pain

NP is defined as pain caused by a lesion or disease of the somatosensory nervous system. NP is diagnosed commonly with up to 25% to 35% presenting to facial pain centers across the United States and Europe.[12–14] Etiologies of NP include trauma, infection, chemotherapy, surgery, neurotoxins, inflammation, and tumor infiltration. Studies have described NP as dysfunctional pain due to afferent stimulation that can be both spontaneous and stimulus-dependent.[12] The trigger can be perioral stimuli and/or environmental like ambient cold and touch. NP commonly presents on the face along the dermatome of the trigeminal nerve. Further classification separates NP into episodic and continuous. Episodic is characterized by sudden electric-like, as well as shooting pains that can last over seconds to minutes. Continuous NP is pain originating in neural structures constant and varies in intensity without total remission. Episodic disorders include TN and glossopharyngeal neuralgia, whereas continuous pain disorders can arise because of injury of nerves in both the peripheral and CNS, that is, neuromas and atypical odontalgia.[12–14]

An understanding of the pathophysiology of episodic and continuous NP provides the clinician with a strong rationale for choices of pharmacologic therapy. **Box 1** lists the pharmacologic therapies broken into 3 main tiers that vary in the mechanism of action due to site of neurologic innervation, that is, synapses, membrane stabilizing agents, and receptor agonists/antagonists. Each agent can be administered either by topical application or systemically. All agents may be preceded by the use of local anesthesia to localize peripheral versus central origin.[10,14–16]

TRIGEMINAL NEURALGIA

Trigeminal neuralgia (TN), or tic douloureux, is an uncommon syndrome characterized by chronic, recurrent attacks of intense, lancinating pain localized to the dermatome of the trigeminal nerve. The trigeminal nerve is the fifth cranial nerve (CN V) that provides both motor and sensory functions of the face distributed by the 3 main branches, the ophthalmic, maxillary, and mandibular nerves.[17] One or multiple branches of the trigeminal nerve can be involved, with the maxillary nerve involved the most and the ophthalmic nerve the least.[18] A focal vascular compression of the trigeminal nerve root close to its point of entry into the pons is the most common cause of TN. The International Headache Society (INS) divides TN into 2 categories. The typical type I TN (TN1) presents as a sporadic but severely burning facial pain with each episode lasting up to 2 minutes. The onset of pain may occur in clusters that persist for several hours at a time. In contrast to TN1, the atypical type II TN (TN2) presents as a constant stabbing pain with less severity.[17,18] Any type of stimuli such as eating, drinking, light touching, washing, talking, smiling, draughts of wind, and applying make-up can trigger TN. The cutaneous perception of temperature and light touch can be slightly impaired within the affected area.[19]

The annual incidence of TN is reported as 4.3 per 100,000 population, with slight female predominance. The male-to-female prevalence ratios range from 1:1.5 to 1:1.7. The overall prevalence is 0.015%. Advanced age is a risk factor. The peak incidence is at 60 to 70 years of age, and is unusual before age 40 years. However, it can occur

---

Box 1
Pharmacologic agents by location/etiology of drug action

Synaptic cleft

  Benzodiazepines

  Clonidine

  Tricyclic antidepressants:

  - Amitriptyline
  - Nortriptyline
  - Imipramine

  Serotonin reuptake inhibitors/Norepineph-rine selective reuptake inhibitors:

  - Venlafaxine
  - Duloxetine
  - Trazodone
  - Milnacipran

Membrane stabilizing drugs

  Anticonvulsants:

  - Carbamazepine
  - Oxcarbazepine
  - Phenytoin
  - Gabapentin
  - Pregabalin
  - Lamotrigine
  - Valproic acid
  - Topiramate
  - Tiagabine
  - Zonisamide

Additional pharmacologic agents

  Opioids

  Local anesthetics

  Corticosteroids

  NSAIDs:

  - Aspirin

  Acetaminophen

  Antifungal agents

  Antiviral

  BOTOX

  Antioxidants:

  - Alpha lipoic acid

  Salivary stimulants:

  - Pilocarpine
  - Cevimeline

Topical agents

  Lidocaine patches

  Proparacaine

  Streptomycin/Lidocaine

  Capsaicin

  Topical NSAIDs

  Antidepressants

  Anticonvulsants

  Botulinum toxins

---

at any age, including rare cases in children. TN is predominantly unilateral, though rarely can be bilateral. No racial predilections are associated with the disease. Most cases are sporadic with rarely reported familial inheritance.[17,20]

The main theory of pathophysiology of TN involves neurovascular compression of the nerve root at the prepontine cistern. Primary compression results from the direct compression of the nerve without a secondary cause, whereas secondary compression can be caused by meningiomas, vestibular schwannomas, aneurysms, arteriovenous malformations, or epidermoid cysts. Compression of the trigeminal nerve root may be mediated by the tumor itself, by an interposed blood vessel, or by distortion of the contents of the posterior fossa with displacement of the nerve root against a blood vessel or the skull base.[17,21]

The NP caused by TN is also believed to be caused by nerve demyelination leading to ephaptic transmission of impulses, which may transfer from nearby light touch to pain fibers.[18] Certain conditions such as multiple sclerosis can lead to a plaque of demyelination encompassing the root entry zone of the trigeminal nerve in the pons. Carcinomatous deposits within the nerve root and trigeminal amyloidomas can both contribute as infiltrative disorders of the trigeminal nerve. Nondemyelinating lesions such as infarct or angioma can also lead to TN. Although familial TN is rare, there is a reported association between Charcot-Marie-Tooth disease and TN.[21]

The International Classification of Headache Disorders categorizes TN into classical, secondary, or idiopathic types. In classical TN, paroxysmal attacks of noncontinuous pain last from a fraction of a second to 2 minutes involving one or more divisions of the trigeminal nerve. The pain is caused by neurovascular compression without any other neurologic defects. Secondary TN is associated with continuous pain triggered by underlying pathologies such as arteriovenous malformation, certain brain tumors, or multiple sclerosis. Idiopathic TN is diagnosed when there are no other clear causes. MRI is the standard imaging study to evaluate any neurovascular compression, brain tumors, or AV malformations.[17,18]

PAINFUL POST-TRAUMATIC TRIGEMINAL NEURALGIA

Painful post-traumatic trigeminal neuralgia (PTTN) is one variant of TN which occurs secondary to trauma, brought about by common dental procedures. It is described as a "moderate-to-severe continuous burning pain" and can have a significant impact on daily function and a significant psychological impact on the affected patient. The domain of the trigeminal nerve encompasses the face, eyes, tongue, nose, and therefore heavily impacts our social lives. The pain may be similar to a toothache and lead to dental treatments that are not necessary. In many cases, it is overwhelming and relentless for the patient. From all cases of TN about 40% may be classified as PTTN. It has been described under several names including "phantom tooth pain," "atypical facial pain," or "atypical odontalgia." The term "painful post-traumatic trigeminal neuralgia" is the most recent description by the International Headache Society.[22]

Pulp extirpation, apicoectomy, other routine endodontic procedures, and tooth extraction can all precede the finding of PTTN. During a tooth extraction, iatrogenic trauma can be imposed upon the inferior alveolar nerve, lingual nerve, and branches of the maxillary nerve. Various reasons regarding the etiology of PTTN are brought to attention in current literature. Some noted reasons are self-explanatory and include poor surgical protocol being used during tooth extraction, and poor technique when administering injection of local anesthetic.[23] Other causative factors include a long preoperative pain duration, previous chronic pain issues, and a history of pain during other treatments.

Some observational studies of PTTN found a higher distribution in males (60.4%) compared to females (39.6%) and found a large incidence of PTTN related to extractions of the mandible (79.2%). The reason for this is likely due to mandibular molars being close to the inferior alveolar nerve, lingual nerve, and other branches of the mandibular nerve.[24]

The nature of severity of symptoms a patient is encountering (pain, psychological issues) will define the approach taken toward management. Treatment (medical or surgical) is often dependent on the nature of injury, the patient's symptomatic findings, and length of injury.[25] There is known to be a limited time to optimize IAN injury resolution as a result of implants, endodontic procedures, or extraction. One report suggests that removal of implants that impose injury to the IAN within 30 hours may assist in neuropathy resolution.[26] The current indicated therapies for acute neuropathy include corticosteroids and anti-inflammatory medications.[27] For those patients suffering from chronic NP due to injury, possible treatment options include topical local anesthetic, anticonvulsants for stimulus or spontaneous pain, TCAs, or serotonin reuptake inhibitors for constant/elicited burning pain.[28] Of all patients who suffer from PTTN, 15% are using long-term systemic medications and 18% of patients are using topical medications. Botulinum toxin injections are sometimes poorly tolerated and can pose a risk of facial palsy as a side effect of treatment.[29]

CARBAMAZEPINE AND OXCARBAZEPINE

The first-line medications for long-term treatment of TN are the antiepileptic medications carbamazepine and oxcarbazepine.[30] There is controversy regarding which of the 2 medications is more efficacious and better tolerated by patients; however, there is substantial evidence that there is substantial variability of responses by patients taking the medications. This suggests and indicates that if one medication is not effective, the other should be tried next. However, there is caution indicating that cross-reactivity may occur in instances where one of the medications causes an allergic reaction. These medications are typically titrated slowly to the optimal symptom-eliminating dose while patients are monitored for any side effects that may arise. Patients taking these medications are instructed to alter the dosage in variance with pain severity and side effects. It is possible for patients to experience either partial or complete remission of symptoms.[31]

In cases where there is a poor patient response to carbamazepine or oxcarbazepine, many alternatives exist. Lamotrigine, gabapentin, botulinum toxin type A, pregabalin, or phenytoin are all recognized treatments that may be adjunctive or used as monotherapies.[29] The use of botulinum toxin type A is the most recent addition to the medical treatment portion found in the European Academy of Neurology guidelines, although studies are still pending and treatment results have not been finalized. Local anesthetics, greater occipital nerve blocks, and topiramate are considered second-line options; however, the evidence is limited and trials are needed (**Table 1**).

Nonsteroidal Anti-inflammatory Drugs

Nonsteroidal anti-inflammatory drugs (NSAIDs) are best used orally for continuous NP conditions

Table 1
The drugs and principles of titration and tapering are based on recommendations from the European Academy of Neurology guidelines and expert opinion

Treatment	Starting Dose	Dose Range	Typical Daily Dose Needed	Frequency	Titration	Tapering	Comments, Side Effects
Carbamazepine (First-line)	200–400 mg	200–1800 mg	200–1800 mg	2–4 times a day	Increase by 200 mg every third day	Decrease by 100 mg every 7–14 d	Laboratory work and ECG are mandatory before initiating treatment. A slow-release preparation is also available. If there is no efficacy from carbamazepine, treatment can be switched directly to the equipotent dose of oxcarbazepine (200 mg carbamazepine = 300 mg oxcarbazepine). There can be allergic cross-reactivity between carbamazepine, oxcarbazepine, and lamotrigine. Long-term treatment is associated with low bone mineral density. Consider vitamin D and calcium supplements. Carbamazepine decreases the plasma concentration of warfarin and oral contraceptives (and other drugs) and can cause hyponatremia. Measure sodium after 1 mo and then regularly. Consider decreasing the dose in patients with reduced liver function. Exert caution with drug combinations with other anticholinergic drugs, especially in older people or people with dementia, as there is a cumulative effect

of central and peripheral side-effects when using multiple anticholinergic drugs. Do not combine with monoamine oxidase inhibitors. It is contraindicated in atrioventricular block (and other rarer conditions). Common side-effects include, but are not limited to, tiredness, dizziness, ataxia, nausea, and leukopenia. Carbamazepine can affect the ability to drive.

| Oxcarbazepine (First-line) | 300–600 mg | 300–2700 mg | 300–2700 mg | 2–4 times a day | Increase by 300 mg every third day | Decrease by 150 mg every 7–14 d | Laboratory work and ECG are mandatory before initiating treatment. If there is no efficacy from oxcarbazepine, treatment can be switched directly to the equipotent dose of carbamazepine (200 mg carbamazepine = 300 mg oxcarbazepine). There can be allergic cross-reactivity between carbamazepine, oxcarbazepine, and lamotrigine. Long-term treatment is associated with low bone mineral density. Consider vitamin D and calcium supplements. Exert caution in cardiac insufficiency and conduction disorders. Oxcarbazepine might decrease the plasma concentration of oral |

(continued on next page)

Table 1
(continued)

Treatment	Starting Dose	Dose Range	Typical Daily Dose Needed	Frequency	Titration	Tapering	Comments, Side Effects
							contraceptives. Oxcarbazepine often causes hyponatremia. Measure sodium after 1 mo and then regularly. Decrease dose in patients with severe liver disease. Titrate slowly in patients with reduced kidney function. Exert caution at drug combinations with other anticholinergic drugs, especially in older people or people with dementia, as there is a cumulative effect of central and peripheral side effects when using multiple anticholinergic drugs. Common side effects include, but are not limited to, tiredness, dizziness, headache, double vision, ataxia, and nausea. Oxcarbazepine can affect the ability to drive.
Pregabalin (Second-line)	150 mg	150–600 mg	150–600 mg	Twice a day	Increase by 150 mg every 7 d	Decrease by 150 mg every 7–14 d	Decreased dose recommended in patients with decreased kidney function. Exert caution advised in patients with cardiac insufficiency. Extreme caution when combined with opioids or

other CNS depressants. Common side effects include headache, dizziness, and gastrointestinal symptoms.

Titration: increase dose until sufficient pain relief or intolerable side effects is achieved; titration can be done slower than suggested in the table to avoid severe and sudden side effects. Unlike epilepsy, measuring serum concentrations of antiepileptics is not relevant to monitor efficacy.

Tapering: decrease dosage until the lowest sufficient dose for pain relief or tolerable side effects is achieved; in remission periods, tapering can continue until treatment is fully stopped; tapering can be done slower than suggested in the table to allow the patient to detect recurrence of pain. Frequency of dosing varies depending on whether slow-release formulations are used.

From Bendtsen L, Zakrzewska JM, Heinskou TB, Hodaie M, Leal PRL, Nurmikko T, Obermann M, Cruccu G, Maarbjerg S. Advances in diagnosis, classification, pathophysiology, and management of trigeminal neuralgia. Lancet Neurol. 2020 Sep;19(9):784-796. Reprinted with permission of Elsevier, Inc.

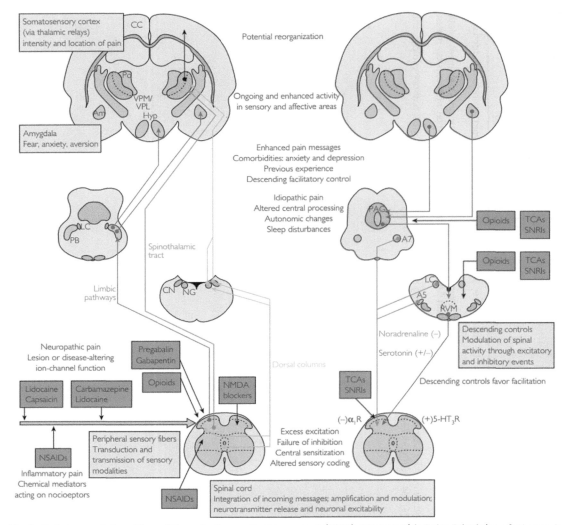

Fig. 1. Pain transmission. (*From* Gilron, I., Baron, R., & Jensen, T. (2015). Neuropathic Pain: Principles of Diagnosis and Treatment. Mayo Clinic Proceedings, 90(4), 532–545.)

such as peripheral neuritis, atypical odontalgia, or PHN. Neuropathy due to inflammation mediated by the production of cytokines, such as due to implant placement in the case of orofacial NP, is described as peripheral neuritis. A commonly used delivery method is topically, like for peripheral trigeminal neuritis. Using topical drug delivery method can be effective locally, but also minimizes the possibility for undesired systemic adverse events. Topical NSAIDs have been shown effective in treating pain due to TMJ disorder without producing the typical gastric side effects seen with NSAIDs. Topical diclofenac (Voltaren Gel 1%) was shown equally as effective compared to 100 mg oral diclofenac.

Lyrica—Pregabalin

Pregabalin (Lyrica) is an anticonvulsant that inhibits the release of excitatory neurotransmitters like glutamate by combining with the $\alpha2\delta$ subunit of the voltage-gated calcium channel, also used to relieve continuous NP. It is considered to be a first-line agent for the treatment of NP.[8,32,33] The total daily dose recommended is 300 to 600 mg divided into two daily doses. The dosage should be titrated up over 1 to 2 weeks from 150 mg per day divided into 2 to 3 doses. Major adverse effects of pregabalin include sedation, dizziness, weight gain, edema, and blurred vision.[8,32] It may be prudent to track a patient's weight, especially

Table 2
Classification of neuropathic pain

Pathology	Peripheral	Spinal	Brain
Genetic	Fabry neuropathy	Syringomyelia	Syringobulbia
Metabolic	Painful diabetic neuropathy	B_{12} myelopathy	
Traumatic	Nerve injury	Spinal cord injury	Multiple sclerosis
Vascular	Vasculitic neuropathy	Spinal cord stroke	Brain stroke
Neoplastic	Tumor compression neuropathy	Tumor compression	Tumor compression
Immunologic	Guillain-Barré syndrome	Multiple sclerosis	Multiple sclerosis
Infectious	HIV, Borreliosis	Infectious myelitis	Encephalitis
Toxic	Chemotherapy neuropathy		

From Gilron, I., Baron, R., & Jensen, T. (2015). Neuropathic Pain: Principles of Diagnosis and Treatment. Mayo Clinic Proceedings, 90(4), 532–545.

if they are diabetic. Owing to the dose-dependent sedation and dizziness effects, it is wise to start at lower doses and titrating up as needed. Renal insufficiency should also be taken into account when dosing, which can be made in relation to creatinine clearance.[34] A combination therapy of duloxetine (SNRI) with pregabalin or gabapentin can be considered for second-line therapy of TN. Pregabalin has linear pharmacokinetics, making dosing easier than with gabapentin. Pregabalin and gabapentin are also effective in treating postherpetic TN pain and numbness, and diabetic neuropathy[35,36] (**Fig. 1**; **Table 2**).

NONSURGICAL PHARMACOLOGIC THERAPY FOR TN

The pharmacologic paradigms for TN typically consist of first-line and second-line therapies.[14,16,37,38]

Anticonvulsive Agents

First-line therapy consists of antiepileptic medications such as carbamazepine, oxcarbazepine, and gabapentin.[39–42] Systematic reviews have supported the use of carbamazepine (200–1200 mg/d) as a prognostic marker for definitive therapy because when it eliminates the symptoms, the clinician has successfully diagnosed TN.[11] Carbamazepine inactivates voltage-gated sodium channels and depresses postsynaptic reflex arcs in the spinal cord. Although it is very effective in resolving pain, it does not address the etiology of this neuralgia. The use of carbamazepine requires judicious dosing because this medicine has numerous side effects, that is, leukopenia, agranulocytosis, aplastic anemia, drowsiness, and ataxia. Therapeutic levels must be followed to

avoid adverse events, especially thrombocytopenia. Oxcarbazepine is a newer agent that has been used, which has fewer side effects and has become the drug of choice for treating TN unless it fails.

Another group of anticonvulsive agents, gabapentin and pregabalin, are now being used to treat NP with even fewer side effects.[43] The mechanism of action resides in their ability to increase GABA in the CNS and therefore increase the inhibition of pain sensors.[44] The main side effect of this group is drowsiness and the requirement of good kidney function. Baclofen and Lamotrigine are two other agents that have fewer side effects and are used for the treatment of TN. Baclofen has less effect on blood cells but does have GI sequelae, vomiting and cramping. Lamotrigine is a phenothiazine derivative and also acts by stabilizing sodium channels and inhibiting the release of neurotransmitters.[11,43] Caution must be used when this agent is chosen because it elicits a Steven-Johnson syndrome. The latter, if present, must be discontinued at a tapering dose. Topiramate is another agent that can act at the voltage-sensitive sodium channels, as well as, modulating GABA. It is derived from the sulfonamide group and has side effects such as nephrolithiasis, somnolence, anxiety, and drowsiness. This agent must also be tapered if discontinuing its use. **Table 3** depicts the dosing for anticonvulsant medications that may benefit patients with TN.

Antidepressants

The use of TCAs in the treatment of NP has spurred debate because of their potential side effects, including anticholinergic effects, cardiac

Table 3
Pharmacologic agents for neuropathic pain: dosing guide

Drug/Condition	Dosing
Episodic NP: *Trigeminal Neuralgia/Glossopharyngeal* *Neuralgia/Occipital Neuralgia*	
First Line	*Maximum dosing per day administration protocols vary*
• Carbamazepine • Oxcarbazepine	200–1200 mg/d 600–1800 mg/d
Second Line	
Combination of first line with: • Lamotrigine • Baclofen	400 mg/d 40–80 mg/d
Third line	
Phenytoin Gabapentin Pregabalin Valproate Tizanidine Tocainide Local anesthetics	300 mg orally daily 300–1600 mg/d 25–300 mg/d

Continuous NP:
Peripheral Neuritis/Postherpetic
  Neuralgia/Atypical
  Odontalgia/Burning
  Mouth Syndrome)	

Peripheral Neuritis/Postherpetic *Neuralgia*	*Maximum dosing per day administration protocols vary*
NSAIDs • Ibuprofen • Aspirin • Naproxen Corticosteroids	800–3200 mg/d (4×/d) 2000–4000 mg/d (4–6×/d) 500–1500 mg/d (2×/d) 40–60 mg/d tapered over 3 wk
Atypical Odontalgia	
Antivirals • Acyclovir • Valacyclovir • Famciclovir Acetaminophen NSAIDs Opioids • Oxycodone ER • Tramadol TCAs Anticonvulsants	800 mg 5×/d 1000 mg 3×/d 500 mg 3×/d 4000 mg/d See above 10–40 mg 2×/d 50–400 mg/d 150 mg/d See above
Burning Mouth Syndrome	

Benzodiazepines:
  Clonazepam
  Chlordiazepoxide
	0.5–2 mg/d
	10–30 mg/d

Anticonvulsants:
  Gabapentin
  Pregabalin
	300–1600 mg/d; mg dosing varies depending on side effects seen. Can start with 100 mg at night and then increase to 3×/d
	25–300 mg/d: start with 25 mg at night and then increase by 25 mg over 7 d to 3x/day

(continued on next page)

Table 3
(continued)

Drug/Condition	Dosing

Antidepressants:
  Amitriptyline
  Nortriptyline
	10–150 mg/d: 10 mg at night and increase by 10 mg over 7 d not exceeding 4×/d
	10–150 mg/day: 10 mg at night and increase as needed 10/d over 7 d not exceeding 4×/d

Selective serotonin
  reuptake inhibitors:
  Paroxetine
  Sertraline
  Trazodone
	20–50 mg/d
	50–200 mg/d: 50 mg initially and can increase by 25 mg every 7 d; max 200 mg/d
	100–400 mg/d: 5–0 mg initially and increase by 50 mg 4–7 d; max 400 mg/d

Selective norepinephrine
  reuptake inhibitors:
  Milnacipran
  Duloxetine
	100 mg/d: 50 mg BID; 12.5 initially then BID; max 200 mg/d
	60–120 mg/d; PO QID

Antioxidants: Alpha lipoic acid	600–1200 mg/d; 300–600 mg BID

This table provides a guide for exploring treatment protocols. This is not an exhaustive list of potential pharmacologic therapies for NP.
Abbreviation: NSAID, nonsteroidal anti-inflammatory drug.

side effects, Xerostomia, constipation, urinary retention, and anesthetic drug interactions.

Amitriptyline has been used at doses that result in a membrane-stabilizing effect.[21,22,28] A 10 mg dose of this drug can have a profound effect because of their mechanism of increasing the load of endogenous serotonin and norepinephrine at the synaptic cleft. TCAs can relieve tension headaches and NP. In addition, TCAs are considered first-line agents in the treatment of musculoskeletal pain associated with fibromyalgia.[22,28]

More recently, selective serotonin reuptake inhibitors (SSRIs) have been applied for the treatment of not only NP but also other OFP syndromes such as chronic pain.[22,29] SSRIs (fluoxetine and paroxetine) as well as SRNIs (duloxetine/milnacipran) have been successfully used for fibromyalgia and other centrally mediated pain syndromes (see section on Neurovascular Pain below). See **Table 3** for a dosing guide for antidepressants.

The benzodiazepines have been used in combination with the above groups of agents for TN (see list of references for further information on benzodiazepine therapy for NP).

SSRI/SNRI FOR TREATMENT OF NP
SNRI

Among the most commonly referenced treatment algorithms for NP, serotonin and norepinephrine reuptake inhibitors rank among the most reliable, first-line drugs for NP management. Unlike the 2- to 4-week delay, it takes the antidepressant effect to take effect, the onset of therapeutic effect is faster as treatment for NP suggesting that SNRIs have a different mechanism of action than their use as an antidepressant. Studies have shown that a noradrenaline upswing by reuptake inhibition in the spinal cord inhibits NP at the α2-adrenergic receptors directly. In addition, upswing in noradrenaline improves the function of the descending noradrenergic inhibitory system by acting on the locus coeruleus.[45]

Among SNRIs, duloxetine is the most studied for NP purposes though venlafaxine would be an appropriate SNRI as well. The recommended regimen would be 60 to 120 mg, once a day (duloxetine); 150 to 225 mg, once a day (venlafaxine extended release.)[8] Adverse effects of SNRI include nausea, loss of appetite, constipation, sedation, dry mouth, hyperhidrosis, and anxiety. The added major adverse effect pertaining to venlafaxine would be potential for hypertension and for this reason, it should be used cautiously in the hypertensive patient or contraindicated in the uncontrolled hypertensive. Providers should also caution against the use of SNRI with collateral use of SSRI or tramadol treatment. Duloxetine should be used with caution in the patient with bleeding disorders, concomitant anticoagulant use, and history of seizures or mania. Past studies have shown that plasma concentrations of duloxetine in smokers are about 50% of that in nonsmokers. Patients taking monoamine oxidase inhibitors—MAO inhibitors—are contraindicated for concomitant use of SNRIs.[8]

SSRI

Serotonin-specific reuptake inhibitors are highly effective as antidepressants but considered third-line agents for NP. Taking into consideration the low level of evidence for efficacy against NP, SSRIs may be considered for treatment therapy by pain specialty clinic but typically are not used.[8,45–47] Fluoxetine is the typical SSRI used for NP, whereas other third-line therapies include interventional therapies. Potential adverse effects include hyponatremia, suicide, serotonin syndrome, hepatoxicity, and cardiovascular complication[8,48]

Duloxetine (Cymbalta)

Antidepressant medications such as TCAs and serotonin-noradrenaline reuptake inhibitors have historically been used to medically manage TN. Duloxetine works by inhibiting the reuptake of serotonin and norepinephrine. Although duloxetine is known for its preliminary use in depression as well as peripheral NP secondary to diabetes, there have been reported cases of its therapeutic effect in TN. K S Anand and colleagues reported the use of duloxetine 40 mg daily on 15 patients with TN, and statistically significant pain relief was reported in 9 patients with no significant adverse drug reactions.[49] Chung-Chih H er al reported a rapid and remarkable relief of TN in a patient who had developed major depressive and was thus treated by duloxetine 60 mg daily for depression.[50] It is suggested that in addition to duloxetine's inhibitory modulation of the synaptic availability of norepinephrine and serotonin for depression management, this medication has an analgesic effect where N-methyl-D-aspartate (NMDA) receptors are antagonized, impeding the L-arginine-nitric oxide (NO)-cyclic guanosine monophosphate (cGMP) pathway which is involved in NP.[50] It also postulates that in TN, the pain spreads rapidly through hyperexcitable neurons causing synchronized, continuous after-discharge activity that is associated with paroxysmal lancinating pain. Because duloxetine has been shown to disrupt the synchronized firings of action potential via its antagonism against NMDA receptors in animal studies, it is hypothesized that duloxetine can therefore effectively control the pain manifested in TN.[50,51]

GLOSSOPHARYNGEAL NEURALGIA

Glossopharyngeal neuralgia is another episodic form of NP. It is unilateral with electric-shock-like episodes localized to the tongue, throat, and ear and under the mandible. It is usually provoked with swallowing or speaking and can occur concurrently in 10% of patients with TN.[11,40] Its incidence rate is 0.2/100,000 patients seen yearly and is also seen in patients suffering from MS. There can be other concomitant symptoms such as syncope and cardiac arrhythmias as well as poor nutrition because swallowing food or liquids precipitate severe attacks. Pharmacologic therapeutics are similar to TN. First-line therapy is the use of carbamazepine or oxcarbazepine with second-line therapy use of local anesthetics to direct sites of pain. If medical treatment is unsuccessful then surgical procedures are warranted.[10,40,52]

OCCIPITAL NEURALGIA

Occipital neuralgia presents as a unilateral pain in the posterior scalp area innervated by the greater and lesser occipital nerves. It must be distinguished from referred pain from the neck. It is treated with corticosteroids and local anesthesia.[53]

CONTINUOUS NP

As stated earlier, continuous NP has its causation in central neural regions and is manifested by pain that is constant in awareness and unremitting. There may be refractory periods but never totally resolved. Okeson's classification of facial pain axis 1 maps the 3 types of continuous NP: centrally mediated, peripherally mediated, and metabolic polyneuropathies.

Several examples are described as follows:

1. Peripheral trigeminal neuritis: This type of neuritis is a unilateral facial/OFP that manifests itself as a burning sensation after trauma of the trigeminal nerve. The latency period is about 3 to 6 months and is preceded by allodynia and hyperalgesia. The etiology is often an exposure to dental work like a root canal or dentoalveolar trauma. Chronic pain will persist in 5% of patients who report this event.[32] Diagnostic blocks with local anesthetics can be applied as immediate relief followed by topical medicaments (discussed below) to both alleviate pain and reduce adverse systemic events.[54–56] Pharmacologic management consists of antidepressant therapy and anticonvulsants to control explosive periods of burning and stabbing in the area traumatized. In addition, the use of capsaicin at a concentration of 0.05%

with benzocaine 20% can be applied on a stent.[33] Other topical agents have compounded several drugs such as ketamine, NSAIDs, and anticonvulsants for relief (see below)

2. Peripheral neuritis: Peripheral neuritis describes neuropathy secondary to inflammation usually mediated by the production of cytokines. Perineural inflammation occurs in the orofacial cavity because of dental procedures such as implant placement. Other etiologies include chronic sinusitis, TMJ degeneration, and malignant neoplasms that spread on the nerve trunk.[56–60] Pharmacologic intervention consists of anti-inflammatory agents such as NSAIDs, corticosteroids, and topical agents.[56,61]

3. Herpes zoster (HZ)/PHN: PHN originates after the outbreak of HZ virus. The virus undergoes a dormant period within the dorsal root ganglia; 55% of the time in the thoracic spine and associated with the cranial nerves (CNs); most often CN V and CN VII.[38,62] Ten percent to 15% of cases are localized to CN V3 and 80% of cases are recorded in CNV1. The incidence of disease is greater in the elderly and begins with significant prodromal symptomatology—headache, malaise, abnormal skin sensation, and fever. Once reactivated, the condition is referred to as "shingles." The goals of pharmacologic management are to eliminate pain and accelerate healing. Several prescribed modalities exist to address these concerns.

Medication groupings are as follows:

1. Antivirals: These agents are applied within several days of symptomatology to decrease the rash and pain severity. Examples are acyclovir, valacyclovir, and famciclovir
2. Opioids: Used for severe pain
3. Nonopioids: Acetaminophen or NSAIDs to control inflammation, pain, and fevers.
4. Corticosteroids added to antivirals to relieve pain.
5. Antidepressants: Amitriptyline, desipramine, and nortriptyline are often used in small doses and the gabapentin group has been recently approved by the FDA to treat PHN.[60]

Both HZ and PHN are preventable with vaccinations. The Center for Disease Control (CDC) recommends patients aged 60 years or older receive vaccinations regardless of exposure risk.

ATYPICAL ODONTALGIA/NONODONTOGENIC TOOTHACHE

Atypical odontalgia is a centralized trigeminal neuropathy characterized by an idiopathic pain that is throbbing or burning and misdiagnosed as dental in origin resulting in unnecessary treatment. The age range is usually from 25 to 65 years and the most common tooth is the molar followed by the premolar followed by the incisor with the maxilla as site of origin more often than the mandible. Diagnostic imaging shows no pathology but the teeth can elicit a hyperesthetic response to percussion. Diagnostic blocks with local anesthetics may either relieve the pain temporarily or exhibit an equivocal response. Associated symptomatology includes depression, oral dysesthesia, and problems with oral hygiene.[12,36,63]

Studies have suggested that vascular mechanisms, as well as sympathetic system imbalance, may play a role in the neuropathology of atypical odontalgia. The patient will be frustrated as they may want the specific tooth to be treated in a case of a nonodontogenic toothache.[63–65]

Pharmacologic therapy is challenging because both central and peripheral mechanisms are "misaligned."[66–69] The TCAs are first-line agents because at low doses, they exhibit their analgesic action—25 to 50 mg/d. The reuptake inhibition of serotonin and norepinephrine increases the effectiveness of inhibitory pathways of pain perception.[63,65] The anticonvulsant gabapentin at a moderate dosing of 3600 mg/d is effective with drowsiness as a side effect. Pregabalin can also be a drug of choice to relieve continuous NP. Peripheral components of atypical odontalgia may be treated with topical agents and stent placement. Benzocaine mixed with carbamazepine and/or ketamine may also provide a true benefit in pain relief. Topical agents dosed in patches are now being studied to reduce the symptoms of continuous NP (see section below on pharmacology of topical agents)

Burning Mouth Syndrome

BMS/BM disorder presents as burning sensations within the oral cavity, that is, tongue, lips, and oral mucosa that are continuous with an increase in intensity throughout the day.[70–72] The epidemiology of BMS varies from 1% to 3%. Women are predisposed (6:1 male) to BMS during their perimenopausal to postmenopausal years and up to 50% report a concomitant xerostomia and dysgeusia.[63,71] The greatest frequency of BMS occurs on the anterior one-third of the tongue followed by the gingiva and palate. It is most often a diagnosis of exclusion. As to a definitive etiology, an in-depth HPI is essential before management because BMS can manifest itself in a variety of systemic diseases, that is, GERD, diabetes, HTN, and autoimmune diseases. Deficiencies in certain vitamins, that is, iron, vitamin B12, and folic acid can exacerbate BMS-induced xerostomia and the clinician may consider saliva flow studies as a prerequisite to treating BMS.[72,73]

Pharmacologic strategies for treatment must begin with establishing a definitive diagnosis, followed by a well-tailored treatment schedule that accounts for the multifactorial risk factors. Treatment can be palliative, symptomatic, as well as a combination of both to reach a therapeutic range of pain relief. It is judicious for the clinician to explain why therapy is complex so patient compliance can be achieved. The mainstay of treatment is with the use of topical medications. Random control trials have established that benzodiazepines, clonazepam, should be considered first at a dosing of 0.25 mg to 2 mg/d in wafer or orally disintegrating tablet forms.[74,75] Other topical agents are capsaicin (1:2 dilutions), doxepin (5% cream), and 2% viscous lidocaine, every 4 to 6 hours or prn. Additional choices include artificial sweeteners providing mucosal relief, antimicrobials such as lactoperoxidase rinses TID, and the use of antifungal medications when candidiasis is the etiology.[75] Systemic medications are the next choice of pharmacotherapy. As with NP management, the TCAs, amitriptyline and nortriptyline, can be administered at a dosing of 10 to 150 mg maximum (due to side effects) over 5 to 7 days.[75–77] The use of SSRIs, paroxetine, sertraline, trazadone and the anticonvulsants pregabalin and gabapentin as a combination therapy have had variable success in population studies.[76–78] Studies of clinical outcomes in large populations conclude that only 3% to 5% of patients reach a complete resolution of their symptoms. Although the management of BMS is quite challenging, better strategies for definitive diagnoses will aid clinicians in choosing more efficacious pharmacology to better manage their patients presenting with BMS.[79,80]

Neurovascular Pain

Neurovascular pain is episodic and based on disturbances of the trigeminovascular system and often presents clinically as a headache in patients with OFP.[81] The WHO characterizes headache disorders as the 10th disability in women and the cost of care exceeds 27 billion dollars globally.[63,82,83] The International Headache Society (HIS) divides primary headaches into 4 categories: (1) migraines, (2) tension-type headaches: cluster headaches and paroxysmal hemicranias, (3) trigeminal autonomic cephalgias, and (4) other headaches. The reader is referred to the bibliography for further interest.[81–83]

TOPICAL MEDICATIONS FOR OFP:

Topical medications offer distinct advantages over systemic agents: greater safety, rapid onset of action, and low side effect profile.[84,85] Complete cessation of pain on the application of topical anesthetic may not, however, be possible, as some of the neuronal changes may be central or because of neuropathic changes not easily reached by most topical anesthetics. Nevertheless, topical medications are useful for NP due to peripheral nerve sensitization, as well as for centralized neuropathy that is accompanied by local allodynia. In the latter situation, the topical medication is used over the trigger site to reduce the ongoing neural stimulation that maintains the central sensitization. In cases of mild-to-moderate pain, the local therapy might be the sole intervention. For moderate-to-severe pain, the use of systemic medications as well as local topical medications is more appropriate. A locally applied medication can offer faster relief while a centrally acting medication can be titrated up to effective levels.[56,78,86] Clinicians can manage OFP by applying topical medications that are formulated according to accepted clinical indications, that is, the composition can be modified for individual patient requirements. These medications should be compounded by a pharmacy known to have high standards of quality, manufacturing technique, and reproducibility of compounded products. Topical medications can be applied directly to mucosa, skin, as well as indirectly using a custom-made, stable intraoral carrier referred to as a neurosensory stent to ensure adequate drug delivery at the site of NP. Examples of the most commonly used medicaments are as follows:

Topical Anesthetics

Lidocaine patches
The 5% lidocaine transdermal patch (Lidoderm) is currently FDA approved for the treatment of pain associated with PHN.[60,62] The patch is 10 to 14 cm in area and contains 700 mg of lidocaine, although only about 3% of this dose is absorbed resulting in peak blood levels of 130 ng/mL during the recommended 12-h application. This is slightly more than that achieved following an injection of one-half cartridge of 2% lidocaine with epinephrine.[64,65] According to the manufacturer, the patch can be cut into smaller sizes with scissors before removal from the release liner. In addition to placebo-controlled trials in PHN, the drug has also proven efficacious in other NP states, that is, in patients who have chronic lower back pain and osteoarthritis.[70–72] The systemic absorption

of lidocaine from the patch is minimal in healthy adults even when 4 patches are applied for up to 24 hours per day, and lidocaine absorption is even lower among PHN patients than healthy adults at the currently recommended dose. Because of its proven efficacy and safety profile, the lidocaine patch 5% has been recommended as a first-line therapy for the treatment of the NP of PHN.[73]

Proparacaine

The benefit of the topical anesthetic proparacaine in TN was investigated in a randomized double-blind placebo-controlled trial of 47 patients.[74] Subjects were assigned randomly to either 2 drops of 0.5% proparacaine or buffered saline into the eye on the side of the TN. The results showed no benefit from proparacaine delivered in this way. Further studies are in progress to determine a proper dosing, as well as a combination therapeutic alternative in this group of agents.

Streptomycin and lidocaine

A total of 17 patients with TN were entered into a randomized double-blind study involving weekly injections of 2 mL of 2% lidocaine with or without 1 g streptomycin.[79] The authors concluded that although effective initially, streptomycin is not responsible for any pain relief in the long term.

Vanilloid Compounds (Capsaicin)

Capsaicin is a derivative of chili pepper. Its proposed mechanism of action involves depletion of substance P and calcitonin gene-related peptide from peripheral afferent nerve endings. Several randomized double-blind trials in osteoarthritis and NP have demonstrated efficacy in these chronic pain populations.[81–83] The recently characterized capsaicin receptor is known as the transient receptor potential channel–vanilloid subfamily 1 (TRPV1) whose activation is believed to be necessary for the release of these inflammatory and pain-provoking compounds.[82,83] Although the use of topical capsaicin has been proposed in patients who have TMD surprisingly there are no clinical trials or even case-controlled studies evaluating its therapeutic effect in the TMD population.[82,83] From a safety profile, the topical application of the drug is devoid of systemic toxicity, although patients must be counseled to expect a burning feeling during the initial applications of the drug, with continued application, this unpleasant feeling will dissipate. Combining capsaicin with a topical anesthetic, such as benzocaine 20% in pluronic lecithin organogel may help reduce this burning sensation.[87] Capsaicin is probably best used as an adjunct to

NSAIDs, benzodiazepines, or other systemic modalities. It is an effective treatment for the pain of PHN.

Topical NSAIDs

Ketoprofen

Ketoprofen (Topofen, Achelios Therapeutics) is a fast-acting transdermal gel NSAID that possesses analgesic, antipyretic, and anti-inflammatory properties. Topical application of the active ingredient is locally effective and at the same time minimizes the risk of systemic adverse events. A study at the University of Zagreb, in Croatia, evaluated the use of topical ketoprofen (called Fastum gel in Croatia) with the concurrent use of physical therapy for the treatment of TMD in 32 patients over an 8-month period.[84] They found that in comparing asymptomatic subjects, their active mouth opening was greater postmedication administration than in placebo-treated controls ($P<.0001$).[84]

Diclofenac

In patients with painful TMD, topical diclofenac (Voltaren Gel 1%) was as effective as 100 mg oral diclofenac in reducing symptoms. Di Rienzo Businco and colleagues reported that topically applied diclofenac and oral diclofenac are equally effective in the treatment of TMD symptoms; however, topical diclofenac did not have had untoward effects on the gastric apparatus as the oral diclofenac.[85]

Antidepressants

Topical amitriptyline alone or combined with ketamine relieves peripheral NP.[86,88] Topical application of doxepin significantly relieves chronic NP and when mixed with capsaicin, the effect was observed significantly earlier. TCAs have been used for their central analgesic effect. Although it is known that there are serotonin receptors in peripheral nerves residing outside the CNS, it is unclear if this fact is important to the topical effect of TCAs, which are known to block the reuptake of serotonin. In addition, cyclobenzaprine, a TCA analog, is used as a muscle relaxant. It has been used for peripheral application for muscle trismus and spasm, but adequate studies supporting this use as a standard of care are lacking.

Sympathomimetic Agents

Sympathomimetic agents may be useful in some forms of chronic NP where nociceptor activity is being stimulated by sympathetic fiber release of norepinephrine in the periphery. It has been shown that injured C fibers express α1-receptors on their peripheral membranes. Sympathetic activity then would excite the C fibers, signaling pain. Clonidine, an α2-adrenergic agonist, is thought to relieve pain by decreasing the abnormal excitability of these functional nociceptors. Clonidine is available as a transdermal patch for extraoral use. For intraoral use, it is better to have clonidine compounded into a transdermal penetrating cream and dispensed in a calibrated syringe so that the dose can be better controlled.

NMDA-Blocking Agents

Recent studies have shown that NMDA-receptor antagonists may be useful in the treatment of neurogenic pain.[89] Several studies have been conducted in which orally administered ketamine, an NMDA antagonist, has shown effectiveness in alleviating refractory NP. Although this medication has promise for the treatment of neuropathies, it can cause adverse effects such as hallucinations and dysphoria. Topical ketamine may be useful, but specific studies are needed to evaluate this therapeutic alternative. As with clonidine, this medication would be best compounded into a transdermal penetrating cream and dispensed in a calibrated syringe.

Botulinum A Toxin

Botulinum A toxin is produced by *Clostridium botulinum* which affects the presynaptic membrane of the neuromuscular junction where it prevents acetylcholine release and therefore muscle contraction. Inactivation persists until collaterals form in junction plates on new areas of muscle cell walls. Botulinum toxin has been applied as a strategy for pain management whose mechanism of action is a reduction in spasticity in both dystonias and migraines.[90] BOTOX A injections have been shown to be effective in the prevention of migraines. Headaches must be greater than or equal to 15 days per month with headache lasting 4 hours a day or longer. The BOTOX A is administered via 31 injections into 7 specific head and neck sites.[90,91] When injected at labeled doses in recommended areas, it is expected to produce results lasting up to 3 months depending on the individual patients. Side effects of Botulinum toxin include pain, erythema, and unintended paralysis of nearby muscles.

There has been an increase in the number of studies investigating the use of Botox A to treat TMDs and bruxism; however, it is not considered a first-line treatment option. Before using Botox A as a treatment modality for bruxism, it is imperative that a definitive diagnosis of bruxism is made and that all other noninvasive and commonly validated methodologies are used in an attempt to

manage the condition. The possible clinical effects of Botox A in the treatment of bruxism and TMDs at first appears attractive. Soares and colleagues in a Cochrane Review on the long-term efficacy of Botox A concluded there was not enough evidence to support Botox use for myofascial pain syndrome and that more randomized controlled trials are needed.[90]

OFP can be the result of a diverse set of pain disorders. When general dentists and especially oral and maxillofacial surgeons consult, many OFP patients will require treatment for an NP disorder. Once a definitive diagnosis has been established for the patient's pain disorder, the primary approach of pain management is through astute pharmacotherapy and potentially invasive and noninvasive techniques. The presented therapeutic options will hopefully expand the knowledge and armamentarium for oral health care practitioners to best care for patients with OFP.

CLINICS CARE POINTS

- Orofacial pain can be the result of a diverse set of pain disorders.
- Once a definitive diagnosis has been established for the patient's pain disorder, intelligent pharmacotherapy is a highly effective method of pain management.

DISCLOSURE

The authors have nothing to disclose.

REFERENCES

1. De Rossi SS. Orofacial pain: a primer. Dent Clin North Am 2013;57(3):383–92.
2. Melzack R, Wall PD. Pain mechanisms: a new theory. Science 1965;150(3699):971–9.
3. Okeson JP. The classification of orofacial pain. Oral Maxillofac Surg Clin N A 2008;20(2):133–44.
4. Lipton JA, Ship JA, Larach-Robinson D. Estimated prevalence and distribution of reported orofacial pain in the United States. J Am Dent Assoc 1993;124(10):115–21.
5. Lancer P, Gesell S. Pain management: the fifth vital sign. Health Benchmarks 2001;8(6):68–70.
6. De Leeuw R. Orofacial pain: guidelines for assessment, classification, and management. In: The American Academy of orofacial pain. 4th edition. Chicago: Quintessence Publishing Co, Inc; 2008.

7. International Association for the Study of Pain. IASP Taxonomy. Pain terms. Neuropathic pain 2017.
8. Gilron I, Baron R, Jensen T. Neuropathic pain: principles of diagnosis and treatment. Mayo Clinic Proc 2015;90(4):532–45.
9. Do TM, Unis GD, Kattar N, et al. Neuromodulators for atypical facial pain and neuralgias: a systematic review and meta-analysis. Laryngoscope 2021; 131(6):1235–53.
10. Stacey BR. Management of peripheral neuropathic pain. Am J Phys Med Rehabil 2005;84(Supple): S4–16.
11. Okeson JP. General considerations in managing oral and facial pain. In: Okeson JP, editor. Bell's oral and facial pain. 7th edition. Hanover Park, IL: Quintessence Publishing Co; 2014. p. 181–232.
12. Romeo-Reyes M, Uyanik JM. Orofacial pain management: current perspectives. J Pain Res 2014;7: 99–115.
13. Costigan M, Scholz J, Woolf CJ. Neuropathic pain: a maladaptive response of the nervous system to damage. Ann Rec Neurosci 2009;31:1–32.
14. Spencer CJ, Gremillion HA. Neuropathic orofacial pain: proposed mechanisms, diagnosis, and treatment considerations. Dent Clin North Am 2007;51: 209–24.
15. Katusic S, Williams DB, Beard CM, et al. Incidence and clinical features of glossopharyngeal neuralgia. Rochester , MN, 1945-1984. Neuroepidemiology 1991;10(5–6):266–75.
16. Balsubramaniam R, Klasser GD. Orofacial pain syndromes: evaluation and management. Med Clin North Am 2014;1385–405.
17. Jones MR. A comprehensive review of trigeminal neuralgia. Curr Pain Headache Rep 2019;23(10). https://doi.org/10.1007/s11916-019-0810-0.
18. Krafft RM. Trigeminal neuralgia. Am Fam Physician 2008;77(9):1291–6.
19. Bowsher D. Trigeminal neuralgia: an anatomically oriented review. Clin Anat 1997;10(6):409–15.
20. Katusic S, Beard CM, Bergstralh E, et al. Incidence and clinical features of trigeminal neuralgia, Rochester, Minnesota, 1945-1984. Ann Neurol 1990;27(1): 89–95.
21. Love S, Coakham HB. Trigeminal neuralgia: pathology and pathogenesis [published correction appears in Brain 2002 Mar;125(Pt 3):687]. Brain 2001;124(Pt 12):2347–60.
22. Olesen J, Bendtsen L, Dodick D, et al. Headache Classification Committee of the International Headache Society (IHS). The International Classification of Headache Disorders, 3rd edition (beta version). Cephalalgia 2013;33:629–808.
23. Penarrocha M, Penarrocha D, Bagán JV, et al. Post-traumatic trigeminal neuropathy. A study of 63 cases. Med Oral Patol Oral Cir Bucal 2012;17: e297–300.
24. Kumar S, Kumar A, Rani V, et al. Prevalence of post-traumatic trigeminal neuralgia (PTTN) in Dental OPD at tertiary care center, Bihar: a retrospective cross-sectional epidemiological study. Sch J App Med Sci 2017;5:626–31.
25. Bendtsen L, Zakrzewska JM, Heinskou TB, et al. Advances in diagnosis, classification, pathophysiology, and management of trigeminal neuralgia. Lancet Neurol 2020;19(9):784–96.
26. Khawaja N, Renton T. Case studies on implant removal influencing the resolution of inferior alveolar nerve injury. Br Dent J 2009;206:365–70.
27. Seo K, Tanaka Y, Terumitsu M, et al. Efficacy of steroid treatment for sensory impairment after orthognathic surgery. J Oral Maxillofac Surg 2004;62: 1193–201.
28. Khawaja N, Yilmaz Z, Renton T. Case studies illustrating the management of trigeminal neuropathic pain using topical 5% lidocaine plasters. Br J Pain 2013;7:107–13.
29. Herrero BA, Kapos FP, Nixdorf DR. Intraoral administration of botulinum toxin for trigeminal neuropathic pain. Oral Surg Oral Med Oral Pathol Oral Radiol 2016;121:148–53.
30. Bendtsen L, Zakrzewska JM, Abbott J, et al. European Academy of Neurology guideline on trigeminal neuralgia. Eur J Neurol 2019;26:831–49.
31. Maarbjerg S, Gozalov A, Olesen J, et al. Trigeminal neuralgia–a prospective systematic study of clinical characteristics in 158 patients. Headache 2014;54: 1574–82.
32. Finnerup NB, Sindrup SH, Jensen TS. The evidence for pharmacological treatment of neuropathic pain. Pain 2010;150(3):573–81.
33. Finnerup NB, Kuner R, Jensen TS. Neuropathic pain: From mechanisms to treatment. Physiol Rev 2020. https://doi.org/10.1152/physrev.00045.2019.
34. Dworkin RH, O'Connor AB, Audette J, et al. Recommendations for the pharmacological management of neuropathic pain: an overview and literature update. Mayo Clin Proc 2010;85(3 Suppl):S3–14.
35. Shinoda M, Imamura Y, Hayashi Y, et al. Orofacial neuropathic pain-basic research and their clinical relevancies. Front Mol Neurosci 2021;14:691396.
36. Di Stefano G, Truini A, Cruccu G. Current and innovative pharmacological options to treat typical and atypical trigeminal neuralgia. Drugs 2018;78(14): 1433–42.
37. Shinal RM, Fillingim RB. Overview of orofacial pain: epidemiology and gender differences in orofacial pain. Dent Clin North Am 2007;51(1):1–18.
38. Ohba S, Yoshimura H, Matsuda S, et al. Diagnostic role of magnetic resonance imaging in assessing orofacial pain and paresthesia. J Craniofac Surg 2014; 25(5):1748–51.
39. Mueller D, Obermann M, Yoon MS, et al. Prevalence of trigeminal neuralgia and persistent idiopathic

facial pain: a population based study. Cephalalgia 2011;31(15):1542–8.

40. Rozen TD. Trigeminal neuralgia and glossopharyngeal neuralgia. Neurol Clin North Am 2004;22:185–206.

41. Zakrzewska JM. Medical management of trigeminal neuropathic pains. Expert Opin Pharmacother 2010;11(8):1239–54.

42. Reisner L, Pettengill CA. the use of anticonvulsants in orofacial pain. Oral Surg Oral Med Oral Pathol Oral Radiol Endod 2001;91(1):2–7.

43. Attal N, Crucco G, Baron R, et al. EFNS guidelines on the pharmacological treatment of neuropathic pain: 2010revision. Eur J Neurol 2010;17:1113.

44. Saarto T, Wiffen PJ. Antidepressants for neuropathic pain. Cochrane Database Syst Rev 2005;3:CD005454.

45. Obata H. Analgesic mechanisms of antidepressants for neuropathic pain. Int J Mol Sci 2017;18(11):2483.

46. Bates D, Schultheis BC, Hanes MC, et al. A comprehensive algorithm for management of neuropathic pain. Pain Med 2019;20(Suppl 1):S2–12.

47. Finnerup NB, Attal N, Haroutounian S, et al. Pharmacotherapy for neuropathic pain in adults: a systematic review and meta-analysis. Lancet Neurol 2015;14(2):162–73.

48. Lee Y-C, Chen P-P. A review of SSRIs and SNRIs in neuropathic pain. Expert Opin Pharmacother 2010;11(17):2813–25.

49. Anand KS, Dhikav V, Prasad A, et al. Efficacy, safety and tolerability of duloxetine in idiopathic trigeminal neuralgia. J Indian Med Assoc 2011;109(4):264–6.

50. Hsu CC, Chang CW, Peng CH, et al. Rapid management of trigeminal neuralgia and comorbid major depressive disorder with duloxetine. Ann Pharmacother 2014;48(8):1090–2.

51. Molina LA, Skelin I, Gruber AJ. Acute NMDA receptor antagonism disrupts synchronization of action potential firing in rat prefrontal cortex [published correction appears in PLoS One. 2014;9(7):e104110]. PLoS One 2014;9(1):e85842.

52. Stieber VW, Bourland JD, Ellis TL. Glossopharyngeal neuralgia treated with gamma knife surgery: treatment outcome and failure analysis case report. J Neurosurg 2005;102(Suppl):155–7.

53. Vanelderen P, Lataster A, Levy R, et al. Occipital neuralgia. Pain Pract 2010;10(2):137–44.

54. Bramwell BL. Topical orofacial medications for neuropathic pain. Int J Pharm Compd 2010;14(3):200–3.

55. Kennedy PG. Varicella-Zoster virus latency in human ganglia. Rev Med Virol 2002;12:327–34.

56. LeResche L, Mancl LA, Drangsholt MT, et al. Predictors of onset of facial pain and temporomandibular disorders in early adolescence. Pain 2007;129:269–78.

57. Rodriguez-de Rivera –Campillo E, Lopez-Lopez J. Evaluation of the response to treatment and clinical evolution in patients with burning mouth syndrome. Med Oral Pato Oral Cir Bucal 2013;18:e403–10.

58. Sreebny LM, Yu A, Green A, et al. Xerostomia in diabetes mellitus. Diabetes Care 1992;15:900–4.

59. Heckmann SM, Kirchner E, Grushka M, et al. A double-blind study on clonazepam in patients with burning mouth syndrome. Laryngoscope 2012;122(4):813–6.

60. Thoppay JR, DeRossi SS, Ciarrocca KN. Burning mouth syndrome. Dent Clin North Am 2013;57(3):497–512.

61. Patton LL, Siegel MA, Benoliel R, et al. Management of burning mouth syndrome : systematic review and management recommendations. Oral Surg Oral Med Oral Pathol Oral Radiol 2007;103(Suppl):S39.e1.

62. deMorales M, do Amaral Bezerra BA, da Rocha Neto PC, et al. Randomized trials for the treatment of burning mouth syndrome: an evidence-based review of the literature. J Oral Pathol Med 2012;41(4):281–7.

63. Gorsky M, Silverman S Jr, Chinn H. Clinical characteristics and management outcome in the burning mouth syndrome. An open study of 130 patients. Oral Surg Oral Med Oral Pathol 1991;72:192–5.

64. Comer AM, Lamb HM. Lidocaine patch 5%. Drugs 2000;59(2):245–9.

65. Benoliel R, Sharav Y. Chronic orofacial pain. Curr Pain Headache Rep 2010;14:33–40.

66. Campbell BJ, Rowbotham M, Davies PS, et al. Systemic absorption of topical lidocaine in normal volunteers, patients with post-herpetic neuralgia, and patients with acute herpes zoster. J Pharm Sci 2002;91(5):1343–50.

67. Kim H, Ramsay E, Lee H, et al. Genome-wide association study of acute post-surgical pain in humans. Pharmacogenomics 2009;10:171–9.

68. Rowbotham MC, Davies PS, Verkempinck C, et al. Lidocaine patch: double-blind controlled study of a new treatment method for post-herpetic neuralgia. Pain 1996;65(1):39–44.

69. Galer BS, Rowbotham MC, Perander J, et al. Topical lidocaine patch relieves post herpetic neuralgia more effectively than a vehicle topical patch: results of an enriched enrollment study. Pain 1999;80(3):533–8.

70. Rees RT, Harris M. Atypical odontalgia: differential diagnoses and treatment. Br J Oral Surg 1978;16:212–8.

71. Graff-Radford SB, Solberg WK. Atypical odontalgia. J Craniomandibular Disord 1992;6:260–5.

72. Rhodus NL, Carlson CR, Miller CS. Burning mouth syndrome (disorder). Quintessence Int 2003;34:587–93.

73. Danhauer SC, Miller CS, Rhodus NL, et al. Impact of criteria –based diagnosis of burning mouth syndrome on treatment outcome. J Orofacial Pain 2002;16:305–11.
74. Galer BS, Jensen MP, Ma T, et al. The lidocaine patch 5% effectively treats all neuropathic pain qualities: results of a randomized, double-blind, vehicle-controlled, 3-week efficacy study with use of the neuropathic pain scale. Clin J Pain 2002;18(5):297–301.
75. Galer BS, Gammaitoni AR, Oleka N, et al. Use of the lidocaine patch 5% in reducing intensity of various pain qualities reported by patients with low-back pain. Curr Med Res Opin 2004;20(Suppl 2):S5–12.
76. Galer BS, Sheldon E, Patel N, et al. Topical lidocaine patch 5% may target a novel underlying pain mechanism in osteoarthritis. Curr Med Res Opin 2004;20(9):1455.
77. Davies PS, Galer BS. Review of lidocaine patch 5% studies in the treatment of postherpetic neuralgia Drugs. Drugs 2004;64:937–47.
78. Kondziolka TL, Kestle JR, Lunsford LD, et al. The effect of single-application topical ophthalmic anesthesia in patients with trigeminal neuralgia: a randomized double-blind placebo-controlled trial. J Neurosurg 1994;80:993–7.
79. Stajcic Z, Juniper RP, Todorovic L. Peripheral streptomycin/lidocaine injections versus lidocaine alone in the treatment of idiopathic trigeminal neuralgia: a double blind controlled trial. J Craniomaxillofac Surg 1990;18:243–6.
80. Kopp S. The influence of neuropeptides, serotonin, and interleukin 1ß on temporomandibular joint pain and inflammation. J Oral Maxillofac Surg 1998;56:189–91.
81. Sato J, Segami N, Yoshitake Y, et al. Expression of capsaicin receptor TRPV-1 in synovial tissues of patients with symptomatic internal derangement of the temporomandibular joint and joint pain. Oral Surg Oral Med Oral Pathol Oral Radiol Endod 2005;100:674–81.
82. Padilla M, Clark GT, Merrill RL. Topical medications for orofacial neuropathic pain: a review. J Am Dent Assoc 2000;131(2):184–95.
83. Epstein JB, Marcoe JH. Topical application of capsaicin for treatment of oral neuropathic pain and trigeminal neuralgia. Oral Surg Oral Med Oral Pathol 1994;77:135–40.
84. Tomislav B, Ladislav K, Ivana S, et al. Physical therapy with topical ketoprofen and anxiety related to temporomandibular joint pain treatment. Fiz Rehabil Med 2013;25(1–2):6–16.
85. Di Rienzo Businco L1, Di Rienzo Businco A, D'Emilia M, et al. Topical versus systemic diclofenac in the treatment of temporomandibular joint dysfunction symptoms. Acta Otorhinolaryngol Ital 2004;24(5):279–83.
86. Lynch ME, Clark AJ, Sawynok J. A pilot study examining topical amitriptyline, ketamine, and a combination of both in the treatment of neuropathic pain. Clin J Pain 2003;19:323–8.
87. Klasser GD, Epstein JB, Villines D, et al. Burning mouth syndrome: a challenge for dental practitioners and patients. Gen Dent 2011;59(3):210–20.
88. Lynch ME, Clark AJ, Sawynok J, et al. Topical amitriptyline and ketamine in neuropathic pain syndromes: an open-label study. J Pain 2005;6:644–9.
89. Mathisen LC, Skjelbred P, Skoglund LA, et al. Effect of ketamine, an NMDA receptor inhibitor, in acute and chronic orofacial pain. Pain 1995;61:215–20.
90. Soares A, Andriolo RB, Atallah AN, et al. da Silva Botulinum toxin for myofascial pain syndromes in adults. Cochrane Database Syst Rev 2012;4:CD007533.
91. Kleen JK, Levin M. Injection therapy for headache and facial pain. Oral Maxillofac Clin North Am 2016;28423–34.

An Update on Diagnosis and Pharmacologic Therapy for Headache in the Oral and Maxillofacial Surgery Practice

Leslie R. Halpern, DDS, MD, PhD, FICD[a],*, Paul Gammal, DDS[b], David R. Adams, DDS, FICD[a]

KEYWORDS

- Headache • Pharmacologic management • Migraine • Cluster headache
- Neurovascular headaches • Medication overuse headache

KEY POINTS

- The World Health Organization characterizes headaches among the major etiologies of disability that are underestimated and undertreated throughout the world.
- The International Classification of Headache Disorders provide the most recent description of headache type and diagnosis based on the individual pathologic presentations of primary and secondary headaches.
- Primary headaches refer to those without a clear causation due to pathology, trauma, or systemic etiology. These headaches include migraine, tension-type, and trigeminal autonomic cephalgias.
- Medication overuse headache from either prescribed or over-the-counter drugs is very common in patients with chronic migraine. Preventive strategies and education remain the most important treatment modalities.
- Research into the pharmacology of headache has led to several highly effective new treatments that are targeting the central nervous immune system with less adverse effects and more specific neuron-directed targets for pain relief.

INTRODUCTION

The World Health Organization characterizes headaches among the major etiologies of disability with a global prevalence rate of 47%.[1] Almost one-half of the adult population have had a headache at least once per year, and as such, headaches have been underestimated and undertreated throughout the world.[1,2] Ancient descriptions of headaches date back to 1200 BC and archeologic skull artifacts exhibit areas of surgical exposure for headache treatment in the writings of Hippocrates.[3] The contemporary worldwide prevalence of a chronic daily headache can vary from 3% to 5% diagnosed and most likely represents chronic migraine.[3,4]

Headaches are synonymous with neurovascular pain (cephalalgias), which comprise a heterogeneous group of pain disorders that share a common anatomic region, that is, the head and neck. The oral and maxillofacial surgeon (OMFS) receives consults from many of their medical colleagues to evaluate the chief complaint of a headache. Headaches are often a "universal"

[a] Oral and Maxillofacial Surgery, University of Utah, School of Dentistry, 530 South Wakara Way, Salt Lake City, UT 84108, USA; [b] Department of Dentistry/Oral Surgery, Woodhull Hospital and Mental Health Center, 760 Broadway, Brooklyn, NY 11206, USA
* Corresponding author.
E-mail address: Leslie.halpern@hsc.utah.edu

Oral Maxillofacial Surg Clin N Am 34 (2022) 83–97
https://doi.org/10.1016/j.coms.2021.08.010
1042-3699/22/© 2021 Elsevier Inc. All rights reserved.

disease presentation that is evaluated by the OMFS because many referral physicians equate symptomatology with either an odontogenic nidus or temporomandibular disorder (TMD). There is a new paradigm shift in the understanding of the pathophysiology of headaches based on neuropathic mechanisms that warrant traditional and innovative pharmacologic management strategies. The objective of this article is to describe the epidemiology of neurovascular headaches, their pathophysiologic mechanisms/presentation, the workup of patients, and an up-to-date overview of pharmacologic as well as nonpharmacologic approaches that can be applied in the oral and maxillofacial surgical practice.

LITERATURE SEARCH

A literature search was undertaken using Medline within the PubMed Portal to choose articles within the last 25 years. Only articles in English were chosen for inclusion. Each article's bibliography was evaluated for relevant publications and reviewed by the authors for inclusion. The keywords chosen include "Headache," "Primary and secondary headaches," "International Classification of Headache Disorders (ICHD)," "Neurovascular headache/pain," "Migraine," "Adult and pediatric headache," "Pharmacologic therapy for headaches," "Non-pharmacologic headache therapy," "Pathology of headaches," "medication headache overuse," and "medications for headache treatment." The level of evidence chosen was based on Sacket's hierarchy of evidence and was predominantly level 1A, 2A, 3A, 4, and 5.[5] Sixty articles that were relevant to this review were chosen. Additional references were chosen to support a paradigm shift in the pharmacology of headache therapy moving forward.

EPIDEMIOLOGY

The lifelong prevalence of headaches is at 96% in men and women are disproportionately affected 3:1.[6] The global prevalence rate of a tension-type headache (TTH) is 40% followed by the migraine at 15% to 18%.[7–9] The common neurovascular headache type of migraine occurs more commonly in women (3:1) between the ages of 23 and 55 years.[4,6] Approximately, 44.5 million adults in the United States have experienced a migraine and the cost of treatment is at 17 billion dollars and 13 billion dollars in lost productivity.[7,8] The trigeminal autonomic cephalgias (TACs; ie, cluster headaches [CHs]) are the third most common type of headache with a prevalence rate of 0.1% and a gender ratio of male to female at 3:5

to 7:1.[6] The International Classification of Headache Disorders (ICHD) provide the most recent description of headache type and diagnosis based on the individual pathologic presentations. The ICHD are further classified into primary versus secondary headaches. A primary headache is without a known underlying cause. The most common types of primary headaches include migraine, CHs, and TTHs. Secondary headaches are most often the result of another etiology, that is, inflammation, infection, trauma, vascular diseases, psychiatric disorders, and drugs (**Box 1**).[6,7] A timely diagnostic workup is of the urgency if the patient's clinical presentation is significant for a secondary headache. The latter aids in preventing a serious misdiagnosis because management strategies rely on time from initial presentation (see below). Painful cranial neuropathies that include other facial pains and other headaches comprise the

---

Box 1
Primary and secondary headache classification

Primary Headache Classification:

Migraine type

Tension type

Trigeminal autonomic hemicrania: cluster type and paroxysmal hemicrania

Other: unilateral neuralgiform type

Stimulus-induced headache: "ice-cream headache"

Thunderclap headache:

Primary; idiopathic

Secondary Headache Classification:

Trauma

Infection

Disorders of the sinus/teeth/eyes/ears/facial structures

Vasospasm/vascular diseases of the cranium

Withdrawal from substance abuse

Disorders that originate from psychiatric disease

Thunderclap headache: subarachnoid hemorrhages

Giant cell arteritis/Temporal arteritis

Medication overuse headache

Data from Headache Classification Committee of the International Headache Society (IHS). The International Classification of Headache Disorders, 3rd edition (beta version). Cephalalgia. 2013 Jul;33(9):629-808.

third group of headaches classified by the ICHD (the reader is referred to references for further interest).

PATHOPHYSIOLOGIC MECHANISMS OF HEADACHES

Contemporary reviews define a headache as encompassing the entire head including the orofacial region.[7–11] This evidence has important implications for the OMFS practitioner when patients present with orofacial symptoms. An example is a common neurovascular presentation of a "toothache" in patients with a history of migraine.[7,10] Neurovascular pain can arise in extracranial tissues via a pathway through the dental pulp, which is characterized as a "vascular toothache."[7,11]

All somatosensory information from craniovascular structures including nociceptive reflex arcs are relayed through anatomic connections of the trigeminovascular pain pathway, specifically through the trigeminal nucleus caudalis and its cervical extensions.[9] **Fig. 1** depicts pathways for

innervation by the trigeminal sensory system. This complex network of reflex arcs function based on the properties of trigeminal afferents innervating distinct target tissues. Most are transmitted by somatic, motor, and autonomic nerve networks. These target tissue interactions with trigeminal neuron terminals contribute to the awareness and degree of pain perceived. Trigeminal pain conditions can arise from injury secondary to dental procedures, infection, neoplasia, or other diseases/dysfunction within the peripheral and/or central nervous system. Neurovascular disorders, such as primary headaches, can present as chronic orofacial pain, such as in the case of facial migraine, where the pain is localized in the second and third division of the trigeminal nerve. Cranial nerves 7, 9, and 10 also contribute to afferent input of the head and neck precipitating and/or exacerbating orofacial pain. Their afferent pathways converge on the trigeminal system at the level of the brainstem. This complex network can cause dilemmas in diagnosing the origin of pain. The clinician must differentiate heterotopic pain,

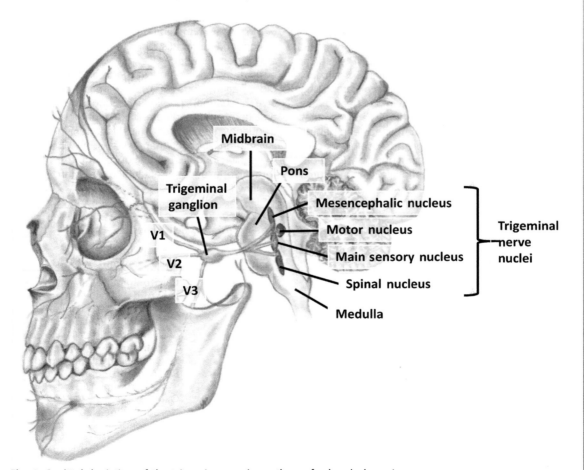

Fig. 1. Sagittal depiction of the trigeminovascular pathway for headache pain.

source of pain not localized at the site of pain, or from referred pain; pain at one area that is supplied by afferents from another source of nociception. This explains why a patient may complain of shoulder and neck pain when describing intraoral pain. Examples of these pathways include peripheral connections, central and ascending connections, brainstem modulation, and hypothalamic modulation. All communicate with the trigeminovascular pain pathway via specific neuropeptides that contribute to autonomic, cognitive, endocrine, and affective symptoms. These pathways exhibit the pathology seen with headaches such as migraine and cluster types (**Box 2** and the reader is referred to reference 9 for an in-depth review of the physiologic mechanisms described earlier).[9]

PATIENT HISTORY AND WORKUP

Pain associated with a headache is a common presenting symptom seen every day and so the physical examination should include paradigms based on anatomic and physiologic correlations. The history of the present illness (HPI) will give the practitioner an accurate diagnosis 90% of the time, and therefore it is essential to allow the patient to describe his/her symptomatology. The common algorithm—chief complaint/HPI/medical history, physical examination, radiologic images, and a psychosocial profile—will facilitate ruling out certain pathology and hone in on specific patterns of pain onset. Other medical disorders, lifestyle features such as diet, caffeine, sleep habits, work, and personal stress provide useful risk predictors. Frequency of headache duration, location, triggering factors, severity, and alleviating features can lead to a well-thought-out differential and definitive diagnosis. The physical examination follows a generalized neurologic approach. Head and neck examination includes palpation of superficial scalp and other vessels of the head and neck, an orofacial examination that includes temporomandibular function, examination of the occlusion, bite, and an in-depth examination of the musculature for evidence of any myofascial pain dysfunction. The latter is most often associated with TTHs (**Box 3**).[12]

Radiologic imaging can be a valuable adjunct depending on the HPI and associated "red flags," that is, new-onset headache in geriatric patients, an abnormal neurologic examination with cranial nerve testing, associated systemic illness with fevers or stiff neck, "worst headache" of one's life or first headache, headaches triggered by coughing, Valsalva upon exertion, and patients who suffer from immunocompromised disease states like HIV. Dodick (2003) introduced the SNOOP mnemonic to characterize "red flags," which may help distinguish primary and secondary headaches.[13,14] These criteria were further revised and adapted to the emergency room setting by Nye and Ward to include systemic illness (eg, fever, chills, human immunodeficiency virus, history of cancer), neurologic signs (eg, change in mental status, asymmetric reflexes), onset (eg, acute, sudden or split second thunderclap headache), older patients (eg, >50 years with new or progressive headache), previous headache history (eg, first headache or different headache changing in frequency, severity, or clinical features), headache in children younger than 5 years, and headache worsening under observation.[15] Some investigators also use an additional expression entitled "yellow flags."[14]

Box 2
Craniovascular nerve fibers and vasoactive neuropeptides in primary headaches

Nerve Fiber Location	Neuropeptide/ Neurotransmitter
Trigeminal sensory nerve	Calcitonin gene-related peptide Substance P/Neurokinin A/ Pituitary adenylate Cyclase activating/Nitric oxide synthase
Parasympathetic fibers	Vasoactive intestinal peptide PACAP/Neuropeptide Y/ Acetylcholine/Nitric Oxide
Sympathetic nerve fibers	Noradrenaline/Neuropeptide Y/Adenosine triphosphate

Adapted from Hoffmann J, Baca SM, Akerman S. Neurovascular mechanisms of migraine and cluster headache. J Cereb Blood Flow Metab. 2019 Apr;39(4):573-594.

Box 3
Diagnostic elements in a history of headache
1. Family history of primary and/or secondary headache symptoms
2. Childhood symptoms of car sickness/Migraine symptoms/Gastrointestinal symptoms
3. Features of an aura
4. Comorbid diseases
5. Age of onset of the first headache
6. Therapies either prior or current to treat symptoms
7. Lifestyle, ie, diet, drugs, alcohol, tobacco
8. Frequency of headache events
Adapted from Rizzoli P, Mullally WJ. Headache. Am J Med. 2018 Jan;131(1):17-24.

The application of neuroimaging to diagnose the aforementioned diseases can be costly and there have been several studies that report a low rate of identifiable intracranial pathology in patients presenting with headaches.[14] A retrospective review by Ifediora examined the rate of intracranial findings following imaging of headache symptomatology over a 7-year period in a catchment of patients seen at a general practice medicine clinic.[16] All forms of headaches and migraines with variations were examined with a mean patient age of 38 years and no gender predilection. This study concluded that regardless of imaging type, that is, CT or MRI, positive intracranial findings were uncommon following imaging. Larger studies, however, are needed especially when comorbidities of psychological disease are also present to validate the findings in this study.[16] Several national and international guidelines exist and most agree that neuroimaging is usually not indicated in patients with a normal neurologic examination in the setting of migraine, CH, and TTH presentation.[14]

PHARMACOLOGIC MANAGEMENT OF HEADACHES BY PRESCRIPTION

Pharmacologic therapy of headaches is most often based on the severity of symptoms and the degree of disability experienced by the patient. The practitioner must be judicious in his/her approach because drug therapy forms a part of an overall algorithm in patient management. Triggers of headache onset are often precipitated by lifestyle issues such as sleep patterns, inadequate hydration, and stress. Correction of these risk predictors can avoid the need for medication,

especially in patients who suffer from TTHs. The latter may also be treated by over-the-counter (OTC) medications (see below). Drug therapy, however, can become the mainstay for the treatment of headaches based on the principles of proper diagnosis and subsequent effective choices of medication. The use of prescription medication, as such, is predicated upon whether its use will be abortive during an acute attack or preventive to reduce the frequency and severity of attacks. This preventive therapy can also decrease or avoid medication overuse headaches (MOHs; see below).

Acute and preventive medications have a broad spectrum of effect, and are specific to particular types of headaches. Abortive (acute) is often administered when symptomatology is mild and often is used in combination with antinausea medications. There is, however, a high potential for medication overuse (see below).[17] Preventive treatment reduces severity, frequency, and avoids medication overuse and is often the treatment applied in patients whose attacks result in disability lasting 3 days or more, patients where acute therapy may be contraindicated or when there exists a combination of headache presentation, that is, hemiplegic migraine or CHs. The latter may require both abortive and preventive therapy.[17]

The following sections focus on current prescription medications for the treatment of acute and chronic headaches (HA). The main types of headaches include migraine, cluster, and tension-type headaches. Each headache type described will aid the provider in determining the proper medications that are evidence-based such as triptans and ergotamine derivatives, as well as OTC medications. The following common primary headache disorders are presented with respect to pharmacologic and nonpharmacologic management. **Fig. 2** provides an algorithm to guide the provider in determining the type of medication(s).

Migraine

Migraine is a common primary headache that affects 10% to 12% of the adult population; 6% of men and 18% of women that peaks between ages 35 and 45 years. The cost of treatment can exceed 19.6 billion dollars per year[18,19] Symptomatology is preceded by triggers such as stress, foods, loss of sleep, and menstruation. Clinical presentation is separated into 4 phases: (1) prodromal, (2) an aura or without aura, (3) the actual headache, and (4) postdrome phase.[1,6,17] A careful differential diagnosis includes tension headache, orodental pain, other vascular disorders,

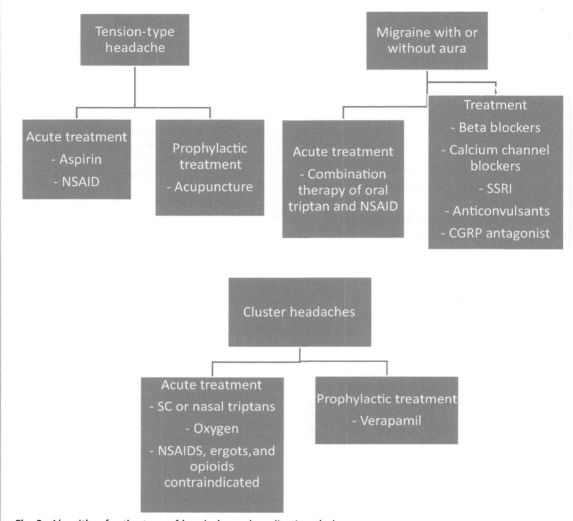

Fig. 2. Algorithm for the type of headache and medication choices.

and intracranial tumors.[20] Although the pathophysiology is not completely clear, it originates from the trigeminovascular system that receives nociceptive afferents from the dura, meningeal blood vessels, and innervation from V1. Cervical innervation also forms part of this network and migraines pain is most often referred to the neck. These afferents cause release of inflammatory mediators (substance P, calcitonin-gene-related peptide, and neurokinins; see **Box 2**) that facilitate the pain transmission.[20,21]

The therapeutic interventions of migraine headaches are either nonpharmacologic (biofeedback, hypnosis, and psychological therapies) or pharmacologic and are predicated upon whether the migraine has an aura phase (A) or not (WA).[20,21] Facial migraines (WA) present with a typical migraine that is localized to the face and is unilateral, associated with nausea, phonophobia, and photophobia.[20–22] Once diagnosed, pharmacologic treatment can be either abortive or preventive based on the timeline of the headache symptomatology. Migraines that occur less than 2 times/mo can be treated with abortive medications, whereas those that occur more frequently need preventive therapy.

Abortive medications

Box 4 lists the pharmacologic abortive agents by type and mechanism of action. Abortive treatment is for acute symptomatic events as well as supplemental therapy for preventive medications during a migraine event. Nonsteroidal anti-inflammatory drugs (NSAIDS) and selective COX-2 inhibitors—naproxen sodium, ibuprofen, and rofecoxib—are effective but not over an extended daily regimen

Box 4
Pharmacologic abortive agents based on type and mechanism of action

Triptans—5-HT1B and 5-HT1D serotonin receptor agonist

- Includes alomtriptan, eletriptan, frovatriptan, naratriptan, rizatriptan, sumatruptan, and zolmitriptan

Ergot derivatives—5HT1 and 5HT2 serotonin receptor agonist

- Ergotamine and dihydroergotamine

Midodrine—α1-receptor agonist

- Midrin
- FDA approval withdrawn in 2017, no longer in use

Drug	Indication	Dose	Adverse effects
Sumatriptan (Imitrex)	Migraine, cluster	Oral: 25, 50, 100 mg capsule, maximum dose 200 mg in 24 h. Subcutaneous: 1–6 mg SC, maximum dose 12 mg in 24 h period, Intranasal: 5 mg, 10 mg, 20 mg, spray into one nostril, maximum dose 40 mg in 24 h period	Coronary artery spasm
Dihydroergotamine (DHE)	Migraine, cluster	1 mg IM/IV/SC, additional 1 mg dose given at hourly intervals as needed, maximum daily dose: IV; 2 mg/24 h, IM/SC 3 mg over 24 h	Nausea/Vomiting

due to adverse systemic effects.[21,23] Ergotamine derivatives (DHE) have been quite effective for severe acute migraine episodes because of their significant effect on vasoconstriction of blood vessels. DHE can be administered intranasally, intravenously, and subcutaneously.[23,24]

Another group, the triptans, has replaced DHE derivatives because of better tolerability and efficacy.[1,22] Serotonin 5-HT receptor agonists are very specific for inhibiting the release of calcitonin gene-related peptide (CGRP), as well as acting at the receptors of meningeal blood vessels and desensitizing the trigeminovascular system by decreasing neurogenic inflammation.[1,9,21,24] The selective serotonin reuptake inhibitor (SSRI) inhibitors—sumatriptan, rizatriptan, and almotriptan—although quite effective, must be carefully tailored to patients who do not suffer from cardiovascular and cerebrovascular anomalies.[25] Combination therapy using sumatriptan with naproxen sodium has been shown to elicit additive effects and another 5-HT receptor agonist; lasmiditan was quite effective in random controlled trails (RCTs) for acute migraine relief. Future research is examining CGRP antagonists as well as other neurogenic inflammatory antagonists in relieving symptoms with minimal side effects.[15]

Preventive medications
Box 5 and **Table 1** list the pharmacologic agents for preventive therapy. More frequent migraine episodes, that is, greater than 5 headaches/mo, are treated with preventive medications that aim to reduce severity, duration, and frequency. When taken on a regular basis, the frequency of attacks is least likely to occur. Their mechanism of action may be different than for acute episodes but medications that are beneficial include beta-adrenergic blockers (propranolol and atenolol), calcium channel blockers (verapamil), and the tricyclic antidepressants (TCSs: amitriptyline and serotonin antagonists [SSRIs]). The comorbidity of migraines and depression support the use of these medications.[7] In addition, the TCAs increase the availability of serotonin and norepinephrine by inhibiting their reuptake.[15,23,25] The antiepileptic agents (gabapentin and pregabalin) are equivocal in their ability to exert a prophylactic effect on the prevention of frequency of attacks.[23] Topiramate and valproate may be beneficial as a prophylactic approach for chronic migraines.[21,23] More recent treatment strategies include the use of botulinum toxin injections for the treatment of migraine headaches (see the section on botulinum below).[26] Outcome studies do support a 50% reduction in

> **Box 5**
> **Pharmacologic preventive agents based on type and mechanism of action**
>
> CGRP receptor antagonist
>
> - Atogepant, rimegepant, and ubrogepant
>
> Anti-CGRP monoclonal antibodies
>
> - Fremanezumab, erenumab, galcanezumab, and eptinezumab
>
> Inhibition of release of CGRP
>
> - Botulinum toxin A
>
> Blockade of voltage-gated sodium channel and neurotransmitter release
>
> - Topiramate and valproate
>
> Beta blocker
>
> - Propanolol, atenolol, metoprolol, and timolol
>
> Calcium channel blockers
>
> - Flunarizine
>
> Tricyclic antidepressants
>
> - Nortriptyline and amitriptyline
>
> Serotonin antagonist
>
> - Pizotifen and methysergide
>
> Antihypertensives
>
> - Lisinopril and candesartan

headache frequency with preventive therapies and hold promise for chronic migraine sufferers.[26,27]

Tension-Type Headache

TTTHs are the most common type of headache in the population with a 1-year prevalence rate of 80%.[6,23] Age range is from 20 to 30 years and they can be episodic or chronic (<12 or >100/y).[6,28,29] Episodic forms are brought on by stress, fatigue, loss of sleep, and alcohol, whereas chronic TTH can be preceded by depression, anxiety, or episodic periods. TTHs have the potential for significant disability with a concomitant socioeconomic impact. The probable mechanism involves an interaction among the limbic system, and peripheral afferents from the intracranial vasculature and skeletal musculature (myofascial input). The TTH is bilateral, dull, nonpulsating and the patient complains of a tight band around the head with myofascial trigger points; most often seen with TMD.[6,28] The duration can last from 30 minutes to 72 hours and there may be associated photophobia, phonophobia, nausea, and

parafunctional habits. Pharmacologic management includes the use of NSAIDS, as well as, low dosing of TCAs. Newer methods for chronic TTH relief include the use of onabotulinum toxin injections because the pain associated with muscle contraction is resolved with the paralytic effect of botulinum toxin.[6,29] Nonmedication management of TTH can include manual manipulation by physical therapy, local anesthetic injections, relaxation therapy, and biofeedback techniques. A Cochrane database review in 2016 found data to support the use of acupuncture in reducing the frequency of TTH attacks.[6,30]

Trigeminal Autonomic Cephalalgias

TACS are a group of headache disorders that are not only associated with headache/facial pain but also manifest themselves with parasympathetic autonomic sequelae.[6] TACS are classified as follows: (1) CHs, (2) paroxysmal hemicranias (PH), (3) unilateral neuralgiform, and (4) hemicrania continua type. They are located in the orbital, temporal, supraorbital, orofacial regions, temporomandibular joints (TMJ), and intraoral structures. A careful differential diagnosis must be made because misinterpretation of clinical symptoms can result in unnecessary treatment interventions.[1,31]

Cluster headaches

CH is the most common headache in the TAC classification with up to 300 cases/100,000 patients, ages of 20 to 30 years, and affecting men more than women (6:1).[32,33] CHs most likely have an autosomal dominant gene with low penetrance, with first-degree relatives having a prevalence rate of 14 to 18 times greater than the general population.[27] Most of the occurrences are usually 2 clusters over several months to a chronic form with greater frequency and no remissions.[23,32] Headaches are unilateral with ipsilateral autonomic features: conjunctival injection, miosis, ptosis, rhinorrhea, and facial sweating. The intensity of autonomic sequela requires the need for an MRI to rule out any organic anomalies, as well as, sleep studies because many who suffer from CH also have obstructive sleep apnea.[33] CHs can recur annually at about the same time of the year, although significant variation is reported.[5,34]

Pharmacologic therapeutics are again either abortive or preventive, that is, oxygen and sumatriptan at dosing of 6 mg subcutaneous or 10 to 20 mg intranasal (IN); DHE, 0.5 to 1.0 mg (IN); and lignocaine, 1 mL 4% to 10% solution IN.[23,33] Preventive pharmacology includes verapamil, 360 to 720 mg/d; lithium, 300 to 1200 mg/d; and/or prednisone, 60 to 80 mg and taper over 4 weeks.

Table 1
Preventive pharmacologic agents with dose and adverse effects

Drug	Indication	Dose	Adverse Effects
OnabotulinumtoxinA	Migraine	31 injections across 7 head and neck muscles, injections repeated every 3 mo	Allergic reaction, rash, itching, headache, neck or back pain, and muscle stiffness
Topiramate	Migraine	Week 1 25 mg at night Week 2 25 mg morning and night Week 3 25 mg morning 50 mg night Week 4 50 mg morning and night	Anxiety, ataxia, confusion, diarrhea, diplopia, dizziness, drowsiness, dysphasia, fatigue, lack of concentration, memory impairment, nausea, nervousness, paresthesia, psychomotor disturbances, depression, visual disturbances, weight loss, dysgeusia, mood changes, and anorexia
Propranolol	Migraine	Initial dose 80 mg orally/d Maintenance dose 160–240 mg/d	Bradycardia, diarrhea, dry eyes, hair loss, nausea, weakness, and fatigue
Pizotifen and methysergide	Migraine	1.5 mg daily initially, 4.5 mg maximum dose	Weight gain and drowsiness
Nortriptyline and amitriptyline	Migraine	10 mg days 1–5 then ramp up dose to 25 mg daily	Nausea, vomiting, nightmares, tiredness, constipation, increased sweating, and dry mouth.
Fremanezumab, erenumab, galcanezumab, and eptinezumab	Migraine	70–140 mg subcutaneously once a month	Injection site pain, redness, and itching
Atogepant, rimegepant, and ubrogepant [a]Will come on the market in Q3 2021	Migraine	Studies conducted with doses of 10, 30, and 60 mg daily	Constipation, nausea, and upper respiratory infection

[a] Personal communication to Dr. Paul Gammal.

Anticonvulsants such as valproic acid, 600 to 2000 mg/d; gabapentin, 900 mg/day; and topiramate, 25 to 200 mg/d can contribute to a remission based on the individual. The clinician must advise that adverse reactions can occur based on the specific drugs, as well as drug-drug interactions, and the risk of medication overuse (the reader is referred to the following sections for further explanation).

Paroxysmal hemicranias

PH presents as a unilateral headache with ipsilateral autonomic sequelae, that is, nasal congestion, lacrimation, and facial flushing. It affects 1 per 50,000 patients presenting for orofacial pain evaluation and is often elusive in diagnosis due to localization in the face.[27,33] It can be episodic or chronic and is triggered by alcohol and head and/or neck pain. Both episodic and chronic are often described with the chronic form which is more prevalent in women.[27,33,34] Pharmacologic intervention involves the use of indomethacin, a well-used anti-inflammatory for PH and whose side effect is dyspepsia whose symptomatology can be controlled with an H2 blocker.[6,23,35] The dosage can vary from 25 to 250 mg/d. If symptoms resolve within 24 hours, it is definitively diagnosed as PH (for further interest in the treatment of TAC, the reader is referred to references).

Vascular Headaches

Vascular headaches have their etiology within the veins and arteries of the head and neck that are somatic in origin. Inflammatory cascades will precipitate either phlebitis or arteritis in the veins or arteries, respectively. Several vascular pains *refer* to the orofacial region, that is, cranial arteritis and carotidynia.

Cranial arteritis

The most common artery inflamed within the head and neck is the temporal artery. Temporal arteritis (TA), giant cell arteritis, and/or polymyalgia rheumatica are common diagnostic terms.[23,36] TA is most often diagnosed during the 6th decade, Caucasian women are at greatest risk, and the risk for TA increases with age. Symptoms include a headache in the temporal region with throbbing, burning, and lancinating sequelae. It can occur bilaterally and palpation of the region elicits a severe tenderness that is exacerbated by constant jaw movement, that is, jaw claudication.[37] Pain related to TA is distributed in the cranial nerve V1 distribution, and can also radiate to V2 and V3. Pain is referred to the shoulder, hip, with other symptoms such as malaise, poor eating, and diplopia, 30% of the time leading to a loss of vision. Blood workup of erythrocyte sedimentation rate (ESR) shows a value > 100 mm/h and C-reactive protein can also be significantly elevated. The definitive diagnosis is obtained with an incisional biopsy of the artery that identifies multinucleated giant cells.[36,37] These inflammatory sequelae contribute to a granulomatous reaction and resultant optic neuropathy.[36–38] TA is considered a medical emergency, and treatment with high doses of glucocorticoids should be initiated as early as possible to rapidly control inflammatory symptoms and prevent inflammatory complications, such as jaw claudication, visual loss, and stroke.[39,40] The burden of high-dose glucocorticoids is, however, considerable, especially in the elderly, with over 80% of the patients experiencing significant treatment-related side effects. Studies reported a high number of major adverse advents related to long-term glucocorticoid use in giant cell arteritis (GCA): posterior subcapsular cataract (41%), bone fractures (38%), infections (31%), hypertension (22%), diabetes mellitus (9%), and gastrointestinal bleeding (4%).[40] The dosing schedule is 40 to 60 mg of prednisone daily that is gradually tapered based on symptomatology and decreased ESR. The timeline for treatment will vary based on the individual.[37–39]

Carotidynia

Carotidynia is a unilateral vascular pain that originates from the cervical carotid artery and radiates to the ipsilateral side of origin, that is, ear, face. Facial pain is reported with overlying edema at the site affected and palpation at the common carotid bifurcation elicits severe pain. Pain is referred to the eye, malar region, and back of the ear. Two types of pain, acute and chronic, are diagnosed. The acute form can manifest itself over several weeks as a result of a single illness, whereas the chronic form may be a variant of the acute episode. Women are predisposed with a 4:1 ratio and diagnosis is during middle age.[23] The mechanism may be similar to TA and it resolves over several weeks. Pharmacologic therapy is similar to TA. 30 mg/d dosing of prednisone can be followed by a tapering dose over 4 days. Chronic therapy mimics pharmacologic prescribing for chronic migraines (see the section on migraine pharmacologic treatment above).[23,41]

OVER THE COUNTER MEDICATIONS TO TREAT HEADACHE

OTC medications such as acetaminophen, ibuprofen, naproxen, aspirin, and combinations of these medications with caffeine make up the first-line therapies for many mild to moderate headaches. The lower costs of these medications compared with prescription medications makes them widely available to many patients. When used as directed, most of these medications have relatively low occurrences of significant adverse effects and have low abuse potential. **Tables 2** and **3** list these medications as described in the following sections.

Acetaminophen

Acetaminophen (APAP) is known to act through inhibition of the cyclooxygenase (COX-1 and COX-2) causing inhibition of prostaglandin synthesis. Prostaglandins are significant mediators of the inflammatory response and play a large role in pain, fever, and inflammation. Unlike NSAIDs, acetaminophen only inhibits the COX pathways in the central nervous system and not in the peripheral tissues.[42] When taken as advised, acetaminophen has a low risk of adverse events and nearly negligible risk for severe events. It is metabolized in the liver and its breakdown products are recovered in the urine. A secondary pathway metabolizes acetaminophen to a reactive intermediate which is reduced by glutathione. If liver glutathione

Table 2
Over-the-counter medications for headache pain relief

Generic Name	Brand Name	Use	Precautions	Possible Side Effects
Acetaminophen	Tylenol, Panadol	Pain relief Headache		Few side effects if taken as directed but may include changes in blood counts and liver damage
Aspirin	Bayer, Bufferin	Pain relief Headache	Do not use in children younger than 19 y with viral illness due to potential for Reye's Syndrome	Gastritis, GI bleeding, bronchospasm, anaphylaxis, and gastric ulcers
Ibuprofen	Advil, Motrin	Headaches Migraines		GI upset, drowsiness, dizziness, vision disturbances, and ulcers
Naproxen	Aleve	Prevention of tension headaches Treatment of migraines		Similar to other NSAIDs
Acetaminophen-Aspirin-caffeine	Excedrin	Treatment of migraines Tension-type headaches		Same as acetaminophen and aspirin

Table 3
Success rate[a] of various OTC medications and combinations in relieving at least 50% maximum pain relief (f)

Drug	Dose (mg)	Success Rate (%)
Ibuprofen + paracetamol	400 + 1000	70
Ibuprofen + paracetamol[b]	200 + 500	67
Ibuprofen (fast acting)	400	57
Ibuprofen + caffeine	200 + 100	54
Ibuprofen (fast acting)	200	52
Ibuprofen	400	45
Naproxen	500/550	44
Naproxen	400/440	43
Paracetamol	500	43
Paracetamol	975/1000	34
Aspirin	1000	31
Aspirin	600/650	28
Paracetamol	600/650	26
Naproxen	200/220	21
Aspirin	500	11

[a] Success rate is calculated by taking the proportion of participants who get good pain relief with analgesic minus the proportion who get good pain relief with placebo and expressing this as a percentage of the maximum possible success rate for the analgesic, that is, 100% minus the positive rate with placebo.
[b] Paracetamol is the outside-of-the-United States equivalent to acetaminophen.
Adapted from Moore RA, Wiffen PJ, Derry S, Maguire T, Roy YM, Tyrrell L. Non-prescription (OTC) oral analgesics for acute pain - an overview of Cochrane reviews. Cochrane Database Syst Rev. 2015 Nov 4;2015(11):CD010794.

is depleted as in alcoholism, hepatotoxicity can develop. Acetaminophen should be avoided in patients with liver disease and a history of high alcohol consumption.[42,43] In some studies, data have shown that this medication was not effective for headaches at doses below 1000 mg and was less effective than NSAIDs.[17]

Nonsteroidal Anti-inflammatory Drugs

Ibuprofen

Ibuprofen (IBU) is the most commonly used NSAID. It nonselectively inhibits COX-1 and COX-2 and acts both in the central nervous system and in the peripheral tissues. The most common side effects are gastrointestinal. The inhibition of prostaglandin in the stomach can lead to inflammation, bleeding, and ulceration.[43] In chronic use of NSAIDs, the inhibition of COX-1 in the kidneys can contribute to acute renal failure, especially in patients with CHF, hepatic cirrhosis, and renal disease. In several studies, ibuprofen was shown to be more effective than acetaminophen in controlling acute pain (see **Table 2**).

Naproxen

Naproxen mode of action is similar to ibuprofen. Its half-life is 15 hours, which is much longer than ibuprofen. There is a higher risk of gastric ulcers than is seen with ibuprofen. As with other NSAIDs, these medications should be avoided in patients with a known hypersensitivity to aspirin, NSAID/aspirin-induced asthma, significant history of active GI bleeding or ulcers, or in the third trimester of pregnancy.[42]

Aspirin

Aspirin (ASA) irreversibly inhibits COX-1 and COX-2 as in the other NSAIDs. This inhibition also hinders thromboxane synthesis, resulting in a decrease in platelet function.[42] Chronic use of aspirin is well known to be associated with gastric bleeding and nephrotoxicity. Children under the age of 19 years recovering from viral illnesses such as flu or chickenpox should avoid aspirin because of the potential for Reye's syndrome.[44]

Combination of over the counter drugs with caffeine in the treatment of headaches

In the treatment of headaches, notably migraine and TTHs, commonly used OTC medications may be combined with caffeine which acts as an analgesic adjuvant. Analgesic adjuvants do not have analgesic properties themselves but they do augment the actions of specific analgesics including APAP, ASA, and IBU. When combined with ASA and/or APAP, the analgesic effect is enhanced by about 40%.[44] Caffeine promotes the adsorption of these analgesics by lowering the gastric pH. It also increases gastric motility. At doses in the range of 10 to 35 mg per kg, it enhances the pain relief with APAP and several different NSAIDs.[45,46]

MEDICATION OVERUSE HEADACHE

Studies have shown that medications to treat headaches can cause a paradoxic effect by increasing the frequency and intensity of headache occurrence.[47] MOH is defined as headaches that occur greater than 15 d/mo in patients with re-existing primary headaches who regularly use drugs for acute headache treatment.[1] The epidemiology of MOH indicates that 1% of the population who suffer from headaches can be susceptible, usually in those with daily chronic headaches.[1,48] The pathophysiology is not well-understood but can be based on the complexity of the genetics, central nervous system networks involved in chronic pain, and triggers of stress within the individual at risk.[1,48] The ICHD classifies MOH specifically as a disorder in patients with chronic migraine headache. Genetic studies have determined that MOH occurs 3 to 4 times more in women during their fourth decade of life and comorbidities include depression and anxiety, low education, gastrointestinal complaints, smoking, caffeine, and use of tranquilizers. MOH can occur on withdrawal of analgesics which exacerbates more analgesic usage and a cycle of adverse events. This is more prevalent with the use of triptans and opiates. Adverse events due to withdrawal of these medications include nausea, gastrointestinal disturbances, and changes in behavior.

The sequelae described warrant a careful diagnosis of MOH as other diagnoses need to be ruled out, that is, intracranial hypertension, vasculitis, malignancy, depression, and anxiety. Treatment strategies, as such, need to be tailored to the individual. Education is the first step in a series of strategies for prevention.[48,49] Patients with migraines and TTHs are advised to keep a diary that records the frequency of medications used, as well as dosing as the latter can exacerbate the headache event. Other strategies include a careful algorithm for drug withdrawal. Triptans, for instance, can be abruptly discontinued, as well as simple analgesics.[1,48,49] Patients must be counseled, however, that withdrawal headaches are to be expected over a period of 2 to 10 days with side effects of nausea, vomiting, anxiety, and possible insomnia. Those on triptans will improve over 7 to 10 days, whereas those on simple analgesics improve over 2 to 3 weeks.[48,49] Medication overuse with opioids require possible supervision with inpatient hospital admission and a detoxification protocol and pharmacotherapy by intravenous administration of lidocaine, antiemetics, benzodiazepines, hydration, and dexamethasone. Adjunctive psychotherapy may be warranted using cognitive-behavioral therapy in order to encourage patients to not consider themselves as "addicts" but suffer from an illness that requires these therapeutic approaches for the resolution of MOH. These patients may also benefit from adjunctive therapy with topiramate and botulinum toxin (the reader is referred to the references for further interest).[1,48,49]

SUMMARY

The pharmacologic treatment of primary and secondary headaches continues to be an area of increasingly intense interest and focus. Potential challenges, however, still need to be addressed. Additional therapeutic modalities continue to be discovered without clinical trial methodology or rationale. Therapeutic decisions require large clinical trials to support the emerging therapies specifically targeting headache pain pathways. An example is botulinum toxin and its success in resolving "chronic migraine" via a mechanism that is a paradox not normally seen. Research in the pharmacology of headache has led to several new treatments that target the central nervous immune system without the typical CNS adverse events. They exert their action through neuron-directed mechanisms. Examples mentioned in this article include efficacious preventive drugs that suppress excitatory nervous signaling via sodium and/or calcium receptors, facilitate GABAergic inhibition, reduce neuronal sensitization, block cortical spreading depression, and/or reduce circulating levels of CGRP.

The OMFS clinician must be judicious in crafting a differential diagnosis when their patients complain of headache pain, specifically that which nonodontogenic in nature is. The complexity of the anatomy, neurobiological physiology, and variable presentations of toothache can make potential pitfalls of diagnosis inevitable. Premature surgical intervention can precipitate/exacerbate neurovascular symptomatology and mask comorbid diseases such as migraine, depression, seizures, and cerebrovascular accidents. As such, there needs to be flexibility in the categorization of various headaches so that the resolution of symptoms can be tailored for disease resolution. A practical approach using existing evidence-based guidelines can enable the OMFS practitioner to effectively treat the common presentations of headache seen in practice.

CLINICS CARE POINTS

- The etiology of headaches resides within the anatomic connections of the trigeminovascular pain pathway, and present anywhere within trigeminally innervated tissues.
- Greater than 90% of patients who present to their oral health care provider for evaluation of headache have a primary headache disorder characterized as migraine, cluster, or tension-type headache.
- Migraine headache is characterized as the third most prevalent and the seventh most common cause of disability throughout the globe.
- Medication overuse headache often coexists with migraine type and needs to be addressed to avoid medication adverse events.
- Emerging pharmacologic therapies and methods of delivery are now being used to target specific neuronal pathways without concomitant adverse medication sequelae.

ACKNOWLEDGMENT

The authors thank Yuliya Petukhova (Petukhova, DDS) for figure 1 artwork.

DISCLOSURE

The authors have nothing to disclose.

REFERENCES

1. Sinclair AJ, Sturrock A, Davies B, et al. Headache management: pharmacological approaches. Pract Neurol 2015;15:411–23.
2. Available at: https://www.who.int/news-room/fact-sheets/detail/headache-dsiorders. Accessed March 20 2021.
3. Magiorkinis E, Diamantis A, Mitsikostas DD, et al. Headaches in antiquity and during the early scientific era. J Neurol 2009;256:1215–20.
4. Burch RC, Loder S, Loder E, et al. The prevalence and burden of migraine and severe headache in the United States updated statistics from government health surveillance and studies. Headache 2015;55(1):21–34.
5. Burns PB, Rohrich RJ, Chung KC. The levels of evidence and their role in evidence-based medicine. Plast Reconstruct Surg 2011;128(1):305–10.
6. Rizzoli P, Mullally WJ. Headache. Amer J Med 2018; 131:17–24.
7. Nixdorf DR, Velly AM, Alonso AA. Neurovascular pain: Implications of migraine for the oral and

maxillofacial surgeon. Oral Maxillofac Clin North Am 2008;20(2):1–24.

8. Hu XH, Markson LE, Lipton RB, et al. Burden of migraine in the United states. Arch Int Med 1999; 159(8):813–8.

9. Hoffmann J, Baca SM, Akerman S. Neurovascular mechanisms of migraine and cluster headache. J Cereb Blood flow Metabol 2019;39(4):573–94.

10. Namazi MR. Presentation of migraine as odontalgia. Headache 2001;41(4):420–1.

11. Czenisky R, Benoliel R, Sharav Y. Orofacial pain with vascular-type features. Oral Surg Oral Med Oral Pathol Oral Radiol Endod 1997;84(5):506–12.

12. Headache classification committee of the International Headache society (HIS). The International Classification of Headache disorders. 3rd edition (beta version). Cephalalgia 2013;33(9):629–808.

13. Dodick D. diagnosing headache: clinical clues and clinical rules. Adv Study Med 2003;3(2):87–92.

14. Gadde JA, Cantrell S, Patel SS, et al. Neuroimaging of adults with headache: Appropriateness, utilization, and an economical overview. Neuroimaging Clin North Am 2019;29:203–11.

15. Silberstein SD, Holland S, Freitag F, et al. Evidence-based guideline update: Pharmacologic treatment for episodic migraine prevention in adults: Report of the quality standards subcommittee of the American Academy of Neurology and the American Headache Society. Neurology 2012;78:1337–45.

16. Ifediora CO. Insights into radiographic investigations for headaches in general practice. Fam Pract 2018;35(4):412–9.

17. Weatherall M. Drug therapy in headache. Clin Med 2015;15(3):273–9.

18. Hu XH, Markson LE, Lipton RB, et al. Burden of migraine in the United States: Disability and economic costs. Arch Intern Med 1999;159:813–8.

19. Stewart WF, Ricci JA, Chee E, et al. Lost productive work time costs from health conditions in the United States: results from the American Productivity Audit. J Occup Environ Med 2003;45(12):1234–46.

20. Karli N, Zarifoglu M, Calisir N, et al. Comparison of pre-headache phases and trigger factors of migraine and episodic tension-type headache: do they share similar clinical pathophysiology? Cephalalgia 2005;25(6):444–51.

21. Romeo-Reyes M, Uyanik JM. Orofacial pain management: current perspectives. J Pain Res 2014;7:99–115.

22. Mayans L, Walling A. Acute migraine headache: treatment strategies. Amer Fam Physician 2018;97(4):243–51.

23. Okeson JP. General considerations in managing oral and facial pain. In: Okeson JP, editor. Bell's oral and facial pain. 7th edition. Hanover Park, IL: Quintessence Publishing Co; 2014. p. 181–232.

24. Silberstein S, Kori S, Dihydroergotamine. a review of formulation approaches for the acute treatment of migraine. CAN Drugs 2013;27(5):385–94.

25. Dodick D, Lipton RB, Martin V, et al. Triptan Cardiovascular Safety Expert Panel: consensus statement: cardiovascular safety profile of triptans (5-HT agonists) in the acute treatment of migraine. Headache 2004;44(5):414–25.

26. Dodick DW, Turkel CC, DeGryse RE, et al. PREEMPT Chronic migraine study. Onabotulinum toxin A for treatment of chronic migraine: pooled results from the double blind, randomized, placebo-controlled phases of the PREEMPT clinical program. Headache 2010;50(6):921–36.

27. Benoliel R, Eliav E. Primary headache disorders. Dent Clin North Am 2013;57(3):513–39.

28. Freitag F. Managing and treating tension-type headache. Med Clin North Am 2013;97:281–92.

29. Wheeler A, Smith HS. Botulinum toxins: mechanisms of action, anti-nociception and clinical applications. Toxicology 2013;306:124–46.

30. Linde K, Allais G, Brinkhaus B, et al. Acupuncture for prevention of migraine. Cochrane Database Syts Rev 2016;(6):CD001218.

31. Prakash S, Patel P. Hemicrania continua: clinical review, diagnosis and management. Pain Res 2017;10:1493–509.

32. Leone M, Bussone G. Pathophysiology of trigeminal autonomic cephalalgias. Lancet Neurol 2009;8(8):755–64.

33. Balasubramaniam R, Klasser GD, Delcanho R. Trigeminal autonomic cephalalgias: a review and implications for dentistry. J Am Dent Assoc 2008;139(12):1616–24.

34. Nesbitt AD, Goadsby PJ. Cluster headache. Br Med J 2012;344:e2407.

35. Cittadino E, Matthau MS. Goads by PJ. Paroxysmal hemicranias: a prospective clinical study of 31 cases. Brain 2008;131(Pt4):1142–56.

36. Ponte C, Rodrigues AF, O'Neill L, et al. Giant cell arteritis: current treatment and management. World J Clan Cases 2015;3(6):484–94.

37. Kraemer M, Metz A, Harold M, et al. Reduction in jaw opening: a neglected symptom of giant cell arteritis. Rheumatol Int 2011;31:1521–3.

38. Renton T. Tooth-related pain or not? Headache 2020;60:235–46.

39. Redillas C, Solomon S. Recent advances in temporal arteritis. Curr Pain Headache Rep 2003;7:297–302.

40. Proven A, Gabriel SE, Orces C, et al. Glucocorticoid therapy in giant cell arteritis: duration and adverse outcomes. Arthritis Rheum 2003;49:703–8.

41. Comacchio F, Bottin R, Brescia G, et al. Carotidynia: new aspects of a controversial entity. Acta Otorhinolaryngol Ital 2012;32:266–9.

42. Peck J, Urits I, Zeien J, et al. A Comprehensive review of over-the counter treatment for chronic migraine headaches. Curr Pain Headache Rep 2020;24:19.

43. Abbott F. Use and abuse of over-the -counter analgesic agents. J Psychiatry Neurosci 1998;23(1): 13–34.

44. FDA. Federal Register, vol. 68, 2003. No 74.

45. Lipton RB, Diener H-C, Robbins MS, et al. Caffeine in the management of patients with headache. J Headache Pain 2017;18(1):107.

46. Moore RA, Wiffen PJ, Derry S, et al. Non-prescription (OTC) oral analgesics for acute pain – an overview of Cochrane reviews. Cochrine Database Syst Rev 2015;2015(11):CD010794.

47. Rolan PE. Understanding the pharmacology of headache. Curr Opin Pharmacol 2014;14:30–3.

48. Wakerley BR. Medication –overuse headache. Pract Neurol 2019;19:399–403.

49. Schwedt TJ, Chong CD. Medication overuse headache: pathophysiological insights from structural and functional brain MRI research. Headache 2017;57:1173–8.

Pharmacological Management of Common Soft Tissue Lesions of the Oral Cavity

Guillermo Puig Arroyo, DMD*, Ashley Lofters, DDS*, Earl Clarkson, DDS

KEYWORDS

- Aphthous lesions • Oral herpes • Candidiasis • Ulcerative diseases • Pemphigus • Pemphigoid

KEY POINTS

- The diagnosis of soft tissue lesions in the oral cavity requires a thorough clinical evaluation; therefore, avoiding confusion between similar appearing lesions.
- Topical medications have been proven to be the most effective management of certain oral mucosal lesions.
- When managing candidiasis it is important to address any underlying factor when possible.
- Patients with ulcerative diseases may have superimposed candidiasis altering the clinical appearance of a lesion.
- The overall objective of steroidal therapy is to decrease the number, size, and discomfort of lesions.

Lesions of the oral cavity can arise from many different etiologies, inflammatory, infection, traumatic, immunologic, or neoplastic. Obtaining a detailed patient history and physical examination of the lesion may give us suspicion of associated conditions or diseases; whether or not there is a triggering factor; new or recurrent lesion; pain or painless, length of time the lesion has been present; and rate of growth of the lesion over time. Neoplastic ulcerated lesions are notorious in the oral cavity for their ability to mimic benign ulcerative lesions, highlighting the essential nature of biopsy to establish a diagnosis in cases that are not clinically identifiable or do not respond as expected to treatment.[1] Additional physical evaluations, laboratory tests, or adjunctive tests may be required for final diagnosis. This article divulges a selection of the most common oral lesions providers are likely to encounter and the recommended pharmacologic management.

COMMON SOFT TISSUE ORAL LESIONS
Recurrent aphthous stomatitis

Aphthous lesions are one of the most common oral lesions, they can affect up to 25% of the general population. Three month recurrence rates are as high as 50% with a predilection for women. Although it is unclear what causes aphthous ulcers, factors such as trauma, nutritional deficiency, stress, tobacco, food hypersensitivity, hormonal changes, and drugs, can contribute to the disease.[2,3] These lesions can occur as a single, isolated event, or in groups of 2 or more that may reoccur at intervals.[4] In such cases, the condition is known as recurrent aphthous ulcers or recurrent aphthous stomatitis (RAS). The lesions emerge in 4 stages, in first stage or prodromal stage, the individual will experience tingling and burning in the normal-appearing site; during the second stage or preulcerative stage, red oval papules appear

Department of Oral and Maxillofacial Surgery, Woodhull Medical Center, 760 Broadway, Room 2C319, Brooklyn, NY 11206, USA
* Corresponding authors.
E-mail addresses: guillermo_puig@outlook.com (G.P.A.); ashley.lofters@gmail.com (A.L.)

Oral Maxillofacial Surg Clin N Am 34 (2022) 99–114
https://doi.org/10.1016/j.coms.2021.08.013
1042-3699/22/Published by Elsevier Inc.

that intensifies; in the third stage or ulcerative stage, classic ulcer appear. The 4 stages are the healing stage, in which granulation tissue followed by epithelialization occurs.[5]

Minor aphthae is the most common form of RAS and approximately 85% of patients have lesions of this type.[6] Minor aphthae are superficial mucosal ulcers with variable shape and size typically 4 to 5 mm diameter but less than 1 cm. Minor aphthae involve the nonkeratinized movable oral mucosa of the oral cavity (the labial and buccal mucosa (**Fig. 1**), the floor of the mouth and the ventral, or lateral surface of the tongue).[3] (**Fig. 2**) They tend to heal within a period of 10 to 14 days, at this stage, granulation tissue followed by epithelial migration and epithelial migration incurs in healing without a scar.[5]

Major aphthae have identical developmental stages in their general appearance except that are larger (exceeding 10 mm), deeper (extending to submucosal layers and underlying muscle at times), and longer lasting (can last up to 6 weeks).[5]

Herpetiform ulcerations are characterized by multiple recurrent small size ulcers from 2 to 3 mm in diameter. Multiple lesions may coalesce to form large irregular ulcers that last for about 10 to 14 days. These herpetiform ulcers, unlike herpetic lesions, are not preceded by vesicles and do not contain virally infected cells. Herpetiform aphthae are more common in women and have a later age of onset than other clinical variants.[2]

Treatment

The treatment of aphthous ulcers is palliative, the goal being to reduce the duration, size, and recurrence of lesions. Most individuals can endure minor levels of discomfort and are preferable to risking therapy with agents that can have potential side effects.[5]

First-line treatment options comprise antiseptics, such as chlorhexidine, antiinflammatory drugs, and analgesics for as long as the lesions persist.[7] A mixture often called magic mouthwash, which often consisting of diphenhydramine hydrochloride, viscous lidocaine, Kaopectate, and corticosteroids[8] may be useful in controlling the number, frequency, and duration of lesions. The patient is instructed to use 1 tsp at a time and swish, hold the solution in his or her mouth as long as possible, and swallow, three times daily.[5]

Topical steroids can decrease the symptoms and improve healing time, but do not affect the recurrence rate. If multiple lesions are present, an aqueous solution is preferred. A dexamethasone rinse can be considered or in isolated lesions, a high potency topical steroid (kenalog, clobetasol, or fluocinonide) for no more than 2 weeks[9,10] (**Table 1**). A trial with the antibiotic minocycline, which has immunomodulatory effects suppressing neutrophils, T lymphocytes, and collagenase activity, can be used. A blind crossover study shows a significant reduction in duration and severity of pain compared with placebo.[11]

In severe cases, whereby these regimens fail and the number, size, and discomfort of the lesions increases, and lesions, an injectable or systemic steroid, such as prednisone, are recommended. It is started at 1 mg/kg/d as a single dose in patients with severe lesions and tapered after 1 to 2 weeks. The recommendation is to use less than 50 mg per day, preferably in the morning, for 5 days.[9,12]

When managing patients with RAS, a thorough medical history and further work-up should be

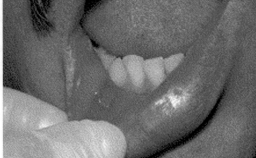

Fig. 1. Aphthous lesions in the mucosal surface of the lower lip. (*From* Saunders WB. Chapter 2: Ulcerative Conditions. In: Regezi JA, Sciubba JJ, Jordan RCK, eds. Oral Pathology. 6th ed. Elsevier; 2012: 22-78.)

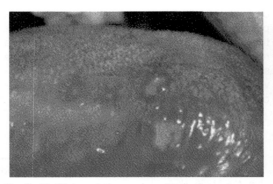

Fig. 2. Multiple aphthous ulcers in the lateral surface of tongue. (*From* Saunders WB. Chapter 2: Ulcerative Conditions. In: Regezi JA, Sciubba JJ, Jordan RCK, eds. Oral Pathology. 6th ed. Elsevier; 2012: 22-78.)

Table 1
Topical medications for the treatment of aphthous ulcers

Topical Medications for the Treatment of Aphthous Lesions	
Drugs	**Use**
Chlorhexidine 0.12%	5 mL swish and spit TID for 14 d
Dexamethasone 0.2%	5 mL swish and spit TID for 10 d
Kenalog 0.1%	Apply to affected areas TID for 10 d
Minocycline 0.5%	5 mL swish and spit QID for 10 d
Fluocinonide 0.05%	Apply ointment to affected areas TID for 10 d

conducted to rule out any systemic conditions associated with aphthous ulcers. Systemic conditions such as Behcet syndrome, hand-foot-and-mouth,[5] cyclic neutropenia, periodic fever with aphthae, pharyngitis and adenitis syndrome, Reiter syndrome, and Sweet syndrome, gluten-sensitive enteropathy, Crohn's disease, ulcerative colitis, and immune deficiencies, may all have oral manifestations; thus, need to be considered at the time of diagnosis.[12,13]

ORAL HERPES (HERPES SIMPLEX VIRUS)
Primary herpetic gingivostomatitis

Primary herpetic gingivostomatitis are caused by herpes simplex virus (HSV) and can be seen most commonly in children and young adults. Infection can be asymptomatic or can cause painful vesicular lesions on all mucosal surfaces and rupture and produce foul smell. Patients can become febrile and have significant malaise and tender cervical lymphadenopathy.[14] Lesions and acute illness can last from 5 to 10 days and resolve with scar formation. The clinical course is limited by the synthesis of viral-specific antibodies (IgM, days 3–5; IgG, days 5–21).[5] HSV gains access via direct or airborne water-droplet transmission. The lesions in mucosal membranes represent direct viral infection and the virus then ascends along the epineurium of the trigeminal nerve, establishing latency in the Gasserian ganglion, where it develops dormant existence within ganglion cell bodies (**Fig. 3**). It can become reactivated under various stimuli: stress, fever, ultraviolet light, trauma, or menstruation.[15]

Recurrent herpes infection

On reactivation of herpes lesions, the patient first experiences the prodromal symptoms of pain, itching, burning, or paresthesia.[16] Viral shedding occurs mostly during the time of active lesions and therefore, the time of greatest transmissibility. Recurrent secondary lesions may be more frequent and intense within the initial few years after primary infection and decrease in severity and increased intervals as time passes.[5]

Treatment

Herpes labialis is frequently occurring and self-limiting thus, many patients do not consult their general practitioners and use over-the-counter medication. Treatment with indifferent (zinc oxide and zinc sulfate), anesthetic, or antiviral cream has a small favorable effect on the duration of the symptoms, if applied promptly. A randomized controlled study with zinc oxide as a treatment showed that after 5 days, 50% of the patients in the treatment group were symptom-free compared with 35% in the placebo group.[17]

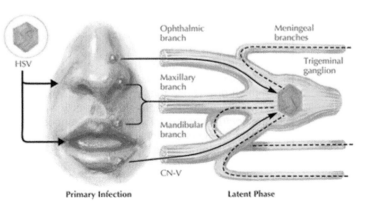

Primary Infection   Latent Phase

Fig. 3. Pathogenesis and clinical course of Herpes Simplex Virus. (*From* Traub M. Chapter 177: Herpes Simplex. In: Pizzorno JE, Murray MT, eds. Textbook of Natural Medicine. 5th ed. Churchill Livingstone/Elsevier; 2020: 1368–1371.e1.)

When using antiviral therapy, the aim is to block viral replication. Peak viral titers occur in the first 24 hours after lesion onset when most lesions reach the vesicular stage. Thus, for the treatment to be effective, it should be started at the first signs. Some topical agents include penciclovir 1% cream, acyclovir 5% cream, and docosanol cream. Penciclovir is inactive until it is phosphorylated within the virus, whereby it selectively inhibits herpes viral DNA synthesis and replication. Therefore, it has low toxicity and good selectivity.[18] Acyclovir 200 mg oral for 5 days can be started at first prodromal signs. Antivirals are used in primary and recurrent infections to decrease pain, viral shedding, and duration of symptoms. Prophylactic use of antivirals has proven useful in decreasing the frequency of recurrences, especially in immunocompromised patients and immunocompetent persons who experience frequent recurrences of oral or genital HSV infections[19] (**Table 2**).

For primary herpetic gingivostomatitis, the clinician might recommend only supportive care consisting of hydration, antipyretics, nutrition, and if secondary bacterial infections arise the use of antibiotics. However, severe cases may require systemic antiviral therapy.[5]

CANDIDIASIS

Oral candidiasis is caused by an overgrowth of the normally present organism *Candida albicans*. The infection is associated with alterations in the host's defense mechanisms. The incidence varies depending on age and certain predisposing factors. Some of the predisposing factors include impaired salivary gland function, drugs, dental prosthesis, high carbohydrate diet, and extremes of age, smoking, diabetes mellitus, Cushing's syndrome, malignancies, prolonged antibiotic use, and immunosuppressive conditions or agents

Table 2
Topical medications for the treatment of oral herpes lesions

Topical Medications for the Treatment of Oral Herpes	
Drugs	**Use**
Zinc Oxide 1% gel	Apply to affected area q 2 h for 5 d
Acyclovir 5% Ointment	Apply to affected area q 3–4 h for 4 d
Penciclovir 1%	Apply to affected area q 2 h for 4 d

Oral candidiasis can have multiple clinical presentations that vary greatly according to the predisposing factors.[20,21] Classifications of oral candidosis include Pseudomembranous form, hyperplastic form, and atrophic form. The symptoms of the acute form are rather mild and the patients may complain only of a slight tingling sensation or foul taste, whereas the severe chronic forms may involve the esophageal mucosa leading to dysphagia.[22,23]

Pseudomembranous candidiasis

Pseudomembranous candidiasis often referred to as *thrush*, can present as both acute and chronic forms. The affected mucosal surface becomes tender with red and white to whitish-yellow creamy plaques resembling milk curds or cottage cheese. These white plaques consist of cellular debris mixed with Candida organisms. The red areas correspond to the areas whereby organisms have invaded into the upper layers of the mucosa, resulting in parakeratinization, hyperemia, atrophy, and inflammation.[5] The white plaques or pseudomembrane characteristically can be easily removed, leaving behind an underlying erythematous and hemorrhagic area.[21] The oral surfaces frequently involved include labial and buccal mucosa, tongue, hard and soft palate, and oropharynx. The involvement of both oral and esophageal mucosa is prevalent in AIDS patients. Few lesions mimicking pseudomembranous, candidiasis could be white-coated tongue, thermal and chemical burns, lichenoid reactions, leukoplakia, secondary syphilis, and diphtheria.[24]

Atrophic (erythematous) candidiasis

Clinically, atrophic candidiasis manifests as a painful localized erythematous area. The chronic form usually involves the dorsum of the tongue, palate, and occasionally the buccal mucosa. Red lesions are seen on the dorsum of the tongue typically presenting as depapillated areas. Other forms of atrophic candidiasis includes *denture stomatitis, angular cheilitis,* and *median rhomboid glossitis* (**Fig. 4**).

Denture stomatitis, commonly known as "chronic atrophic candidiasis" is a chronic inflammation of mucosa that involves the denture area. Here the high-frequency, low-intensity trauma of the denture compressing the palatal mucosa alters the barrier mechanism allowing for the overgrowth of *candida* organisms.[5,25]

Angular cheilitis, also known as perleche, presents as erythematous or ulcerated fissures affecting the commissures of the lip unilaterally or bilaterally. This form is commonly associated

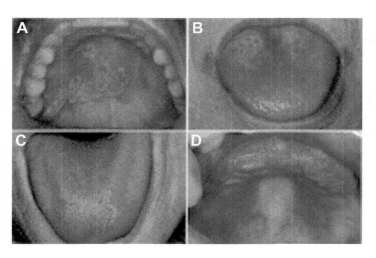

Fig. 4. Variations in clinical manifestation of oral candidiasis. (*A*). Thrush (pseudomembranous candidiasis). (*B*). Chronic erythematous candidiasis and angular cheilitis. (*C*). Chronic atrophic candidiasis. (*D*). *Candida*-associated denture stomatitis. (*From* Hu L, He C, Zhao C, Chen X, Hua H, Yan Z. Characterization of oral candidiasis and the Candida species profile in patients with oral mucosal diseases. Microb Pathog. 2019 Sep;134:103575.)

with patients with chronic lip-licking habit or loss of the occlusal vertical dimension. The constant moisture and cracking at the commissure and predispose the tissue to Candida proliferation and invasion.[5]

Median rhomboid glossitis appears as a well-demarcated, symmetric, depapillated area arising anterior to the circumvallate papillae typically located around the midline of the dorsum of the tongue. Although most cases are asymptomatic, some patients may report persistent pain, irritation, or pruritus. The lesion is believed to be a localized chronic infection by *C. albicans*. It is commonly seen in tobacco smokers and inhalation-steroid users.[26]

Hyperplastic candidiasis

Hyperplastic candidiasis also referred to as "candidal leukoplakia", mainly presented in chronic form. Clinically, it will present as a well-demarcated, raised lesion that may vary from small translucent whitish areas to large opaque plaques less likely to be scraped off. Unlike the pseudomembranous type, the hyperplastic type seems to have a positive association with immunosuppression, malnutrition, smoking, and in addition, may present with varying degrees of dysplasia.[27] The whitish lesion surface may often present localized erythematous areas.[28]

Treatment

Diagnosis of oral candidosis includes the physical examination of clinical signs and symptoms, presence of the candida organisms on the direct examination of a smear from the lesion or biopsy examination showing hyphae in the epithelium,

positive culture, and serologic test. The concern of non–candida albican candida species is a concern in certain mucosal lesions, oral cancer, and elderly hospitalized patients, this is due to NCAC species to be naturally resistant to some of the common antifungal drugs.[29]

When managing all forms of candidiasis, it is important to address any underlying factor when possible. Specific therapy for mild oral disease remains the standard nystatin oral suspension, 100,000 U/mL to be taken 5 mL (1 teaspoon) at a time as an oral swish and spit or swish and swallow 4 times daily. For chronic, candidiasis limited to the oral cavity and upper digestive tract, nystatin as noted above combined with clotrimazole troches, 10 mg five times daily, or the vaginal suppositories used as an oral troche three times daily, is very effective. In addition, the oral solution of itraconazole 10 mg/mL as 10-mL swish and swallow twice daily, is also effective, as is the oral solution of posaconazole 20 mg/mL as 5-mL swish and swallow twice daily (**Table 3**). Regular dental evaluation is recommended as the clotrimazole troches contain sugars that may stimulate active caries, especially in xerostomic patients. Patients with dentures can also benefit from sprinkling nystatin powder into their dentures twice a day, and those with angular cheilitis may also want to apply nystatin cream to the skin 4 times a day.[5]

For patients with refractory candidiasis, mucocutaneous candidiasis, women with concurrent candida vaginitis, or patients in whom compliance is a problem, a systemic antifungal therapy with ketoconazole or fluconazole 200 mg first day, followed by 100 mg daily for 2 weeks is recommended.[30,31]

Table 3
Topical medications for the treatment of oral candidiasis

Drugs	Use
Nystatin Suspension 100,000 IU/mL	5 mL swish and spit for 14 d
Clotrimazole Troche 10 mg	Dissolve in 10 mL and swish and swallow BID for 14 d
Nystatin-Triamcinolone Acetonide 15g	Apply to corners of mouth after meals and at bedtime for 14 d

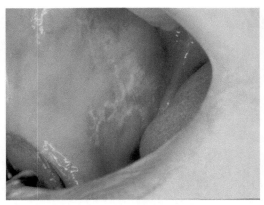

Fig. 5. Classical clinical presentation of reticular oral lichen planus in a 42-year-old asymptomatic woman. The lesions occurred bilaterally on the buccal mucosa. The disease was discovered during a routine dental examination, and the disease duration was estimated to be about 1 year. (*From* Chainani-Wu N, Silverman S Jr, Lozada-Nur F, Mayer P, Watson JJ. Oral lichen planus: patient profile, disease progression and treatment responses. J Am Dent Assoc. 2001 Jul;132(7):901-9.)

AUTOIMMUNE VESICULOBULLOUS AND ULCERATIVE DISEASES

Lichen planus (LP), the spectrum of pemphigus, pemphigoid, and lupus erythematosus are a gamut of autoimmune vesiculobullous and ulcerative diseases which are responsible for an onslaught of oral soft tissue lesions which affect the entire mucosa. It would behoove all practitioners to be well versed in recognizing and treating these lesions as they can prove to be difficult to differentiate. For that reason, it is imperative that the provider biopsy lesions when an autoimmune process is suspected. When selecting a site for biopsy, the target site should be a clinically involved area with an intact surface and some adjacent normal-appearing tissue.[5]

Lichen planus

LP is a mucocutaneous disease that manifests as a result of a delayed T cell-mediated hypersensitivity whereby the basal layer of skin and/or mucosa is attacked.[5] This disease corporealizes as one of the 3 clinical forms which have a global prevalence of ~0.1–2.2% and tend to present in patients older than 40 with a predilection for women.[32,33] All forms have a predilection for the buccal mucosa, tongue, and buccal surface of the attached gingiva. In order of advancing severity and symptomatology, LP has a reticular, plaque, and erosive form.

The reticular form (**Fig. 5**) is most notably characterized by the pathognomonic Wickham's striae which are lacy, white, interlacing lines found mostly on the characteristic sites of the posterior bilateral buccal mucosa, attached gingiva, and tongue.[34] The aforementioned striae are usually asymptomatic; they wax and wane over a period of weeks to months while assuming a limited rather than disseminated territory of oral mucosa.[5]

The plaque form is characterized by a slightly elevated, homogenous hyperkeratotic white patch with irregular borders that closely resemble leukoplakia. These patches are usually asymptomatic and present on the characteristic sites (bilateral buccal mucosa, attached gingiva, tongue). Rarely, this form may be associated with some discomfort. Given the striking resemblance to leukoplakia, the biopsy of this form is required to differentiate from premalignant or malignant mucosal changes. Differential diagnosis includes nonspecific benign hyperkeratosis, a spectrum of epithelial dysplasias, verrucous hyperplasia, verrucous carcinoma, invasive squamous cell carcinoma, or hypertrophic candidiasis.[5,35]

Erosive lichen planus (ELP) is the most severe in symptomatology and presentation. It is characterized by intense pain and erythematous mucosal inflammation. When involving the buccal mucosa or tongue, lesions present as fibrinous based ulcers in an atrophic erythematous background with occasional white, hyperkeratotic foci and borders of fine, white radiating striae. If involving the attached gingiva, presentation is often a boggy, red, and friable tissue that bleeds easily (**Fig. 6**). This reaction pattern is known as desquamative gingivitis.[34] If the erosive component is severe, the basal layer is compromised by the immune cells resulting in vesicle formation with a positive Nikolsky sign. This is a particularly rare presentation known as bullous LP.[5,34] These lesions must undergo biopsy. Differential diagnosis includes

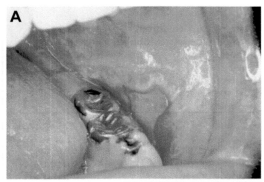

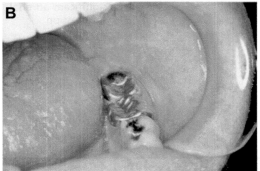

Fig. 6. (*A*) Painful, erosive oral lichen planus, or OLP, of the left buccal mucosa in an otherwise healthy 60-year-old man. He had no other complaints or findings, and the results of a recent physical examination were within normal limits. The gold crowns were placed after the OLP appeared, because the dentist thought that the lesion might have been due to some old molar amalgam restorations, although this was unlikely. (*B*). Daily doses of prednisone (60 mg) for 1 week led to complete remission. After 1 month, the disease recurred, but was controlled indefinitely with topical corticosteroid treatment. (*From Chainani-Wu N, Silverman S Jr, Lozada-Nur F, Mayer P, Watson JJ. Oral lichen planus: patient profile, disease progression and treatment responses. J Am Dent Assoc. 2001 Jul;132(7):901-9.*)

lupus erythematosus, chronic ulcerative stomatitis, dysplasia, squamous cell carcinoma, and pemphigoid. ELP may progress to squamous cell carcinoma in approximately 2% to 3% of cases as a function of disease duration (15 years or more).[5,34]

Treatment

Treatment for the reticular and plaque forms is reassurance and follow-up.[5,34] In some cases, patients may have superimposed candidiasis and complain of a burning sensation in the mouth. These instances necessitate treatment with antifungal therapy such as miconazole gel or chlorhexidine mouthwash rinses.[34,36] Some authors

have suggested topical retinoids (isotretinoin 0.1%) and other vitamin A analogs (etretinate, 0.05% tretinoin, retinoic acid in orabase 0.05%, tazarotene 0.1%); however, almost all reticular LP is asymptomatic and nonprogressive; additionally, almost all striae return if the drug is discontinued. Common side effects of topical retinoids include transient burning sensation and taste abnormalities. Typically, improvement in lesion presentation is noticeable after 3 weeks.[37] Dapsone has also been effective for mild cases of LP involving skin. If used, the patient's serum should be tested for the presence of glucose-6-phosphate dehydrogenase because dapsone may precipitate a G6PD-deficiency hemolytic episode. Dapsone can be given in a dose of 50 mg per day and may be continued for several weeks.[5]

Milder forms of erosive LP can be treated with topical corticosteroids, usually 0.05% clobetasol propionate gel, 0.1%–0.05% betamethasone valerate gel, 0.05% clobetasol ointment or cream, 0.1% triamcinolone acetonide ointment in orabase or lozenge, or 0.05% fluocinonide gel (Lidex gel) 4 times daily.[38] Fluocinonide gel may be combined with antifungal agent griseofulvin 250 mg twice daily. Efficacy of the agent is related to the side effect of promoting epithelial differentiation and maturity. Topical 0.1% tacrolimus cream (Protopic) also may be used.

Resistant or extensive lesions may be treated 2 to 4 times weekly with intralesional subcutaneous injections of 0.2–0.4 mL of a 10 mg/mL solution of triamcinolone acetonide by means of a 1.0 mL 23 or 25 gauge tuberculin syringe.[39]

Most severe erosive LP are resistant to topical and intralesional approaches and require systemic corticosteroids, prednisone is typically the drug of choice given as recommended by Regimen I or II or less commonly IIIA or IIIB (**Tables 4–7**).[5] Oral griseofulvin, topical 0.05% fluocinonide, or 0.1% protopic can be added to either regimen to reduce the prednisone requirements or help maintain a remission. In refractory cases, systemic tacrolimus or rituximab can be effective.[5]

It is imperative to educate patients on the side effects of prolonged corticosteroid use (sodium and water retention, hypertension, hypernatremia/hypokalemia, hyperglycemia, infections including iatrogenic candidiasis, mood changes, increased risk for peptic ulcer disease, muscle wasting/fat deposit, delayed wound healing, osteoporosis, cataracts, and increased risk for cancer). Complete treatment at low doses of prednisone (5–10 mg every other day) may be extended for up to 3 years.[5] A milder, residual clinical disease usually persists. Consequently, a drug-free total

Table 4
Systemic corticosteroid regimen I for autoimmune vesiculobullous and ulcerative diseases

Systemic Corticosteroid Regimen I	Rationale
Prednisone 100–120 mg qd (1.5 mg/kg/d) x 2 wk	Objective: Gain rapid suppression with an initial high loading dose
A tapering schedule reduces prednisone by 20 mg per day each week over several weeks until a dose of 20 mg/d is reached. This dose is continued for 1 month followed by 10 mg per day for 3 mo.	Objective: taper off dose rapidly enough to avoid serious side effects of high dose prednisone
Dose reduced to 10 mg every other day for 3 mo followed by 5 mg every other day for 6 mo	Tapered dose extended in length to avoid exacerbation at the time of dose reduction or after drug discontinuation
After 6 mo, a 5 mg dose of prednisone every other day, the drug may be discontinued a high possibility of an extended remission in a drug-free state.	Designed to permit the hypophyseal-adrenal cortical axis to regain its function

Data from Marx RE, Stern D. Oral and Maxillofacial Pathology: A Rationale for Diagnosis and Treatment. 2nd ed. Quintessence Publishing. 2012; 200.

remission is less common than a maintenance-control remission. Often, the disease can be suppressed with prednisone to a point at which topical fluocinonide and/or griseofulvin can maintain remission without continued prednisone or with only a low, every other day prednisone schedule. Any ELP that does not respond to therapy, especially prednisone, should be viewed with suspicion for malignant transformation to squamous cell carcinoma.[5]

Pemphigus vulgaris

Pemphigus vulgaris is a potentially fatal painful autoimmune mucocutaneous disease that

Table 5
Systemic corticosteroid regimen II for autoimmune vesiculobullous and ulcerative diseases

Systemic Corticosteroid Regimen II	Rationale
Prednisone 100–120 mg qd (1.5 mg/kg/d) x 2 wk, drug then abruptly discontinued	Objective: Gain rapid suppression with initial dose and discontinue before side effects or significant adrenal suppression develop Advantage: approach is effective and straightforward Disadvantage: exacerbations are more frequent, disease process is less controlled

Data from Marx RE, Stern D. Oral and Maxillofacial Pathology: A Rationale for Diagnosis and Treatment. 2nd ed. Quintessence Publishing. 2012; 200.

Table 6
Systemic corticosteroid regimen IIIA for autoimmune vesiculobullous and ulcerative diseases

Systemic Corticosteroid Regimen IIIA	Rationale
Prednisone 100–120 mg qd (1.5 mg/kg/d) × 2 wk	Objective: Gain rapid suppression with an initial high loading dose
A tapering schedule reduces prednisone by 20 mg per day each week over several weeks until a prednisone level is reached without exacerbating the disease. T	Many individuals remain on 20 mg/d or higher doses due to disease exacerbation with lower doses Appropriate for cases of disease intensity and organ involvement that lower doses of prednisone cannot control

Data from Marx RE, Stern D. Oral and Maxillofacial Pathology: A Rationale for Diagnosis and Treatment. 2nd ed. Quintessence Publishing. 2012; 200.

Table 7
Systemic corticosteroid regimen IIIB for autoimmune vesiculobullous and ulcerative diseases

Systemic Corticosteroid Regimen IIIB	Rationale
Prednisone 100–120 mg qd (1.5 mg/kg/d) × 2 wk	Objective: Gain rapid suppression with initial high loading dose
A tapering schedule reduces prednisone by 20 mg per day each week over several weeks until a prednisone level is reached at which the disease is exacerbated. This and slightly higher prednisone levels may still be associated with disease activity ergo other immunoregulatory drugs (cyclophosphamide, azathioprine, methotrexate, mycophenolate, rituximab, infliximab) are added	Objective: Attack disease with double or triple drug therapy in order to reduce drug dosage and side effects. Reserved for refractory cases and persons in whom corticosteroid complications pose a greater risk (diabetics, history of tuberculosis, peptic ulcer disease, cataracts, osteoporosis).
Dose reduced to 10 mg every other day for 3 mo followed by 5 mg every other day for 6 mo	Tapered dose extended in length to avoid exacerbation at the time of dose reduction or after drug discontinuation
After 6 mo, a 5 mg dose of prednisone every other day, the drug may be discontinued a high possibility of an extended remission in a drug-free state.	Designed to permit the hypophyseal–adrenal cortical axis to regain its function

Data from Marx RE, Stern D. Oral and Maxillofacial Pathology: A Rationale for Diagnosis and Treatment. 2nd ed. Quintessence Publishing. 2012; 200.

manifests as a result of a B-cell mediated process whereby autoantibodies develop against the epidermal cell surface glycoproteins desmoglein 1 and 3 or against desmoglein 3 only. Desmogleins are components of desmosomes, the structures which bond squamous epithelial cells together.[5,34] The consequence is a cascade of events that results in the destructive fixation of complement followed by a bout of inflammation which causes a suprabasilar split and intraepithelial blisters (**Fig. 7**). Ultimately, individual squamous cells lose their desmosomal attachment and become rounded polygonal acantholytic cells known as *Tzanck* cells.[5,34]

The clinical ramification of this process is the formation of a fragile vesicle that is superficial in nature and thus rapidly ruptures (**Fig. 8**). Exposed is a basal layer that is in close proximity to free nerve endings whereby fixation of complement initiates inflammation and pain. Oral lesions form on all mucosal surfaces and may exhibit a Nikolsky sign. Individuals may present with irritability due to pain, fever from secondary infection, dehydration, and cervical lymphadenitis from secondary

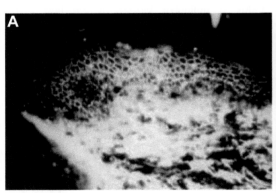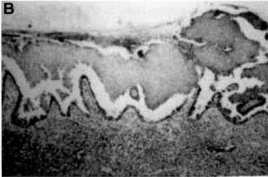

Fig. 7. (*A*). Direct immunofluorescent staining (immunoglobulin G) revealing pemphigus vulgaris antigen distribution in the oral epithelium. Note the "spider-web" distribution of reaction product in the spaces between squamous epithelial cells (obtained from perilesional biopsy specimen containing intact epithelium). (*B*). Hematoxylin-and-eosin–stained section revealing acantholysis, mononuclear infiltrate, and suprabasilar separation. (*From* Sirois D, Leigh JE, Sollecito TP. Oral pemphigus vulgaris preceding cutaneous lesions: recognition and diagnosis. J Am Dent Assoc. 2000 Aug;131(8):1156-60.)

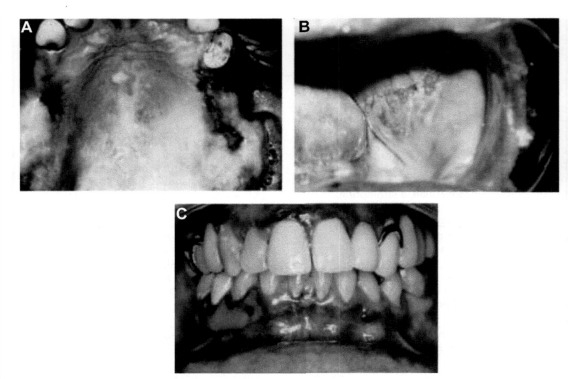

Fig. 8. A. variety of clinical presentations of oral pemphigus vulgaris, which generally appears in the form of shallow, irregular nonspecific ulcers. (*A*). The palate. (*B*). The buccal mucosa. (*C*). The gingivae. (*From* Sirois D, Leigh JE, Sollecito TP. Oral pemphigus vulgaris preceding cutaneous lesions: recognition and diagnosis. J Am Dent Assoc. 2000 Aug;131(8):1156-60.)

infections of numerous oral ulcers. This primarily affects individuals in their fourth to sixth decade, blacks, south Asian, and those of Ashkenazic Jewish descent. The estimated incidence is 1 to 5 cases per million people diagnosed each year. These lesions have the notoriety of "first to show, last to go" as the oral lesions are the first sign of the disease and are the most difficult to treat.[5,34]

Skin lesions are more likely to show vesicles or even bullae due to increased thickness of skin epithelium and keratin layer as compared with mucosa. The lesion will frequently form on otherwise normal-appearing skin which subsequently becomes inflamed and then ruptures leaving a denuded surface. Ocular involvement is rare and is manifested as bilateral conjunctivitis without any incidence of scarring and symblepharon formation (**Fig. 9**).[5,34]

Treatment

As mentioned previously, individuals will often present with dehydration secondary to poor oral intake and frequently with a secondary infection. Therefore, appropriate initial management includes starting hydration with intravenous fluids,

beginning antibiotic therapy, and pain control measures. Lesions should be biopsied in the interim and direct immunofluorescent studies will demonstrate intercellular deposition of IgG.[40] Pemphigus is a systemic disease, therefore, this disease responds well to systemic corticosteroids. Initiation of corticosteroid therapy should not preclude a definitive biopsy. If the first biopsy

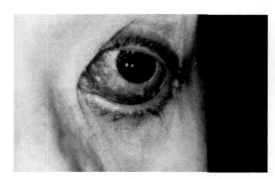

Fig. 9. Corneal erosion due to pemphigus vulgaris. (*From* Sirois D, Leigh JE, Sollecito TP. Oral pemphigus vulgaris preceding cutaneous lesions: recognition and diagnosis. J Am Dent Assoc. 2000 Aug;131(8):1156-60.)

specimen is nondiagnostic, a second biopsy would have an altered tissue response which will obscure diagnosis and complicate treatment.[5,34]

The accepted treatment is with high doses of systemic steroids (prednisone 1–2 mg/kg/d). Once the disease is under control, prednisone can be reduced to the lowest possible maintenance levels.[40] About a small percentage of cases respond incompletely to and require the addition of rituximab 375 mg/m² of the body surface, cyclophosphamide 50–100 mg po twice daily or azathioprine 50 to 100 mg twice daily to reduce corticosteroid doses and mortality from the side effects of systemic corticosteroids. If refractory, methotrexate 25 mg per week may be substituted for azathioprine or rituximab. Plasmapheresis may also be used as an adjunctive method to reduce corticosteroid dosage. Isolated oral lesions may be treated with injectable corticosteroids.[5,34]

If untreated, pemphigus vulgaris is fatal in 2 to 5 years. Treatment of cutaneous pemphigus results in a residual 10% to 15% mortality rate at 15 years because of complications from long-term prednisone therapy and other immunosuppressive drugs. The most common cause of death is *Staphylococcus aureus* septicemia which is often difficult to detect because of immunosuppression caused by concomitant corticosteroid therapy.[5,34]

Paraneoplastic pemphigus

Paraneoplastic pemphigus is a severe variant of pemphigus vulgaris that represents a heralding sign of an undiscovered or uncontrolled malignancy. The most frequent culprits are Hodgkin's lymphoma, non–Hodgkin's lymphoma, chronic lymphocytic leukemia, and thymoma.[5,34,40] One may expect to see the rapid onset of numerous painful lesions on oral mucosa, skin, conjunctiva, and progressive pulmonary involvement in up to 40% of patients. Lesions may resemble a lichenoid drug reaction, erythema multiforme, LP, or pemphigus clinically and histologically. Unfortunately, despite steroid and/or immunosuppressive therapy, the disease course is rapidly progressive over weeks to months and is often fatal. The oral lesions most commonly manifest as large erosive lesions covering the lips, tongue, and soft palate.[5,34,40] To date there are no definitive diagnostic criteria, but the most accepted conditions include painful, progressive stomatitis with preferential involvement of the tongue, identification of circulating antibodies to envoplakin or periplakin and the presence of a neoplasm.[5] The gold standard for diagnosis is immunoprecipitation.

Treatment

A combination of prednisone and immunosuppressive drug therapy may be used to help control the severity of the skin lesions, but the oral, conjunctival, and pulmonary diseases are frequently resistant to treatment.

Pemphigoid group

This is a group of B-cell-mediated autoimmune diseases that characteristically form vesicles and bullae in the skin and mucous membranes. There are classically 2 subtypes of the pemphigoid group: bullous (cutaneous) pemphigoid and mucous membrane (cicatricial) pemphigoid. In cases of overlapping clinical presentations, patients may present with skin, oral mucosa, ocular mucosa, and other mucous membrane involvement.[5] Direct immunofluorescence will show a homogenous band of IgG in the basement membrane zone as well as C3.[5] With the advent of specific direct immunofluorescent markers, it has been made clear that the presentation of cutaneous and mucous membrane pemphigoid is due to autoantibodies to at least 3 different molecules in the lamina lucida region of the basement membrane and on the hemidesmosomes of epithelial basal cells.[5,40]

Bullous pemphigoid (BP) is the most commonly occurring in the pemphigoid group, it usually presents in the 6th decade and greater with an equal affliction for both sexes.[40] BP usually emerges on the skin (scalp, axilla, arms, legs, groin) with the oral mucous membranes involved ~30% of the time. When compared with pemphigus vulgaris, the oral lesions of BP are smaller, less extensive, less painful, and form more slowly. Desquamative gingivitis has been reported to be the most common and often the only oral presentation of BP.[40] BP occurs as a result of the production of autoantibodies (IgG) against 2 proteins (BPAG1 and BPAG2) in the basal cell-basement membrane zone junction and the basement membrane proper. When the IgG type autoantibodies attack the BPAG1 and BPAG2, the antibody–antigen complex fix complement and initiate a series of steps which lead to the degradation of the basement membrane at the lamina lucida level. This generates pain by the formation of bradykinin, kallikrein, and substance P.[5] As a result, the separation occurs within the basement membrane zone and the skin lesions formed are characteristically large bullae (3–15 cm in diameter) which are tense, erythematous, pruritic, and painful. The disease process usually waxes and wanes with periods of remission over a period of 2 to 3 years with the disease usually subsiding into remission or mild symptomatology after 5 to 6 years.

Mucous membrane (cicatricial) pemphigoid is chronic and typically has a predilection for the oral and ocular mucosa with the skin involved ~ 20% of the time and with lesser severity.[5] This disease is often seen in individuals in their fifth decade and occurs twice as frequently in women. The lesions initially blister, ulcerate, and then form scars due to the deeper subepithelial location.[40] The oral mucosa and ocular conjunctiva are most commonly affected in order of decreasing frequency. Oral lesions are most commonly a bright red desquamative gingivitis (**Fig. 10**).[40] When the conjunctiva is involved, if not treated, there is a high incidence of the development of scarring and adhesions between the bulbar and palpebral conjunctiva known as symblepharon. This may progress to corneal damage and blindness in 15% of the affected population.[40] Laryngeal involvement may result in pain, hoarseness, difficulty breathing; esophageal involvement may cause dysphagia which may lead to debilitation and death in severe cases.[40]

Treatment

The treatment of choice for mild or localized oral lesions is a high potency topical corticosteroids or intralesional corticosteroids such as 0.05% clobetasol in orabase, 0.1% triamcinolone acetonide, 0.05% fluocinonide, or betamethasone applied 3 to 4 times daily for 9 to 24 weeks[40,41] If there is no response to topical therapy alone or if the patient cannot tolerate corticosteroids, a regimen of tetracycline, or erythromycin 500 mg twice daily alone or combined with nicotinamide 500 mg twice

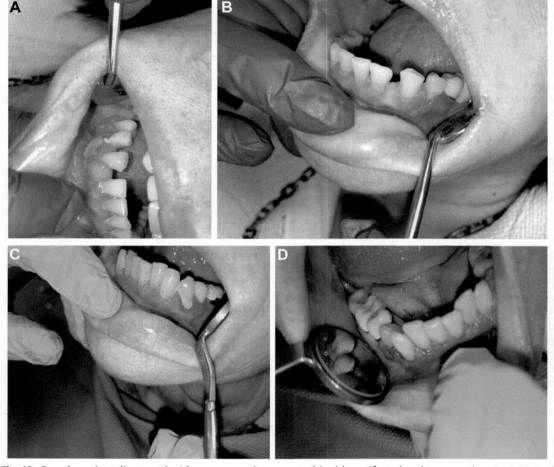

Fig. 10. Female patient diagnosed with mucus membrane pemphigoid manifested as desquamative gingivitis and buccal mucosal ulcerations. (*A*) Grey ulcerative lesion with erythematous borders on the buccal attached gingiva. (*B-D*) Generalized tender, erythematous, sloughed buccal attached gingiva representing desquamative gingivitis. (*Courtesy of* Scott M Peters, New York, NY.)

Table 8
Alternative drugs to corticosteroid therapy for treating immune-based diseases

Drug	Mechanism of Action	Dose
Cyclophosphamide (Cytoxan, Bristol-Myers Squibb)	Biotransformed principally in the liver to active alkylating metabolites by a mixed-function microsomal oxidase system. These metabolites interfere with the growth of susceptible rapidly proliferating malignant cells. The mechanism of action is thought to involve cross-linking of tumor cell DNA.	IV: 40–50 mg/kg given in divided doses over 2–5 d (when used alone in a patient without hematologic deficiency); or 10–15 mg/kg every 7–10 d or 3–5 mg/kg twice weekly Oral: 1–5 mg/kg/d
Tacrolimus	Inhibits T-lymphocyte activation, although the exact mechanism of action is not known.	0.1 mg/kg per day for 1 mo, then reevaluate
Methotrexate	Inhibits dihydrofolic acid reductase, interferes with DNA synthesis, repair, and cellular replication. Actively proliferating tissues such as malignant cells, bone marrow, fetal cells, buccal and intestinal mucosa, and cells of the urinary bladder are in general more sensitive to this effect of methotrexate.	Immune-based disorders: Starting dose of 10 mg/m2 once weekly, followed by 7.5–10 mg weekly; doses may be adjusted by no more than 30 mg/wk to achieve optimal clinical response
Etanercept (Enbrel, Amgen)	Binds specifically to tumor necrosis factor (TNF), a naturally occurring cytokine involved in normal inflammatory and immune responses, and blocks its interaction with cell surface TNF receptors.	50 mg given as one subcutaneous injection using a single-use, prefilled syringe or autoinjector; may also be given as two 25-mg injections
Rituximab (Rituxan, Genentech)	Binds specifically to the antigen CD20. The Fab domain of rituximab binds to the CD20 antigen on B lymphocytes, and the Fc domain recruits immune effector functions to mediate B-cell lysis in vitro. Possible mechanisms of cell lysis include complement-dependent cytotoxicity (CDC) and antibody-dependent cell-mediated cytotoxicity (ADCC). The antibody has been shown to induce apoptosis in the DHL-4 human B-cell lymphoma line.	First infusion: 50 mg/h, but may be increased by 50 mg/h every 30 min (max 400 mg/h) if no toxicity Subsequent infusions: 100 mg/h, but may be increased by 100 mg/h every 30 min (max 400 mg/h) if no toxicity

(continued on next page)

Table 8 (continued)		
Drug	**Mechanism of Action**	**Dose**
Azathioprine (Imuran, Azasan)	Inhibits purine synthesis which results in decreased production of DNA and RNA for the synthesis of white blood cells, thus causing immunosuppression	Oral: 1–2 mg/kg/d
Mycophenolate Mofetil	Exhibits a cytostatic effect on B and T lymphocytes by means of inhibiting inosine monophosphate dehydrogenase which in turn inhibits de novo guanosine nucleotide synthesis, a pathway needed by B and T lymphocytes for proliferation.	Oral: 750 mg - 1 g twice daily

Data from Marx RE, Stern D. Oral and Maxillofacial Pathology: A Rationale for Diagnosis and Treatment. 2nd ed. Quintessence Publishing. 2012; 200.

daily may slowly and gradually decrease the disease activity. In severe cases, systemic corticosteroids (prednisone 1–2 mg/kg/d) alone or combined with adjuvant immunosuppressive agents such as azathioprine, cyclophosphamide or mycophenolate may be beneficial (**Table 8**).[5,40,42] Treatment often reduces symptoms, alleviates large bullae formation induces, and/or hastens remission.[5]

Lupus erythematosus

Lupus erythematosus is an immunologically mediated condition with 3 clinical forms: systemic, chronic cutaneous, and subacute cutaneous. Systemic lupus erythematosus (SLE) is a multisystem disease whereby there is a combination of increased activity in B lymphocytes and abnormal function of T lymphocytes which in conjunction result in a variety of cutaneous and oral presentations. Chronic cutaneous lupus erythematosus (CCLE) is a different but related process that primarily affects the skin and oral mucosa, those afflicted face a good prognosis. Subacute cutaneous lupus erythematosus (SCLE) has clinical features which are intermediate between that of SLE and CCLE.[34]

SLE affects women ~8 to 10 times more frequently than men and is often diagnosed in the third decade of life. SLE initially is nonspecific with patients presenting with constitutional symptoms of fever, weight loss, malaise, fatigue, and arthritis with periods of remission or disease inactivity. 40% to 50% of affected patients have a characteristic butterfly patterned rash over the malar area and nose with sparing of the nasolabial folds. Renal and cardiac involvement is a common complication. Oral lesions develop in 5%–40% and tend to affect the palate, buccal mucosa, and gingiva. Lesions may have a lichenoid, nonspecific, or granulomatous appearance in addition to varying degrees of ulceration, pain, erythema, and hyperkeratosis.[34]

Individuals with CCLE are usually spared from systemic signs or symptoms with a disease course limited to lesions appearing on skin or mucosa. Skin lesions are termed discoid lupus erythematosus (DLE)—this describes the scaly, erythematous patches usually distributed on sun-exposed skin with a concentration in the head and neck area. DLE lesions are often exacerbated by sun exposure. Lesions are notorious for healing in one area spontaneously and then appearing in another. The healing process results in cutaneous atrophy and hypo- or hyperpigmentation and scarring. Oral manifestations of CCLE seem clinically identical to that of ELP (painful, ulcerated or atrophic erythematous central zone surrounded by fine, white radiating striae) (**Fig. 11**). However, unlike ELP, CCLE oral lesions seldom occur in the absence of skin lesions.[34]

The disease course of SCLE is characterized by prominent, photosensitive skin lesions which do not show the induration and scarring that is seen with CCLE. The systemic manifestations are usually limited to arthritis or musculoskeletal abnormalities. SCLE is typically triggered by one of a variety of medications.[34]

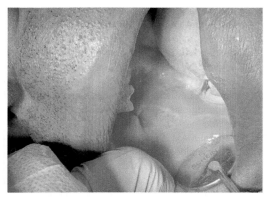

Fig. 11. CCLE oral lesion on the buccal mucosa. (*Courtesy of* Scott M Peters, New York, NY.)

Treatment

Patients should be counseled to avoid sunlight as this may precipitate and exacerbate disease activity. A mild disease course can be effectively managed with a combination of nonsteroidal anti-inflammatory drugs (NSAIDs) and antimalarial drugs such as hydroxychloroquine. More severe episodes, including those with oral presentations, are effectively managed with systemic steroids. Topical steroids appropriately manage CCLE lesions. Potent topical steroids such as clobetasol propionate gel 0.05%, betamethasone dipropionate 0.05%, or fluticasone propionate spray 50 mg aqueous solution are usually required. The treatment may begin with applications 2 to 3 times a day followed by a tapering during the next 6 to 9 weeks. Lesions resistant to topical steroids may be managed with systemic antimalarial drugs or low-dose thalidomide.[34] The overall objective is to use a minimum of steroids to obtain relief.

From this article, one can appreciate that soft tissue lesions commonly seen in the oral cavity tend to overlap in their onset, presentation, and location making it difficult to appreciate whether the etiology is inflammatory, immunologic, traumatic, infectious, or neoplastic. This may be overwhelming to the practitioner with an untrained eye who is not typically exposed to such diseases. Furthermore, as one can imagine, the patient who suffers from such lesions requires not only reassurance, but also appropriate management as these lesions may be detrimental physically and emotionally. As such, this article serves as an important resource for the medical and dental professional to understand these lesions, their management, and the necessity of obtaining a thorough history and physical to guide making a correct diagnosis. Many of these soft tissue lesions can be managed effectively with similar pharmacotherapy regimens; however,

many drugs have serious side effects ergo it is imperative that if not pathognomonic, lesions are biopsied to confirm a suspected diagnosis before instituting the suggested treatment. Furthermore, if managed inappropriately, some lesions may progress in a manner that may worsen morbidity or/and mortality.

CLINICS CARE POINTS

- Always obtain a detailed medical history, allergies, drug reactions or other medications contraindications before starting the treatment.
- Monitor and document therapeutic treatment doses, progress, and adjust pharmacologic treatment if necessary.
- In the management of viral or immune-related diseases, set proper expectations before commencing any pharmacologic treatment.
- Close follow-up and biopsy should be considered in nonresolving suspicious mucosal lesions.

DISCLOSURE

The authors have nothing to disclose.

REFERENCES

1. Fitzpatrick SG, Cohen DM, Clark AN. Ulcerated lesions of the oral mucosa: clinical and histologic review. Head Neck Pathol 2019;13(1):91–102.
2. Preeti L, Magesh K, Rajkumar K, et al. Recurrent aphthous stomatitis. J Oral Maxillofac Pathol 2011; 15(3):252–6.
3. Tarakji B, Gazal G, Al-Maweri SA, et al. Guideline for the diagnosis and treatment of recurrent aphthous stomatitis for dental practitioners. J Int Oral Health 2015;7(5):74–80.
4. Porter SR, Hegarty A, Kaliakatsou F, et al. Recurrent aphthous stomatitis. Clin Dermatol 2000;18:569–78.
5. Marx, Robert E. and Stern, Diane, 2012. Oral and maxillofacial pathology: a rationale for diagnosis and treatment, second edition.
6. Rogers RS 3rd. Recurrent aphthous stomatitis: clinical characteristics and associated systemic disorders. Semin Cutan Med Surg 1997;16(4):278–83.
7. Belenguer-Guallar I, Jiminez-Soriano Y, Claramunt-Lozano A. Treatment of recurrent aphtous stomatitis. A literature review. J Clin Exp Dent 2014;6(2): 168–74.

8. Chan A, Ignoffo RJ. Survey of topical oral solutions for the treatment of chemo-induced oral mucositis. J Oncol Pharm Pract 2005;11(4):139–43.

9. Scully C, Gorsky M, Lozada-Nur F. The diagnosis and management of recurrent aphthous stomatitis. A consensus approach. J Am Dent Assoc 2003; 134:200–7.

10. Ship J, Arbor A. Recurrent aphtous stomatitis [review]. Oral Surg Oral Med Oral Pathol 1996;80(2):141–7.

11. Gorsky M, Epstein J, Raviv A, et al. Topical minocycline for managing symptoms of recurrent aphthous stomatitis. Spec Care Dentist 2008;28:27–31.

12. Stanley HR. Aphthous lesions. Oral Surg Oral Med Oral Pathol 1972;33(3):407–16.

13. Healy CM, Thornhill MH. An association between recurrent oro-genital ulceration and non-steroidal anti-inflammatory drugs. J Oral Pathol Med 1995;24:46–8.

14. Messadi DV, Younai F. Aphtous ulcers. Dermatol Ther 2010;23:281–90.

15. Cunningham A, Griffiths P, Leone P, et al. Current management and recommendations for access to antiviral therapy of herpes labialis [review]. J Clin Virol 2012;53:6–11.

16. Fatahzadeh M, Schwartz RA. Human herpes simplex virus infections: epidemiology, pathogenesis, symptomatology, diagnosis, and management. J Am Acad Dermatol 2007;57:737–63.

17. National Center for Biotechnology Information. PubChem Compound Summary for CID 135398748, Penciclovir. Available at: https://pubchem.ncbi.nlm.nih.gov/compound/Penciclovir. Accessed April 24, 2021.

18. Opstelten W, Neven AK, Eekhof J. Treatment and prevention of herpes labialis. Can Fam Physician 2008;54(12):1683–7.

19. Leflore S, Anderson PL, Fletcher CV. A risk-benefit evaluation of aciclovir for the treatment and prophylaxis of herpes simplex virus infections. Drug Saf 2000;23(2):131–42.

20. Patil S, Rao RS, Majumdar B, et al. Clinical appearance of oral candida infection and therapeutic strategies. Front Microbiol 2015;6:1391.

21. Akpan A, Morgan. Roral candidiasis. Postgrad Med J 2002;78:455–9.

22. Farah CS, Lynch N, McCullough MJ. Oral fungal infections: an update for the general practitioner. Aust Dent J 2010;55(Suppl 1):48–54.

23. Axéll T, Samaranayake LP, Reichart PA, et al. A proposal for reclassification of oral candidosis. Oral Surg Oral Med Oral Pathol Oral Radiol Endod 1997;84(2):111–2.

24. Lalla RV, Patton LL, Dongari-Bagtzoglou A. Oral candidiasis: pathogenesis, clinical presentation, diagnosis and treatment strategies. J Calif Dent Assoc 2013;41(4):263–8.

25. Dodd CL, Greenspan D, Katz MH, et al. Oral candidiasis in HIV infection: pseudomembranous and erythematous candidiasis show similar rates of progression to AIDS. AIDS 1991;5(11):1339–43.

26. Aun MV, Ribeiro MR, Costa Garcia CL, et al. Esophageal candidiasis–an adverse effect of inhaled corticosteroids therapy. J Asthma 2009;46(4):399–401.

27. Williams D, Lewis M. Pathogenesis and treatment of oral candidosis. J Oral Microbiol 2011;35771. https://doi.org/10.3402/jom.v3i0.5771.

28. Sitheeque MAM, Samaranayake LP. Chronic hyperplastic candidosis/candidiasis (Candidal Leukoplakia). Crit Rev Oral Biol Med 2003;14(4):253–67.

29. Gutiérrez J, Morales P, González MA, et al. Candida dubliniensis, a new fungal pathogen. J Basic Microbiol 2002;42(3):207–27.

30. Muzyka BC. Update on fungal infections. Dent Clin North Am 2013;57:561–81.

31. Stoopler E, Sollecito T. Recurrent gingival and oral mucosal lesions. JAMA 2014;312(17):1794–5.

32. Parashar P. Oral lichen planus. Otolaryngol Clin North Am 2011;44:89–107.

33. McCartan BE, Healy CM. The reported prevalence of oral lichen planus: a review and critique. J Oral Pathol Med 2008;37:447–53.

34. Neville BW, Damm DD, Allen CM, et al. Oral and maxillofacial pathology. Philadelphia: Saunders Elsevier; 2016.

35. Brown RS, Bottomley WK, Puente E, et al. A retrospective evaluation of 193 patients with oral lichen planus. J Oral Path Med 1993;22:69–72.

36. Carbone M, Conrotto D, Carrozzo M, et al. Topical corticosteroids in association with miconazole and chlorhexidine in the long-term management of atrophic-erosive oral lichen planus: a placebo-controlled and comparative study between clobetasol and fluocinonide. Oral Dis 1999;5:44–9.

37. Petruzzi M, Alberta L, Carlo L, et al. Topical retinoids in oral lichen planus treatment: an overview, 226. Basel, Switzerland: Dermatology; 2013. https://doi.org/10.1159/000346750.

38. Levin C, Maibach HI. Topical corticosteroid-induced adrenocortical insufficiency: clinical implications. Am J Clin Dermatol 2002;3:141–7.

39. Edwards PC, Kelsch R. Oral lichen planus: clinical presentation and management. JCD 2002;68:494–9.

40. Greenberg MS, Glick M, Ship JA, et al. Burket's oral medicine diagnosis and treatment. Hamilton: BC Decker Inc; 2003.

41. Mehdipour M, Taghavi Zenouz A. Role of corticosteroids in oral lesions, state of the art of therapeutic endocrinology, sameh magdeldin, intechopen, DOI: 10.5772/50287. 2012. Available at: https://www.intechopen.com/books/state-of-the-art-of-therapeutic-endocrinology/role-of-corticosteroids-in-oral-lesions. Accessed June 28, 2021.

42. Mondino BJ, Brown SI. Ocular cicatricial pemphigoid. Ophthalmology 1981;88:95–100.

Update on Management of the Oral and Maxillofacial Surgery Patient on Corticosteroids

Michael H. Chan, DDS[a,b],*

KEYWORDS

- Corticosteroids • Adrenal suppression • Dental extractions • Dental implants • Osteoporosis
- Osteonecrosis • Perioperative "stress steroids" dose

KEY POINTS

- Corticosteroids have beneficial therapeutic properties but it also has a wide range of adverse clinical side effects.
- Most clinicians consider 3 weeks of continuous use of 20 mg of prednisone or its equivalent or higher to cause tertiary adrenal insufficiency and this phenomenon will likely cease after 12 months of drug discontinuation.
- Good perioperative pain control, especially during the postoperative phase, is crucial to decrease cortisol demand.
- High-quality randomized control trials are needed to determine if perioperative "stress dose" steroid is necessary for minor, moderate, and major surgeries.

INTRODUCTION

Corticosteroids have been used to treat a variety of anti-inflammatory and immunosuppression conditions such as arthritis (juvenile idiopathic arthritis, psoriatic arthritis, rheumatoid arthritis), polymyalgia rheumatica, autoimmune disease (ie, systemic lupus erythematosus, giant cell arteritis), chronic obstructive pulmonary disease (COPD)/asthma, dermatologic lesions, inflammatory bowel disease, oral mucocutaneous lesions, adjunctive chemotherapy regimen, and organ transplant recipients. It is estimated that 1.2% of the US population is on chronic steroids.[1] With an aging population, OMFS clinicians will likely encounter these patients in their daily practice. Currently, physicians have been reconditioned to prescribe the lowest dose and the shortest course for targeted therapy to avoid numerous undesirable side effects, but unfortunately, some patients may require a lifelong treatment regimen. The purpose of this article is to highlight some of the current adrenal insufficiency classifications, significant drug-to-drug interactions, adverse effects, and current perioperative recommendations for patients taking long-term corticosteroids suffering from these chronic ailments.

PATHOPHYSIOLOGY AND EFFECTS ON THE HYPOTHALAMUS-PITUITARY-ADRENAL AXIS

Daily endogenous cortisol production by the adrenal gland is approximately 8 to 10 mg/d[2] or 20 mg/d[3] with a higher output in the morning than in the evening. Cortisol helps regulate a variety of normal physiologic functions in response to stress. It

---

[a] Oral & Maxillofacial Surgery, Department of Veterans Affairs, New York Harbor Healthcare System (Brooklyn Campus), 800 Poly Place (Bk-160), Brooklyn, NY 11209, USA; [b] Oral & Maxillofacial Surgery, Department of Oral and Maxillofacial Surgery, The Brooklyn Hospital Center, 121 DeKalb Avenue (Box-187), Brooklyn, NY 11201, USA
* 800 Poly Place (Bk-160), Brooklyn, NY 11209.
E-mail address: chanoms@yahoo.com

Oral Maxillofacial Surg Clin N Am 34 (2022) 115–126
https://doi.org/10.1016/j.coms.2021.08.011
1042-3699/22/© 2021 Elsevier Inc. All rights reserved.

provides anti-inflammatory properties by suppressing prostaglandin production. Impairment of chemotaxis and adequate immune cellular recruitment in particular polymorphonucleocytes and leukocytes, respectively. Hyperglycemia results from gluconeogenesis by the liver and the dysfunction of insulin's ability to reuptake serum blood glucose into adipose tissue.[4] Enhancement of the cardiovascular system through catecholamine stimulation resulting in increased cardiac output and blood pressure.[2] Promotion of osteoclasts and prevention of osteoblasts function on bone remodeling.[4]

All 3 forms of adrenal insufficiencies can result in a net decrease in cortisol production. Secondary adrenal insufficiency is related to the inability of the anterior pituitary to produce adrenocorticotropic hormone (ACTH) due to the pituitary gland's dysfunction (ie, tumor, irradiation, surgery, and genetic alterations), whereas tertiary adrenal insufficiency reflects the lack of corticotropin-releasing hormone, and/or arginine vasopressin released by the hypothalamus with chronic steroid administration being the most common etiology.[5] One of vasopressin's roles is to promote vasoconstriction in response to low blood pressure when sensed by the host's baroreceptors.[6] Daily consumption of corticosteroids will trigger a negative feedback mechanism aimed to "halt" the body's natural cortisol production. Currently, most clinicians consider 3 weeks of continuous use of 20 mg of prednisone per day or its equivalent or higher to cause tertiary adrenal insufficiency and this phenomenon will likely cease after 12 months of drug discontinuation.[4,7]

Patients with primary adrenal insufficiency (Addison's disease), however, lack the inability of the adrenal gland to produce 3 major hormones: mineralocorticoid (aldosterone), glucocorticoids (cortisol), and androgens (dehydroepiandrosterone) predominantly from autoimmune disease when a significant amount of the adrenal gland has been destroyed. Mineralocorticoid deficiency causes hyponatremia, hyperkalemia, and low intravascular volume (blood pressure). In a healthy individual, aldosterone normally stimulates the reabsorption of sodium and water and excretion of potassium at the distal and collecting tubules to help increase blood pressure via the renin-angiotensin-aldosterone-system. Cortisol's availability is also devoid of its essential properties which are to maintain cardiac output and increase vascular tone to catecholamine during a stressful response. An inadequate amount of these functioning hormones could result in adrenal crisis—a rare condition with potential for fatal outcome with vasodilation and severe hypotension with eventual cardiovascular collapse[2,3,5] (**Fig. 1**).

MEDICATION DOSAGES

Prednisone is the most commonly prescribed corticosteroid on the market.[8] Relative potency of 5 mg of prednisone is equivalent to 20 mg of hydrocortisone corresponding to the daily endogenous production. Dexamethasone is 25 times more potent than cortisol and only requires 0.75 mg to have the same equivalency or approximately 4 mg = 100 mg of hydrocortisone (**Table 1**).[3] Inhalation preparation is commonly prescribed for asthmatics and COPD patients with recommended adult dosing in metered-dose inhaler preparation provided (**Table 2**).[9]

ADVERSE REACTION/EVENTS OF CORTICOSTEROIDS

There is no Black Box Warning Label associated with corticosteroids.

Glucocorticoids and Nonsteroidal Anti-Inflammatory Drugs

The combination will increase the risk for gastrointestinal (GI) issues (ie, peptic ulcers and GI bleed). Two separate meta-analyses have demonstrated the adverse effects when these 2 drugs are used together. One study showed 4 times relative increased risk with the combination of glucocorticoids and nonsteroidal anti-inflammatory drugs (NSAIDs) when compared to nonusers.[10] Similarly, a second analysis showed a 3 times relative increased risk when this combination is used when compared to nonusers. It also demonstrated an odds ratio of 1.8 when compared to NASIDs user group suggesting approximately twice the relative risk.[11]

Glucocorticoids and Inducers of Cytochrome-450 (CYP3A4)

These inducers of CYP (ie, barbiturate, phenobarbital, phenytoin, carbamazepine, rifampicin, and troglitazone) increase the breakdown of cortisol and therefore will have decreased levels of circulating cortisol. If permissible by physician, these drugs should be discontinued 24 hours before surgery.[3,5]

Glucocorticoids and Inhibitors of Cytochrome-450 (CYP3A4)

The inhibitors of CYP such as the antifungal class of azole (ie, fluconazole and ketoconazole) and antiviral class (ie, ritonavir) decrease the breakdown of cortisol and therefore will have increased levels of circulating cortisol.[5,12]

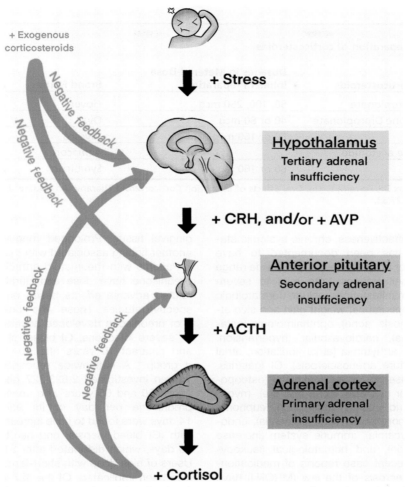

Fig. 1. Hypothalamus-pituitary-adrenal (HPA) axis. The most common cause for tertiary adrenal insufficiency is from chronic exogenous steroids use. This will trigger a negative feedback mechanism to the hypothalamus and anterior pituitary gland creating a shut down in "natural" cortisol production. Secondary adrenal insufficiency reflects the pituitary gland's dysfunction to produce ACTH to stimulate the adrenal gland to make cortisol. While primary adrenal insufficiency is a result of damage from the adrenal gland itself to produce cortisol. Stress is the major trigger for activating the HPA axis. ACTH, adrenocorticotropic hormone; AVP, arginine vasopressin; CRH, corticotropin-releasing hormone.

Table 1
The relative potency of corticosteroids

Name of Drug	Anti-Inflammatory Potency	Mineralocorticoid Potency	Equivalent Dose (mg)	Duration of Action
Cortisol	1	2	20	Short acting < 12 h
Hydrocortisone	0.8	2	20	Short acting < 12 h
Prednisone	4	1	5	Intermediate acting 12–36 h
Prednisolone	4	1	5	Intermediate acting 12–36 h
Triamcinolone	5	0	4	Intermediate acting 12–36 h
Methylprednisolone	5	0.5	4	Intermediate acting 12–36 h
Dexamethasone	25	0	0.75	Long acting > 36 h

Adapted from Little JW, Miller CS, Rhodus NL. Chapter 15: Adrenal Insufficiency. In: Little JW, Miller CS, Rhodus NL, eds. Little and Falace's Dental Management of the Medically Compromised Patient. 9th ed. Elsevier; 2018: 255-267.

Table 2
Inhalation preparation of corticosteroids

Inhalation Corticosteroids	Dosages in Metered-Dose Inhaler Preparation	Brand Names	Adult Dosing
Fluticasone propionate	50, 100, 250 mcg	Flovent	2 puffs BID
Becalometasone Dipropionate	40 or 80 mcg	Qvar	1–4 puffs BID
Ciclesonide	80 or 160 mcg	Alvesco	1–2 puffs BID
Triamcinolone acetonide		Azmacort	
Budesonide	80 or 160 mg	Symbicort	2 puffs BID

Adapted from Cox DP, Ferreira L. The Oral Effects of Inhalation Corticosteroid Therapy: An Update. J Calif Dent Assoc. 2017 May;45(5):227-33.

Despite its effectiveness, chronic systemic steroid therapy has been documented to have numerous major adverse events and a wide range of clinical manifestations from mild to severe forms. These manifestations include dermatologic (cushingoid appearance, weight gain and skin atrophy, ecchymosis, acne), ophthalmologic (cataract, glaucoma), cardiovascular (hypertension, fluid retention, arrhythmia [atrial fibrillation, atrial flutter], premature arteriosclerosis), GI (gastritis, peptic ulcer disease), musculoskeletal (osteoporosis, avascular necrosis, bone fracture), myopathy, psychiatric (mania, depression, euphoria, akathisia, memory impairment, dementia), endocrine (hyperglycemia), immune system (increase risk of infection), and hematological (leukocytosis).[4] Also, recent case reports of medication-related osteonecrosis of the jaw (MRONJ) have been documented.

Chronic inhaled corticosteroids have been shown to induce several intraoral adverse effects such as oral candidiasis, oral hairy leukoplakia, angina bulla hemorrhagic, and Churg-Strauss syndrome with oral candidiasis being the most common finding. The direct local effects of corticosteroids to the oropharyngeal region are from over suppression leading to overgrowth of *Candida albicans* and the condition is fully reversible upon discontinuation of the drug. For those who are reliant on this therapy, oral water rinses after each use and/or attaching a spacer for these inhalers could significantly reduce these occurrences. If needed, nystatin and fluconazole can be prescribed to treat these fungal infections. Angina bullosa hemorrhage are blood-filled lesions with soft palate being the most common site and are self-limiting within 1 weeks with rupture noted within 48 hours of onset. Churg-Strauss syndrome is a rare inflammatory condition of the blood vessels. Patients with a history of asthma or allergies may display intraoral findings commonly seen as "strawberry gingivitis" secondary to inflamed gingival tissue. Prolonged tongue ulceration is another finding associated with this syndrome.[9]

Patients with rheumatoid arthritis on daily oral prednisone have dose and duration-dependent related adverse effects based on several retrospective studies. Those who took 5 to 10 mg/d of prednisone developed adverse effects such as severe infections, GI bleed, skeletal fracture, and cataract 10 years after the 10 to 15 mg/d group.[4] A nationwide retrospective study in Taiwan investigated 2,623,327 people aged between 20 and 65 years who consumed 5 mg of prednisone per day or its equivalent within 14 days were found to have increased association with (GI bleed, sepsis, and heart failure) within 30 days, which dissipated after 31 to 90 days.[13] Users of high dose with short-term duration have also been implicated. Of the 327,452 adults surveyed in the study for the under 65-year-old group, approximately 47% of these patients developed (sepsis, venous thromboembolism, and fractures) within 30 days only after a 6-day course of medrol-dose pack (105 mg of prednisone equivalent).[4]

Glucocorticoid-induced osteoporosis (GIOP) and osteonecrosis has been well-documented in medical literature in the past decade but not within the dental community.[14,15] Specifically, vertebral and hip fractures are directly linked with chronic prednisone users with onset noted as early as 3 months. Excess corticosteroids cause decreased osteoblast production by blocking the Wingless (Wnt)/B-catenin signaling pathway along with osteoblast apoptosis resulting from an increased level of reactive oxygen species. Simultaneously, glucocorticoid exerts a direct effect on osteoblast to increase production of receptor activator of nuclear factor kappa-B (ligand) RANKL available for RANK binding on preosteoclasts cells. Upon forming an RANKL/RANK complex, the osteoclast will differentiate and develop into mature osteoclasts ready for bone resorption.

Additionally, osteoblast decreases the secretion of osteoprotegerin (OPG) making it less available to bind with RANKL further tipping the scale toward bone resorption. Lastly, osteocyte's apoptosis is enhanced thus altering normal bony remodeling resulting in poorer bone quality and increased risk for fracture despite maintaining bone mineral density (BMD) values. The net effect is less bone formation (decrease quantity of osteoblasts, osteocytes, and OPG), more bone resorption (increased osteoclast's action), decreased

vascular endothelial growth factor (less VEGF) resulting in osteoporosis or osteonecrosis bony architecture[14,15] (**Fig. 2**).

As mentioned previously, 2 case reports of MRONJ associated with chronic steroid therapy both resulted from an extraction of a single mandibular premolar. Wong and colleagues reported a 30-year-old female who took prednisone 5 mg and 7.5 mg on alternative days for systemic lupus erythematosus (SLE) for the past 9 years (e-mail communication with the author). Although

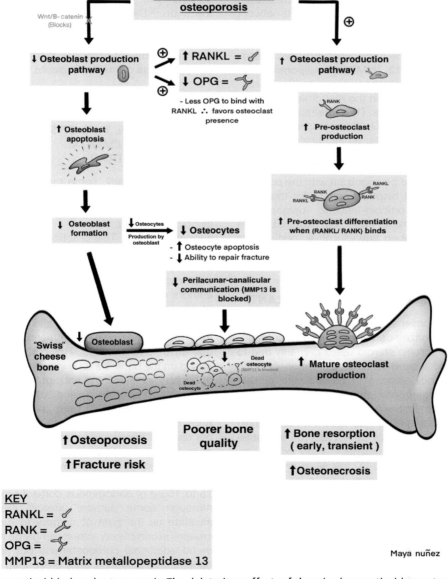

Fig. 2. Glucocorticoid-induced osteoporosis. The deleterious effects of chronic glucocorticoid on osteoblast, osteocytes, and osteoclast with their impact on bone remodeling.

this patient took oral bisphosphonate 2 years after her sequestrectomy was performed from her lower jaw, it was to counteract the osteoporosis diagnosed on her hip which subsequently required a femoral head prosthesis replacement. In this case, BP acted as an adjunctive medication to cause MRONJ.[16] A second case involved a 50-year-old male with a history of psoriatic arthritis on 7.5 mg of prednisone per day for the past 2 years. His mandible was treated with surgical debridement for localized sclerotic bone with complete resolution observed after 30 days.[17]

Recent animal studies on the mandible have demonstrated excess glucocorticoids caused a significant alteration to the osteocyte orchestrated perilacunar-canalicular remodeling (PLR) network within 2 months to incite MRONJ. Osteocyte's cell-to-cell signaling is significantly altered specifically by blocking the perilacunar enzymes (matrix metallopeptidase 13 [MMP13]) responsible for maintenance of normal bony turnover. The disruption of the PLR results in the mandible having the following manifestations: (1) decreased bone volume, (2) decreased BMD, (3) decreased trabecular (marrow) bone thickness, (4) increased incidence of jaw fracture posterior to the molar site, and (5) decreased vascularity[18] (see **Fig. 2**).

Clinicians should be cognizant with the potential concurrent use of bisphosphonate for the treatment of glucocorticoid-induced osteoporosis (GIOP). Alendronate and denosumab are commonly prescribed antiresorptive medications proven to prevent further deterioration of bone loss and prevent skeletal fractures.[14]

CORTICOSTEROIDS AND DENTAL IMPLANTS

The general consensus among the dental community has categorized dental implants as a contraindication for chronic steroid users primarily due to the impaired wound healing, disruption of bone formation, and increase in osteoclastic activity creating an osteoporotic environment.[19,20] However, a recent retrospective study by Petsinis and colleagues in 2017 has shown an osseointegration success rate of 99% (103/104 implants) up to 3 years for 31 patients.[21] Daily corticosteroids ranging from 5 to 60 mg were reported in this group of patients being used to treat various autoimmune disease conditions. Petsinis concluded traditional 2-stage implant surgery without bone grafting could be performed for chronic glucocorticoid users but highlights the importance of future investigation of implant success is warranted.[21] Yet another systematic review with meta-analysis revealed a positive implant survival rate of 100% with a follow-up

period from 4 to 13 years.[22] A variety of autoimmune diseases encompassed this successful group which included Sjogren's syndrome, SLE, polymyalgia rheumatica, scleroderma, and pemphigus vulgaris.[22] He calculated an 88.75% overall implant survival rate for this group (n = 100) being able to be followed for more than 24 months with an average duration of 72.6 months.[22] Furthermore, rheumatoid arthritis patients recorded 92.9% and 100% survival based on 236 implants in 56 patients from 1 prospective and 3 retrospective studies, respectively. Finally, organ transplant recipients on immunosuppressants and chronic steroids had a 100% survival rate up to approximately 4 years of follow-up.[22] Despite these promising data, Duttenhoefer concluded that risk stratification and more randomized control studies are needed to ascertain the validity of immunosuppressants and the clinical effects on dental implants.[22]

PERIOPERATIVE MANAGEMENT OF THE OMFS PATIENT ON CORTICOSTEROIDS (DOSE AND DURATION, TYPE OF SURGERY, AND STEROID SUPPLEMENTAL RECOMMENDATION)

Historically and still, some current surgeons are conditioned to give perioperative "stress dose" steroids for patients with a history of adrenal insufficiency and/or on chronic steroid supplementation. This practice was widely adopted primarily based on 2 historical case reports in the 1950s of adrenal crisis resulting in a fatal outcome.[23,24] Within the past two decades, some authors questioned these guidelines and started to extrapolate data from anesthesia and surgery literature, mainly case series and cohort studies, to formulate their own recommendations for perioperative "stress dose." These formulations are based on the patient's daily intake and the amount necessary to match the anticipated perioperative requirement or the degree of hypothalamus-pituitary-adrenal (HPA) axis suppression. The body normally produces 10 to 20 mg of cortisol per day and this would represent the "physiologic dose." However, patients undergoing minor surgery will require "supra-physiological doses" of 50 mg/d and moderate and major groups needing 75 to 150/d of endogenous cortisol production.[25] Although some authors' steroid requirements escalate as the type of surgery to be done increases in complexity, others simply do not recommend additional corticosteroids but rather have patients maintain their daily prescribed dose. The lack of general consensus for exogenous steroid supplementation guidelines is the reason for various published recommendations ultimately leaving the shared decision between the surgeon and anesthesiologist.

Liu and colleagues' recommendation is based on the risks group stratification (dose and duration) and the anticipated amount of endogenous cortisol needed to respond to the type of surgery performed.[2] The low-risk group for adrenal suppression (those who use steroids <3 weeks and on 5 mg of prednisone per day or less, or prednisone 10 mg every other day) would not require additional supplementation or ACTH stimulation test. However, the intermediate (5–20 mg) and high-risk groups may benefit from the ACTH stimulation test using cosyntropin (ACTH 1–24). High-risk group is defined as (>3 weeks of 20 mg prednisone/day [equal or greater] or with clinical signs of Cushing syndrome). Cushing syndrome is a result of corticosteroid toxicity resulting in numerous undesirable adverse effects mentioned previously (ie, weight gain, round face, etc) with chronic daily use being the most common cause. 250 mcg of cosyntropin either intramuscular (IM)/intravenously (IV) is administered and measurements are taken postinjection at 60 minutes. Normal values of 18 mcg/dL or higher suggest adequate production and therefore no additional stress steroids are needed.[2,26]

Liu and colleagues also categorized 4 types of surgery based on anticipated stress of surgery: (1) routine/superficial, (2) minor, (3) moderate, and (4) major. As dentoalveolar surgery is regarded as "routine" and 8 to 10 mg of cortisol production is expected, continuation of the daily dose without additional further supplementation is suggested. However, patients undergoing minor to major surgery should take their normal daily dose in addition to supplemental hydrocortisone because of the increased demand for physiologic glucocorticoids (**Table 3**).[2]

Hamrahian and colleagues' findings in the most recent UpToDate are very similar to Liu and colleagues' recommendations (**Table 4**). They added long-term use of inhaled and topical corticosteroids can suppress the HPA axis but generally without the same degree of clinical adrenal insufficiency when compared to the oral/parenteral version. They recommended clinical evaluation and ACTH stimulation testing for those who use inhaled, topical preparations, and intraarticular injections with the following parameters:[12]

1. More than or equal to 750 mcg (0.75 mg/d) of daily fluticasone or 1500 mcg (1.5 mg/d) with either beclomethasone, triamcinolone, or budesonide) for more than 3 weeks before surgery.[12,27] This suggests fluticasone is twice as potent.

2. More than or equal to 2 g/d of high potency or super high potency of corticosteroids (class I–III) for more than 3 weeks before surgery.
3. Any individual who has signs of Cushing syndrome.
4. Those who had 3 or more intraarticular or spinal injections within 3 months or have signs of Cushing should be clinically evaluated and tested.

Chilkoti and colleagues proposed a slightly higher threshold for his supplementation regimen. Patients taking more than 10 mg/d prednisone for the last 3 months should be considered adrenally suppressed with supplementation dosage based on surgery type. Minor surgery would only require an additional 25 mg of hydrocortisone during induction, whereas moderate surgery would need an extra 100 mg of hydrocortisone/day for 24 hours and extended up to 72 hours with major surgery (**Table 5**).[25] By supplementing and maintaining a serum level of 100 mg of daily hydrocortisone, the body should be able to withstand succumbing to hemodynamic instability (vasodilation and hypotension) even at critical levels[25].

Little and Falace suggested that secondary or tertiary adrenal insufficiency group do not require additional supplemental steroids regardless of dosage and length of steroid use or type of surgery to be done unless patients have other comorbidities (ie, cancer, infection, trauma, liver dysfunction, and significant pain; **Table 6**). Moreover, additional steroid requirements should be based on the overall health of the patient and the demand required by the body during the perioperative recovery period. Authors also proposed surgical procedures more than 1 hour should be considered as major because of the increased stress and cortisol demand. If the OMFS clinician is still unsure, a physician consultation with ACTH stimulation test may be warranted.[3] Their recommendation was based on a systematic review by Marki and Varon who analyzed 9 studies and found no additional supplementation of steroids was necessary independent of the type of surgery and only recommended a normal daily dose to be taken.[28]

Finally, the latest systemic review performed by Groleau and colleagues in 2018, examined 2 randomized control trials (37 patients), 5 cohort studies (462 patients), and 4 systematic reviews. Despite these low-quality studies and limited evidence, he concluded that the above literature have shown maintenance of daily dose of steroid therapy should meet the cortisol demand in many surgical scenarios. Furthermore, there is no need for perioperative supplementation of exogenous corticosteroids and the use of additional steroids

Table 3
Liu et al's procedure-based stratification for stress dose steroid recommendation

Surgery Type	Endogenous Cortisol Secretion Rate	Examples	Recommended Steroid Dosing
Superficial	8–10 mg/d (baseline)	Dental surgery Biopsy	Usual daily dose
Minor	50 mg/d	Inguinal hernia repair Colonoscopy Uterine curettage Hand surgery	Usual daily dose *plus* Hydrocortisone 50 mg IV before incision Hydrocortisone 25 mg IV every 8 h × 24 h Then usual daily dose
Moderate	75–150 mg/d	Lower extremity revascularization Total joint replacement Cholecystectomy Colon resection Abdominal hysterectomy	Usual daily dose *plus* Hydrocortisone 50 mg IV before incision Hydrocortisone 25 mg IV every 8 h × 24 h Then usual daily dose
Major	75–150 mg/d	Esophagectomy Total proctocolectomy Major cardiac/vascular Hepaticojejunostomy Delivery Trauma	Usual daily dose *plus* Hydrocortisone 100 mg IV before incision Followed by continuous IV infusion of 200 mg of hydrocortisone more than 24 h *or* Hydrocortisone 50 mg IV every 8 h × 24 h Taper dose by half per day until usual daily dose reached *plus* Continuous IV fluids with 5% dextrose and 0.2%–0.45% NaCl (based on degree of hypoglycemia)

Abbreviation: IV, intravenous.
   Data from Axelrod.[4] Salem *et al.*,[13] and Bornstem et al.[6]; and *From* Liu MM, Reidy AB, Saatee S, Collard CD. Perioperative Steroid Management: Approaches Based on Current Evidence. Anesthesiology. 2017 Jul;127(1):166-172.

should be weighed against the adverse effects of the drug during the postoperative course. Lastly, Grouleau recommended high-quality randomized control trials are needed in the future on this topic so a general consensus can be reached.[30]

ANESTHESIA MANAGEMENT

There are no anesthetic technique restrictions for adrenal insufficiency patients except for the use of etomidate (inhibitor of glucocorticoids production). However, OMFS clinicians should be cognizant of the fact that general anesthesia, anxiolytics, and analgesics are also known suppressors of cortisol production. A double-blinded randomized clinical trial has demonstrated the use of 7.5 mg of sublingual midazolam to reduce surgical stress of healthy ASA I patients undergoing wisdom teeth removal. Through saliva collection, they were able to determine plasma cortisol of the control group to be higher than the test group suggesting good sedative effects of midazolam. In addition, he reported cardiovascular stability and mild transient respiratory depression associated with this technique.[31]

All patients under anesthesia should have their vital signs monitored (blood pressure [BP], heart rate [HR], respiration rate [RR], oxygen saturation

Table 4
Hamrahian et al.'s risk stratification for stress dose steroid recommendation

	Dose, Time of day, and Duration	Stress Dose Supplementation Recommendation
Low risk (nonsuppressed HPA axis)	<5 mg/d of prednisone (or equivalent) taken in the AM; or <10 mg of prednisone (or equivalent) every other day	Normal daily dose
Intermediate risk (unknown HPA axis suppression)	5–20 mg/d of prednisone >3 wk (or equivalent); or 5 mg/d of prednisone taken in the PM	Clinical evaluation for Cushing & ACTH stimulation test. If necessary, supplement according to anticipated level of stress of surgery
High risk (suppressed HPA axis)	20 mg of prednisone per day (equivalent) or more >3 wk; or clinical signs of Cushing syndrome	Supplement with steroids according to anticipated level of stress of surgery
History of corticosteroid use in the past year (no evidence to support)	<5 mg/d of prednisone <3 wk (or equivalent) within 6–12 mo	No clinical evaluation or testing required
History of corticosteroid use in the past year (no evidence to support)	>5 mg/d of prednisone >3 wk (or equivalent) within 6–12 mo	Clinical evaluation for Cushing & ACTH stimulation test. If necessary, supplement according to anticipated level of stress of surgery
Inhaled corticosteroids[27]	More than or equal to 750 mcg of daily of fluticasone or (1500 mcg with beclomethasone, triamcinolone, or budesonide) >3 wk before surgery; or signs of Cushing	Clinical evaluation for Cushing & ACTH stimulation test. If necessary, supplement according to anticipated level of stress of surgery
Topical corticosteroids	More than or equal to 2 g/d of high potency corticosteroids (class I–III) >3 wk before surgery; or signs of Cushing	Clinical evaluation for Cushing & ACTH stimulation test. If necessary, supplement according to anticipated level of stress of surgery
Intraarticular and spinal glucocorticoids injection	3 or more intraarticular or spinal injections within 3 mo of surgery; or signs of Cushing	Clinical evaluation for Cushing & ACTH stimulation test. If necessary, supplement according to anticipated level of stress of surgery

Data from Hamrahian AH, Roman S, Milan S. Perioperative glucocorticoids - Uptodate. Walters Kluwer; Feb 2021.

[O_2 sat], and end-tidal carbon dioxide [$ETCO_2$]) with close attention paid to fluid and blood loss. Recognition of adrenal crisis can be challenging while patients are under sedation since altered mental status can be one of the signs of crisis. Although it is a diagnosis out of exclusion, a sudden drop in BP should alert the clinician to be suspicious especially when treatment is refractory to fluid and vasopressor challenge. Immediate steroid supplementation is necessary to prevent mortality.

Good postoperative analgesia either through PO/IM/IV route or long-acting local anesthesia (ie, bupivacaine) should help diminish the host's response to cortisol demand[3]. Interestingly, the highest demand for cortisol is actually during the postoperative phase (ie, during extubation and postoperative recovery).[12] Sustained high levels of plasma cortisol are found even 7 hours after dentoalveolar surgery, indicating increased demand in the postoperative phase mainly in response to pain.[32,33]

Table 5
Chilkoti et al's procedural-based stress dose steroid recommendation

	Patients On Daily Prednisone >10 mg/d or Equivalent in the Last 3 mo (Perioperative Steroid Recommendation)
Minor Surgery (Hernia, Hand Surgery)	25 mg of hydrocortisone at induction
Moderate Surgery (Hysterectomy)	Usual daily dose + 25 mg of hydrocortisone at induction + 100 mg of hydrocortisone for 24 h
Severe Surgery (Major Trauma, Prolonged Surgery)	Usual daily dose + 25 mg of hydrocortisone at induction + 100 mg of hydrocortisone per day up to 72 h

Data from Chilkoti GT, Singh A, Mohta M, Saxena AK. Perioperative "stress dose" of corticosteroid: Pharmacological and clinical perspective. J Anaesthesiol Clin Pharmacol. 2019 Apr-Jun;35(2):147-152.

MANAGEMENT OF ADRENAL CRISIS

Early recognition and treatment of adrenal crisis can prevent morbidity and mortality. Initial management consists of hypotension support, steroid supplementation, and correction of electrolytes.

SIGNS AND SYMPTOMS OF ADRENAL CRISIS[12,25]

1. Hypotension
2. Hypoglycemia
3. Dehydration
4. Nausea/Vomiting
5. Abdominal pain (awake patient)
6. Altered mental status (awake patient)

Table 6
Little and Falace et al's procedural based for stress dose steroid recommendation

	Primary Adrenal Insufficiency (Perioperative Steroid Recommendation)[29]	Secondary & Tertiary Adrenal Insufficiency (Perioperative Steroid Recommendation)[28]
Routine Dentistry	None	None
Minor Surgery	25 mg of hydrocortisone (or equivalent) preoperative dose	Normal daily dose
Moderate Surgery	50–75 mg of hydrocortisone (or equivalent) preoperative dose and up to 24 h. Revert to preoperative dose on postoperative day 2	Normal daily dose
Major Surgery	100–150 mg of hydrocortisone (or equivalent) per day as a preoperative dose and continue for the next 2–3 d. After preoperative dose, hydrocortisone 50 mg IV q8h after initial dose for the initial 2–3 d.	Normal daily dose

Adapted from Little JW, Miller CS, Rhodus NL. Chapter 15: Adrenal Insufficiency. In: Little JW, Miller CS, Rhodus NL, eds. Little and Falace's Dental Management of the Medically Compromised Patient. 9th ed. Elsevier; 2018: 255-267.

TREATMENT OF ADRENAL CRISIS[12,34]

1. Vasopressor
2. Fluid replacement = rapid isotonic saline infusion (1 L) or 5% glucose isotonic saline infusion followed by fluid replacement to match patient's requirement (4–6 L/d)
3. Steroid supplementation = 100 mg of hydrocortisone (bolus) then 200 mg of hydrocortisone for the next 24 hours
4. Transport to hospital for electrolyte correction (hyponatremia, hyperkalemia, hypoglycemia, and possible hypercalcemia)

SUMMARY

OMFS clinicians should be familiar with corticosteroid pharmacology and its wide range of deleterious clinical effects it has on all age groups. With its powerful anti-inflammatory therapeutic properties, the decision to administer perioperative steroids should be weighed against the potential adverse effects on healing capacity. Commonly used medication, such as NSAIDs, can increase the risk for GI bleeding with concomitant use with corticosteroid and should be avoided. Although perioperative recommendations for absolute indication for "stress dose" steroids are still under considerable debate, most researchers are in agreement that good perioperative pain control is essential and will diminish the host's cortisol demand. And with suppression of the cortisol demand, this will also help decrease the chance of precipitating an adrenal crisis. Long-term users of corticosteroids will develop osteoporosis in particular with hip and vertebrae and OMFS should beware of adjunctive use of antiresorptive medications to prevent fragility fractures. Lastly, 2 case reports of MRONJ of the mandible have been reported from chronic steroid use and OMFS are increasingly being challenged by their medical and dental colleagues to evaluate and treat nonhealing surgical sites from either antiresorptives and nonantiresorptive therapies.

CLINICS CARE POINTS OF CORTICOSTEROIDS

- Schedule surgery in the morning to match the body's high cortisol secretion levels.
- Routine dentoalveolar surgery can be performed on patients with secondary and tertiary adrenal insufficiencies while maintaining their normal daily dose.
- High-quality randomized control trials are needed to determine and standardize if perioperative "stress-dose" steroid is necessary for minor, moderate, and major surgeries.

- Good analgesia and sedation perioperatively would decrease the demand for cortisol, therefore, decrease the chances of an adrenal crisis.
- Combination of glucocorticoid and NSAID have 3 to 4 times increased risk for GI bleeds versus nonusers.
- Avoid using medications that are either inhibitors of glucocorticoids or inducers of CYP-450 as both will lower the cortisol level. If permissible by physician, these drugs should be discontinued 24 hours before surgery.
- Early recognition of signs and symptoms of adrenal crisis can prevent a catastrophic outcome.
- Chronic glucocorticoid users will develop skeletal osteoporosis and decreased BMD with resultant fragility fracture (vertebral and hip).
- Beware of adjunctive antiresorptive medications (ie, alendronate and denosumab) used to treat glucocorticoid-induced osteoporosis (GIOP).
- Limited case reports of MRONJ have been linked to chronic steroid use even at low doses.

ACKNOWLEDGMENTS

The author wants to extend a very special thanks to Ms Maya Nunez for her brilliant illustrations for **Figs. 1** and **2**.

DISCLOSURE

The author has nothing to disclose.

REFERENCES

1. Overman R, Yeh J, Deal C. Prevalence of oral, glucocorticoid usage in the United States: a general population perspective. Arthritis Care Res 2013; 65(2):294–8.
2. Liu M, Reidy A, Saatee S, et al. Perioperative steroid management, approach based on current evidence. Anesthesiology 2017;127(1):166–72.
3. Little and Falace's: dental management of the medically compromised patient. 9th edition. St. Louis, Missouri: Elsevier; 2018. p. 255–67.
4. Saag K, Furst D. Major side effects of systemic glucocorticoids. In: Matteson E, Ramirez M, editors. Waltham: UpToDate; 2020. Accessed December 29, 2021.
5. Chamandarin E, Nicolaides N, Chrousos GP. Adrenal insufficiency. Lancet 2014;383:2152–67.
6. Thomas C. Syndrome of inappropriate antidiuretic hormone secretion (SIADH). Medscape; 2019.

7. Nieman L. Pharmacology use of glucocorticoids. In: Lacroix A, Martin K, editors. Waltham: UpToDate; 2021. Accessed December 21, 2021.

8. Fuentes AV, Pineda MD, Venkata KCN. Comprehension of top 200 prescribed drugs in the US as a resource for pharmacy teaching, training and practice. Pharmacy (Basel) 2018;6(2):43.

9. Cox DP, Ferreira L. The oral effects of inhalation corticosteroid therapy: an update. J Calif Dent Assoc 2017;45(5):227–33.

10. Pipper J, Ray W, Daugherty J, et al. Corticosteroid use and peptic ulcer disease: Role of non steroidal anti-inflammatory drugs. Ann Intern Med 1992;114: 735–40.

11. Gabriel S, Jaakkimainen L, Bombardier C. Risk for serious gastrointestinal complications related to use of nonsteroidal anti-inflammatory drugs. Ann Intern Med 1991;115:787–96.

12. Hamrahian AH, Roman S, Milan S. Perioperative glucocorticoids. In: Nieman L, Martin K, editors. Waltham: UpToDate; 2021. Accessed December 21, 2021.

13. Yao TS, Huang YW, Chang SM, et al. Association between oral corticosteroids burst and severe adverse events. Ann Intern Med 2020;173:325–30.

14. Weinstein RS. Glucocorticoids-induced osteoporosis and osteonecrosis. Endocrinol Metab Clin North Am 2012;41(3):595–611.

15. Adami G, Saag K. Glucocorticoidinduced osteoporosis update. Curr Open Rheumatol 2019;31(4): 388–93.

16. Wong LS, Tay KK, Chieng YL. Osteonecrosis of mandible: a rare complication of long-term steroid use. J Oral Maxillo Surg Med Path 2015;27:255–7.

17. Nisi M, Ferla F, Graziani F, et al. Osteonecrosis of the jaws related to corticosteroids therapy: a case report. Ann Stomatol (Roma) 2014;5(2 Suppl): 29–30.

18. Alemi AS, Mazur CM, Fowler TW, et al. Glucocorticoids cause mandibular bone fragility and suppress osteocyte perilacunar-canalicular remodeling. Bone Rep 2018;9:145–53.

19. Fu JH W, Bashutski JD, Al-Hezaimi K, et al. Statins, glucocorticoids, and nonsteroidal anti- inflammatory drugs: their influence on implant healing. Implant Dent 2012;21(5):362–7.

20. Ouanounou A, Hassanpour S, Glogauer M. The influence of systemic medication on osseointegration of dental implants. J Can Dent Assoc 2016;82:g7.

21. Petsinis V, Kamperos G, Alexandridi F, et al. The impact of glucocorticoids administered for systemic diseases on osseointegration and survival of dental implants placed without bone grafting: a retrospective study in 31 patients. J Craniomaxillofac Surg 2017;45(8):1197–2000.

22. Duttenhoefer F, Fuessinger MA, Beckmann Y, et al. Dental Implants in immunocompromised patients: a systematic review and meta-analysis. Int J Implants Dent 2019;5:43.

23. Fraser CG, Preuss FS, Bigford WD. Adrenal atrophy and irreversible shock associated with cortisone therapy. J Am Med Assoc 1952;149:1542–3.

24. Lewis I, Robinson RF, Yee J, et al. Fatal adrenal cortical insufficiency precipitated by surgery during prolonged continuous cortisone treatment. Ann Intern Med 1953;39:116–26.

25. Chilkoti GT, Singh A, Mehta M, et al. Perioperative "stress dose" of corticosteroid: pharmacological and clinical perspective. J Anaesthesiol Clin Pharmacol 2019;35(2):147–52.

26. LabCorp. Available at: http://www.labcorp.com. Accessed January 24, 2021.

27. Lipworth BJ. Systemic adverse effects of inhaled corticosteroids therapy: a systematic review and meta-analysis. Arch Intern Med 1999;159(9): 941–55.

28. Marik P, Varon J. Requirement of perioperative stress dose of corticosteroids. Arch Surg 2008; 143(12):1222–6.

29. Salem M, Tainsh R, Bromberg J, et al. Perioperative glucocorticoid coverage. A reassessment 42 years after emergence of a problem. Ann Sure 1994;219: 416–25.

30. Groleau C, Morris S, Vautour L. Amar-zikin and bessissow a: perioperative corticosteroid administration: a systematic review. Perioper Med (Lond) 2018;7:10.

31. Jerjes W, Jerjes W, Swanson B, et al. Midazolam in reduction of surgical stress: a randomized trial. Oral Surg Oral Med Oral Pathol Oral Radiol Endod 2005;100:564–70.

32. Steer M, Fromm D. Recognition of adrenal insufficiency on the postoperative patient. Am J Surg 1980;139:443–6.

33. Banks P. The adrenal-cortisol response to oral surgery. Br J Oral Surg 1970;8:32–44.

34. Dineen R, Thompson C, Sherlock M. Adrenal crisis: prevention and management in adult patients. Ther Adv Endocrinol Metab 2019;10. 2042018819848218.

Update on Management of the Oral and Maxillofacial Surgery Patient on Selective Serotonin Reuptake Inhibitors

Natasha Bhalla, DDS[a],*, Michael H. Chan, DDS[b,c]

KEYWORDS

- SSRIs • Fentanyl • Serotonin syndrome • NSAIDs • Dental implants • GI bleed • Gastroprotection

KEY POINTS

- Selective serotonin reuptake inhibitors (SSRIs) emerged as the first line of antidepressant medications recommended by the 2011 American Psychiatric Association guidelines.
- SSRIs and fentanyl can precipitate serotonin syndrome—excessive serotonin activity in the central nervous system. Serotonin syndrome presents as a triad of symptoms—mental status changes, autonomic hyperactivity, and neuromuscular abnormalities. Early intervention can prevent morbidity and mortality.
- Several studies have found that implant failure rates are higher in SSRI users versus nonusers. Clinicians can inform patients of mild risk of implant failure in SSRI users.
- Increased gastrointestinal bleeds have been reported with SSRI users, and it doubles when combined with nonsteroidal antiinflammatory drugs versus nonusers.
- Based on the current data, the authors recommend avoiding the combination of ibuprofen and SSRIs. If both medications are deemed to be essential, synthetic prostaglandin, H2-blocker, or PPI can provide gastroprotection.

Depression is a global prevalent disorder affecting millions of people ranging from mild to major forms. It is a medical condition associated with low levels of circulating serotonin, norepinephrine, and dopamine in major depressive disorder, which can be linked with significant disability and reduced quality of life. Antidepressants is a class of medications aimed to treat this condition. Historically, monoamine oxidase inhibitors and tricyclics antidepressants have been used. However, undesirable side effects have many physicians divert to a newer second generation created in the late 1980s namely the selective serotonin reuptake inhibitor (SSRIs). Because of better tolerance and less side effects than its predecessors, SSRIs have emerged as the first line of antidepressant medication recommended by the American Psychiatric Association (APA) in their 2011 guidelines.[1] Six of the top 200 prescribed medications in the United States during 2018 were SSRIs with some of the commercially available ones including citalopram, escitalopram, fluoxetine, fluvoxamine, paroxetine, and sertraline.[1] Between 2015 and 2018, 13.2% of adults in the United States older than 18 years used antidepressants in the past 30 days with women (17.7%) slightly doubled that of men (8.4%).[1] In addition to treatment of depression, they are prescribed for anxiety,

[a] Oral and Maxillofacial Surgery, The Brooklyn Hospital Center, 121 Dekalb Avenue, Brooklyn, NY 11201, USA;
[b] Oral & Maxillofacial Surgery, Department of Veterans Affairs, New York Harbor Healthcare System (Brooklyn Campus), 800 Poly Place (Bk-160), Brooklyn, NY 11209, USA; [c] Oral & Maxillofacial Surgery, Department of Oral & Maxillofacial Surgery, The Brooklyn Hospital Center, 121 DeKalb Avenue (Box-187), Brooklyn, NY 11201, USA
* Corresponding author.
E-mail address: natashaa95@gmail.com

Oral Maxillofacial Surg Clin N Am 34 (2022) 127–134
https://doi.org/10.1016/j.coms.2021.08.009
1042-3699/22/© 2021 Elsevier Inc. All rights reserved.

bulimia nervosa, fibromyalgia, obsessive-compulsive disorder, panic disorder, and post-traumatic stress disorder. The purpose of this chapter is to review pathophysiology, current medications, adverse drug interactions, and management of common OMFS office–based procedures when treating patients on SSRIs.

PATHOPHYSIOLOGY AND MECHANISM OF ACTION OF SELECTIVE SEROTONIN REUPTAKE INHIBITORS

Serotonin (5-hydroxytryptamine [5-HT]) receptors are found in the nervous system, bones, and blood platelets. Hence, SSRIs can have an effect on the nervous, skeletal, and hematological system, respectively.

In the nervous system, there is a wide projection pattern of 5-HT receptors modulating physiologic functions such as sleep, arousal, feeding, pain, emotions, and cognition.[2] Scientists have also found serotonin to play a role in mood enhancement, appetite suppressant, and sleep improvement. The behavioral effects of 5-HT are mediated by a family of 14 5-HT receptor subtypes.[2] The $5-HT_{1A}R$ is one of the best studied subtypes due to its implications in anxietylike behaviors and depression.[2] The most common antidepressant, SSRIs, target the $5-HT_{1A}R$ by inhibiting serotonin reuptake from the synaptic cleft into presynaptic nerve terminals, thereby increasing the concentration of serotonin in the synaptic cleft and enhancing serotonin available for neurotransmission (**Fig. 1**).[2]

In addition, researchers have discovered serotonin to regulate osteoclasts activation and differentiation, as osteoclasts are derived from hematopoietic cell precursors.[3–6] Specifically, serotonin transporters (SERT) and receptors are present in bony microarchitecture.[3–6] An in vivo study has demonstrated significant reduction in osteogenic differentiation and mineralization with concomitant reduction of osteoblast markers including alkaline phosphatase, osterix, and osteocalcin during SSRI administration.[3–6] As a result, SSRIs can have a negative influence on bone mineral density.

The primary role of serotonin in response to vascular injury is to promote vasoconstriction and platelet aggregation for local hemostasis.[7] SERT is responsible for the uptake of serotonin into the platelets specifically into the granular cell compartment. By blocking this site, platelets will be devoid of serotonin rendering it useless from its primary function[12] (**Fig. 2**). Therefore, it may be predicted SSRIs can ultimately reduce platelet aggregation, clot formation, and increased risk of bleeding.[7] Literature reviews have demonstrated a 90% reduction in platelet content of serotonin just after a 2-week course of SSRIs, suggesting clinicians should be aware of the relatively quick onset.[8–12]

MEDICATION DOSAGES

Listed later (**Table 1**) are the starting doses of common SSRI medications along with half-life. This table also touches on the starting dose for different psychiatric conditions.

ADVERSE REACTIONS/EVENTS OF SELECTIVE SEROTONIN REUPTAKE INHIBITORS

SSRIs have only been available in the market for a short period of time. And because of this, knowledge about its adverse effects is emerging through case reports and studies. There is no block box warning label associated with sertraline, fluoxetine, and paroxetine. Citalopram and escitalopram are not approved for the pediatric population, with escitalopram specifically not approved for those younger than 12 years. Safety and efficacy of fluvoxamine in patients younger than 8 years have not been established.

Selective Serotonin Reuptake Inhibitors and Nonsteroidal Antiinflammatory Drugs

Ibuprofen has been ranked as the 34th medication most prescribed in the United States according to the national data from 2018.[13] In addition to prescription sales, ibuprofen is also a commonly purchased over-the-counter (OTC) medicine for treatment of inflammation and pain.[1] Data from the National Consumer League of 2002 showed, of the 4263 individuals that were interviewed, 83% reported OTC analgesic use in the past year.[1] Of these individuals, 15% reported using analgesics daily and 29% reported taking them several times per week, making ibuprofen the most widely used nonnarcotic analgesia only behind acetaminophen.[1]

As a nonselective cyclooxygenase (Cox) 1 and 2 inhibitor, ibuprofen is known to increase the risk of bleeding by causing topical injury to the gastric mucosa by blocking Cox 1 pathway, thus preventing prostaglandin production. By blocking prostaglandin production, the gastric mucosa cannot produce mucous lining and is vulnerable for increased risk in gastrointestinal (GI) bleed.[14] In addition, Cox 1 inhibitor prevents thromboxane A2 production for vasoconstriction and platelet aggregation. Furthermore, these platelets are depleted of serotonin and lack any hemostatic properties seen in normal platelets (see **Fig. 2**).

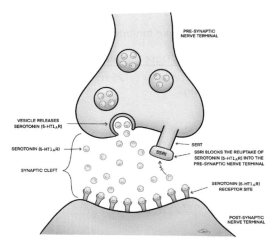

Fig. 1. SSRI blocks the reuptake of serotonin into the presynaptic nerve terminal.

Not all patients will have the same risk of developing GI complications. These risk factors include advanced age (>60 years), existing cardiovascular disease (CV), and concurrent use of other nonsteroidal antiinflammatory drugs (NSAIDs), antiplatelet, or anticoagulant medications. Many of these patients are already taking low-dose aspirin (81 mg Aspirin [ASA]) for prevention of CV events.

And with the addition of ibuprofen, the risk of GI bleed gets elevated to high risk.[14] Also, elderly patients taking SSRIs with concomitant use of ibuprofen have been reported to have a high rate of perioperative GI bleed. One study reported a 3-fold increased risk of GI bleed with a combination of SSRI and ibuprofen when compared with ibuprofen use alone.[1] Other studies have also suggested a similar outcome. There is a 60% risk of a GI bleed with the combination of SSRIs and NSAIDs against non-NSAID/non-SSRI users and a drastic reduction to 30% when SSRI is compared with non-NSAID/non-SSRI users.[1] The risk is doubled by administering NSAIDs to SSRI users.

Anesthesia Case Report of Adverse Drug Interaction Between Selective Serotonin Reuptake Inhibitors and Nonsteroidal Antiinflammatory Drugs

Anesthesia reported a case of a 53-year-old man who underwent a resection of the mandible for treatment of his carcinoma in situ.[15] The surgeon performed primary closure and had established hemostasis at the surgical site.[15] An hour later, in the recovery room, he developed severe dyspnea secondary to hematoma formation from the floor of the mouth.[15] Reintubation was not deemed

NORMAL MECHANISM OF SEROTONIN (5-HT) UPTAKE INTO GRANULAR CELL OF PLATELETS USING SERT	SSRI BLOCKS SERT SITE AND PROHIBITS UPTAKE OF SEROTONIN (5-HT) CAUSING DEPLETION

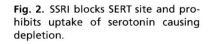

Fig. 2. SSRI blocks SERT site and prohibits uptake of serotonin causing depletion.

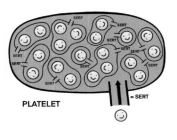
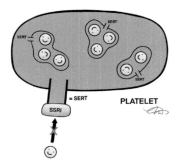

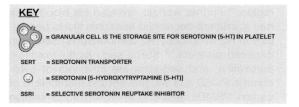

Table 1
Dosages, indications and half-life of common selective serotonin reuptake inhibitors

	Indication	Starting Dose	Half-Life
Sertraline (Zoloft)	Adults		26 h (range 22–36 h)
	Mood depressive disorder (MDD)/ obsessive compulsive disorder (OCD)	50 mg	
	Panic disorder, posttraumatic stress disorder, seasonal affective disorder (PD, PTSD, SAD)	25 mg	
	Pediatric Patients		
	OCD (age 6–12 y)	25 mg	
	OCD (age 13–17 y)	50 mg	
Fluoxetine (Prozac)	Adults		1–3 d
	Depression/OCD/pervasive developmental disorders (PDD)	20 mg	
	Bulimia	60 mg	
	PD	10 mg	
	Pediatric Patients		
	Depression (8–18 y)/depression (lower weight children)/OCD (7–17 y)	10–20 mg	
	OCD (lower weight children)	10 mg	
Paroxetine (Paxil)	Adults		21 h
	Depression/SAD/OCD/PTSD/ generalized anxiety disorder (GAD)	20 mg	
	PD	10 mg	
	PDD	12.5 mg	
	Geriatric Dose		
	OCD/PTSD/SAD/GAD/depression	10 mg	
Citalopram (Celexa)	Adults		36 h
	Depression	20 mg	
	Geriatric patients		
	Depression	20 mg	
Escitalopram (Lexapro)	Adults		27–32 h
	GAD/depression	10 mg	
	Geriatric Patients		
	Depression	10 mg	
	Pediatric Patients		
	Depression	10 mg	
Fluvoxamine (Luvox)	Adults		58 h
	OCD	**50 mg**	
	Pediatrics		
	OCD (8–11 y)	**25 mg**	
	OCD (11–17 y)	**25 mg**	

Data from Refs.[20–24]

possible, and he had to undergo an emergency tracheostomy. Ibuprofen was immediately discontinued, and acetaminophen with codeine was replaced for pain control.[15] On further probing into the patient's surgical history, similar episodes of postoperative bleeding have occurred with procedures such as tooth extraction, correction of deviated nasal septum, and biopsy from the retromolar pad region.[15] Further workup revealed his blood work had significant decreased serotonin levels particularly in his thrombocytes, demonstrating serotonin depleted platelets.[15] SSRIs such as fluvoxamine, paroxetine, and sertraline are inhibitors of cytochrome P-450 and will prevent the metabolism of certain NSAIDs, resulting in NSAID accumulation and the potential increased risk of bleeding.[15]

Selective Serotonin Reuptake Inhibitors and Fentanyl

Fentanyl is a widely used potent analgesic in both inpatient and outpatient settings with its short half-life, making it an appealing choice for many OMFS and anesthesiologists. The interaction between fentanyl, a direct serotonin agonist, and SSRIs could potentially result in an adverse outcome called serotonin syndrome. An excessive serotonin activity in the central nervous system (CNS), typically in the setting of multiple drugs, can result in an overdrive of serotonin neurotransmission.[16–18]

Classically, it presents as a triad of symptoms—mental status changes, autonomic hyperactivity, and neuromuscular abnormalities.[16–18] Clinical manifestations can be rapid or delayed up to 6 hours and is characterized based on severity of the condition: mild (ie, mild hypertension, tachycardia, diaphoresis, myoclonus, tremor), moderate (ie, agitation, clonus, myoclonus, altered mental status), or severe (ie, delirium, seizures, neuromuscular rigidity, hyperthermia, and possible coma leading to death).[17] Diagnosis of serotonin syndrome is based on signs and symptoms, and serum serotonin levels do not correlate with clinical findings.[16–18] Treatment of serotonin syndrome includes early stabilization of vital signs, administration of oxygen, intravenous (IV) fluids, and continuous cardiac monitoring.[17] Patients are typically hospitalized for observation and treatment rendered based on symptoms.[17] Many cases tend to resolve within 24 hours after initiation of supportive care and discontinuation of the offending serotonergic medications.[17]

Management of Serotonin Syndrome

1. Benzodiazepines are given to treat agitation and/or seizures.[17]
2. Serotonergic medication can be flushed out by increasing IV hydration and to protect the kidneys from getting damaged (rhabdomyolysis).[17]
3. In severe cases, cyproheptadine (Periactin) can be used to block serotonin.[17]
4. Cooling blankets can be used for hyperthermia.[17]
5. Hyperthermia may also require immediate sedation and intubation by using a nondepolarizing neuromuscular blocking agent.[17]

Selective Serotonin Reuptake Inhibitors and Local Anesthesia Containing Epinephrine

As per the investigative research, there is currently no contraindications of administering local anesthesia containing epinephrine to patients taking SSRIs.

Selective Serotonin Reuptake Inhibitors and Dental Extractions

There are no case reports of adverse outcomes with this drug and procedure.

Selective Serotonin Reuptake Inhibitors and Dental Implants

Given the interaction among SSRIs, osteoblasts and osteoclasts, several studies have been conducted on SSRIs and osseointegration after dental implant placement.[8–10] In 2014, Wu and colleagues demonstrated implant failure rates were 4.6% for SSRI nonusers and 10.6% for SSRI users.[9] Their study showed failures mostly occurred between 4 and 14 months after implant placement, suggesting implant failure by SSRIs was from the mechanical loading of the implants and not from initial osseointegration.[9] They concluded careful surgical and prosthetic treatment planning were necessary to circumvent these issues.[9] In addition, in 2017, Chrcanovic and colleagues found implant failure rates were 12.5% for SSRI users and 3.3% for nonusers[18] without any statistical differences.[18] Lastly, in 2018, Altay and colleagues discovered implant failure rates for SSRIs users were 5.6% and 1.85% for nonusers.[10] Although the differences between the 2 groups were not statistically significant,[10] patients using SSRIs were found to be 3 times more likely to experience early implant failure than nonusers.[10] The investigators concluded SSRIs may lead to osseointegration failure.[10]

Selective Serotonin Reuptake Inhibitors and Medication-Related Osteonecrosis of Jaw Case Reports

There are currently no case reports of SSRI associated with medication-related osteonecrosis of jaw.

MANAGEMENT OF THE ORAL AND MAXILLOFACIAL SURGERY PATIENTS ON SELECTIVE SEROTONIN REUPTAKE INHIBITORS
Perioperative Management for Intravenous Sedation

Practitioners should weigh the risks, benefits, and alternatives before administering fentanyl to SSRI users. Even though the occurrence is very low, 0.09% in patients who received both fentanyl and a serotonergic agent,[19] the potential of precipitating an iatrogenic serotonin syndrome is real,

---

Box 1
General rules for perioperative management for pain control on selective serotonin reuptake inhibitors

- Use of the lowest effective dose of NSAIDs for the shortest period of time
- Avoid concomitant therapy with corticosteroids, anticoagulants, low-dose ASA (81 mg), or antiplatelet agents.
- Ibuprofen is considered a "safer" NSAID option.
- Eradicate *Helicobacter pylori* infection in patients with prior ulcer therapy.

Prevention Strategies

- No cardiovascular (CV) risk factors and (not on low-dose ASA)
  - No GI risk factors: can use ibuprofen
  - One or more GI risk factors (advanced age, alcohol intake, selective serotonin reuptake inhibitors, corticosteroid, use of antithrombotic drugs and anticoagulants, and a history of complicated peptic ulcer disease): use coxib (standard dose) or ibuprofen + PPI or misoprostol
  - If history of ulcer bleeding: use coxib + PPI. Need to eradicate *H pylori*
- On low dose ASA
  - One or more GI risk factor: use naproxen + PPI or coxib + PPI
  - Avoid combining with ibuprofen since it will increase risk of bleeding with low-dose ASA

Data from Al-Saeed A. Gastrointestinal and Cardiovascular Risk of Nonsteroidal Anti-inflammatory Drugs. Oman Med J. 2011 Nov;26(6):385-91.

---

and early recognition and intervention can prevent morbidity and mortality. The authors also advise clinicians to be aware of the increasing use of SSRIs, especially in the teenage population requiring removal of wisdom teeth under sedation.

Perioperative Management for Dental Implant Surgery

Several studies have demonstrated, although without statistical difference, an increase in failure rate in dental implants performed on patients taking SSRIs. Clinicians can inform these patients of the slight increased risk of implant failure when compared with non-SSRI users, and this does not preclude them from getting the surgery. Future studies are recommended to understand the exact

association between SSRIs and the negative influence on dental implants.

Further studies are also needed to investigate the cause of higher implant failure in SSRI users—osseointegration, prosthetic, or both.

Perioperative Management for Pain Control

The authors recommend avoiding the combination of ibuprofen and SSRIs when possible, to avoid the risk of an upper GI bleed. Alternatively, acetaminophen with or without an additional narcotic can be used. If ibuprofen is deemed to be essential, prevention strategies for GI toxicity should be followed; this is demonstrated on **Box 1** and based on presence of cardiovascular risk factors. If there are no cardiovascular risk factors and if not on daily low-dose ASA, patients can take NSAIDs at normally prescribed dose.[14] When one or more GI risk factors are present, the use of a selective Cox 2 inhibitor (ie, celecoxib) alone or ibuprofen plus a proton pump inhibitor (PPI) or misoprostol can provide gastroprotection.[14] Normally, prostaglandin is produced by both Cox 1 and 2 enzymes, with Cox 1 found in gastric lining and blood platelets. They promote gastric protection and platelets aggregation, respectively. Cox 2 enzyme focuses primarily on inflammation and pain production. By specifically targeting these inflammatory sites by blocking Cox 2, undesirable gastric and bleeding from dysfunctional platelets' adverse effects can be avoided.

Managing Gastrointestinal Toxicity

Patients with GI risk factors, who require nonselective NSAIDs, should receive a gastroprotectant.[14] Misoprostol is a synthetic prostaglandin that stimulates mucous secretion in the upper GI tract.[14] One study showed misoprostol, 200 μg, used 4 times a day orally significantly reduced symptomatic ulcers.[14] However, misoprostol use in clinical practice is limited by its poor tolerability.[14] The required dosing schedule of 4 times per day makes it inconvenient for patients, thereby adversely affecting treatment compliance and outcome.[14] In addition, women of child-bearing age are contraindicated in using this medication due to the increased risk of abortion.[14]

H2-receptor antagonists are gastroprotectants by reversibility interference and blocking histamine receptors in the parietal cell, which reduces acid secretion.[14] High-dose famotidine has been shown to prevent both gastric and duodenal ulcers associated with NSAID use.[14]

Proton pump inhibitors (PPIs) block gastric acid secretion by inhibiting the H+/K + ATPase and are significantly more effective than H2-receptor antagonists for treatment and prevention of acid-related diseases.[14] Studies have confirmed omeprazole (PPI), 20 mg/d, was more effective than ranitidine (H2—antagonist) and low-dose misoprostol in the primary or secondary prevention of gastric and duodenal ulcers in ibuprofen users.[14]

On occasion, clinicians may need to prescribe a lengthy course of NSAIDs for treatment of temporomandibular/myofascial pain; the addition of a gastroprotectant such as misoprostol, histamine-2 receptor antagonist, or a PPI would be recommended.[14]

SUMMARY

With the increasing use of SSRIs in all age groups, the Oral and Maxillofacial Surgeon should be aware of the mechanism of action, medication dosages, and adverse interactions with other common medications.

SSRIs increase the risk of bleeding when used with ibuprofen. Hence, the authors recommend avoiding this combination. Alternatively, acetaminophen with or without an additional narcotic can be used. If ibuprofen use is required, prevention strategies for GI toxicity should be followed. The interaction between fentanyl and SSRIs could result in serotonin syndrome. Early recognition of symptoms and intervention can prevent morbidity and mortality. Last, several studies have demonstrated an increased risk in dental implant failures in those taking SSRIs. Clinicians should inform these patients of the slight increased risk. Whether dental implant failure is due to initial osseointegration or after prosthetic loading, further investigations via randomized controlled trials are needed to elucidate the exact cause.

In conclusion, SSRIs are beneficial to the medical management of patients. Knowledge about the medication will result in appropriate management of patients.

CLINICS CARE POINTS

- Based on the current data, the authors recommend avoiding the combination of ibuprofen and SSRIs. If both medications are deemed to be essential, misoprostol, H2-blocker, or PPI can provide gastroprotection.
- Alternatively, acetaminophen ± narcotic can be used instead of ibuprofen alone for pain control.

- Even though the occurrence of serotonin syndrome is very low, 0.09% in patients who received both fentanyl and a serotonergic agent, the authors advise clinicians to be aware of the increasing use of SSRIs, especially in the teenage population requiring removal of wisdom teeth under sedation.
- Several studies have demonstrated, although without statistical difference, an increase in failure rate in dental implants performed on patients taking SSRIs.

ACKNOWLEDGMENT

The authors want to extend a very special thank you to Ms. Maya Nunez for her brilliant illustrations for **Figs. 1** and **2**.

DISCLOSURE

The authors have nothing to disclose.

REFERENCES

1. Hersh P. Adverse drug interactions involving common prescription and over-the-counter analgesic agents. Clin Ther 2007;29(11):2477–97.
2. Stiedl O, Pappa E, Konradsson-Geuken A, et al. The role of the serotonin receptor subtypes 5-HT1A and 5-HT7 and its interaction in emotional learning and memory. Front Pharmacol 2015;6:162.
3. Serebruany V. Selective serotonin reuptake inhibitors and increased bleeding risk: are we missing something? Am J Med 2006;119(2):113–6.
4. Helin-Salmivaara H. Frequent prescribing of drugs with potential gastrointestinal toxicity among continuous users of non-steroidal anti-inflammatory drugs. Eur J Clin Pharmacol 2005;61(5):425–31.
5. Risser D. NSAID prescribing precautions. Am Fam Physician 2009;80(12):1371–8.
6. LOKE T. Meta-analysis: gastrointestinal bleeding due to interaction between selective serotonin uptake inhibitors and non-steroidal anti-inflammatory drugs. Aliment Pharmacol Ther 2008;27(1):31–40.
7. Dalton S. SSRIs and upper gastrointestinal bleeding: what is known and how should it influence prescribing? CNS Drugs 2006;20(2):143–51.
8. Ouanounou A, Hassanpour S, Glogauer M. The influence of systemic medications on osseointegration of dental implants: a review. J Can Dent Assoc 2016; 82(g7):1–8.
9. Wu A-A. Selective serotonin reuptake inhibitors and the risk of osseointegrated implant failure: a cohort study. J Dent Res 2014;93(11):1054–61.
10. Altay MA, Sindel A, Özalp Ö, et al. Does the intake of selective serotonin reuptake inhibitors negatively

affect dental implant osseointegration? A retrospective study. J Oral Implantol 2018;44(4):260–5.

11. Kirschner R, Donovan JW. Serotonin syndrome precipitated by fentanyl during procedural sedation. J Emerg Med 2010;38(4):477–80.

12. Paton C, Ferrier IN. SSRIs and gastrointestinal bleeding. BMJ 2005;331(7516):529–30.

13. Fuentes AV, Pineda MD, Venkata KCN. Comprehension of top 200 prescribed drugs in the us as a resource for pharmacy teaching, training and practice. Pharmacy 2018;6(2):43.

14. Al-Saeed A. Gastrointestinal and cardiovascular risk of nonsteroidal anti-inflammatory drugs. Oman Med J 2011;26(6):385–91.

15. Van Cann EM, Koole R. Abnormal bleeding after an oral surgical procedure leading to airway compromise in a patient taking a selective serotonin reuptake inhibitor and a nonsteroidal antiinflammatory drug. Anesthesiology 2008;109(3):568–9.

16. Alkhatib AA, Peterson KA, Tuteja AK. Serotonin syndrome as a complication of fentanyl sedation during esophagogastroduodenoscopy. Dig Dis Sci 2010;55::215–216.

17. Greenier E, Lukyanova V, Reede L. Serotonin syndrome: fentanyl and selective serotonin reuptake inhibitor interactions. AANA J 2014;82(5):340–5.

18. Chrcanovic B, Kisch J, Albrektsson T, et al. Is the intake of selective serotonin reuptake inhibitors associated with an increased risk of dental implant failure? Int J Oral Maxillofac Surg 2017;46(6):782–8.

19. Koury KM, Tsui B, Gulur P. Incidence of serotonin syndrome in patients treated with fentanyl on serotonergic agents. Pain Physician 2015;18(1):E27–30.

20. "Sertraline." Drugs.com. 2020. Available at. https://www.drugs.com/ppa/sertraline.html#dosage. Accessed December 1, 2020.

21. "Fluoxetine." Drugs.com. 2020. Available at. https://www.drugs.com/fluoxetine.html#dosage. Accessed December 1, 2020.

22. "Paroxetine." Drugs.com. 2021. Available at. https://www.drugs.com/paroxetine.html#dosage. Accessed December 1, 2020.

23. "Citalopram." Drugs.com. 2019. Available at. https://www.drugs.com/citalopram.html#dosage. Accessed December 1, 2020.

24. "Escitalopram." Drugs.com. 2020. Available at. https://www.drugs.com/escitalopram.html#dosage. Accessed December 1, 2020.

Hyposalivation and Xerostomia and Burning Mouth Syndrome
Medical Management

Jaykrishna P. Thakkar, DDS[a],*, Christopher J. Lane, DDS[b]

KEYWORDS

- Xerostomia • Hyposalivation • Salivary gland dysfunction • Burning mouth syndrome

KEY POINTS

- Xerostomia is the subjective complaint of dry mouth, whereas hyposalivation is the actual decrease in measured salivary outflow.
- Saliva is secreted from major and minor glands of the oral cavity, which serves to lubricate, moisten, protect, and assist in digestion, taste, and smell.
- Saliva is measured through multiple methods such as "spitting and drooling method", modified schirmer test, and sialography among others.
- There are numerous medications that are linked with xerostomia and hyposalivation; the authors describe 10 of the most cited medications and list numerous others.
- Burning mouth syndrome is described as burning in the tongue or other oral mucous membrane that has no medical or dental-related cause.

INTRODUCTION

It is fair to say that the average person does not think about the amount of saliva they have until they notice a decrease and begin to experience the discomfort associated with a decrease in saliva. The lack of saliva can grow to be a devastating experience for a patient's oral health and can diminish their daily quality of life. The role of the oral specialist is to identify the presence, the causes, and the treatment modalities present for such conditions. This chapter helps the practicing oral specialist to review the benefits of saliva and the destructive consequences of its loss. The authors discuss the most common medications used today that are associated with diminished salivary presence and function. It is hoped that this will help their colleagues identify and treat patients even before development of symptoms by identifying high-risk individuals. These preventative measures and treatment modalities can be adapted to the daily practice of the oral specialist. These identifications and recommendations are transcribed from multiple systematic reviews and analyses.

XEROSTOMIA VERSUS HYPOSALIVATION

Xerostomia and hyposalivation are frequently used interchangeably, which is incorrect, and this can cause confusion to the practitioner and the patient and can affect the treatment modalities present. Xerostomia is defined as "the subjective complaint of dry mouth or subjective sensation of oral dryness."[1] The key term in this definition is "subjective." Patients may have normal salivary function but have a feeling of dryness that may be a symptom or a byproduct of a larger a diagnosis. In contrast, hyposalivation is the actual decrease in measured salivary outflow. Several large studies

[a] Oral and Maxillofacial Surgery The Brooklyn Hospital -Brooklyn, 155 Ashland Place, Brooklyn NY 11201, USA;
[b] Oral and Maxillofacial Surgery, St. Barnabas Hospital, 4422 3rd Avenue, Bronx, NY 10457, USA
* Corresponding author.
E-mail address: jthakkarta@gmail.com

oralmaxsurgery.theclinics.com

have reported that the mean flow rate of unstimulated saliva in healthy persons during the day is in the range of 0.3 to 0.4 mL/min. An unstimulated flow of less than 0.1 mL/min is considered evidence of salivary hypofunction.[2] In normal healthy individuals, the total daily salivary production is estimated to be 500 to 600 mL/d.[3]

WHAT IS SALIVA?

Saliva is the watery liquid that is secreted into the oral cavity from the bilaterally paired major salivary glands (parotid, submandibular, and sublingual) as well as the from smaller accessory minor salivary glands found throughout the oral cavity. The parotid gland predominantly produces serous and watery secretions, whereas the sublingual glands produce mucous secretions, and the submandibular glands produce both serous and mucous secretions.

Because saliva has many different functions in the oral cavity, aiding mastication, swallowing, and digestion, its presence goes virtually unnoticed but its absence can be devastating. In the systematic review described by Dawes, saliva has a multimodal role. This role includes lubrication, moistening, and protection of the oral mucosa and esophagus, as well as assisting both taste and smell, and providing enzymes that aid in digestion.[2]

Lubrication, Moistening, and Protection

The benefit of maintaining a moist, lubricated oral mucosa and esophagus prevents abrasion and aids in the removal of bacteria, viruses, fungi, and other microbes. This moist environment also aids in the physical movement of food, making mastication and consumption an easier task. These actions are aided due to mucin production from the submandibular, sublingual, and minor salivary glands. Mucins are heavily glycosylated glycoproteins that coat the oral cavity and act as a lubricant for opposing surfaces encountered during mastication. It is found that patients with decreased mucin will have difficulty in performing common tasks such as speaking, swallowing, or masticating.[2]

Either passively or actively, there is a continuous flow of saliva in the average patient. The continuous outflow of saliva from the salivary ducts in the oral cavity inhibits retrograde flow of harmful microbes into the glands, thus preventing conglomeration of bacteria and the development of infection.[2]

Taste and Smell

Saliva operates as the medium in which taste substances, or tastants, dissolve and interact with chemoreceptors, responsible for taste, located in the oral cavity. "These taste buds are present in the fungiform papillae and in the clefts of the circumvallate and foliate papillae on the tongue, the soft palate, the epiglottis the nasopharynx and esophagus.[2]" There are 5 basic tastes that are recognized, sweet, salty, sour, bitter, and umami/savory. Saliva acts as a protectant against noxious tastes that irritate the oral mucosa and can present a danger to the rest of the gastrointestinal tract. There will be an overproduction of saliva in this circumstance, causing dilution of the noxious taste stimuli, which gives the person the ability to spit out the noxious rich substance.

As the nose, the nasopharynx also contains olfactory receptors that are responsible for perceiving smell. When masticating solid foods, there is a release of aroma. The warmth and the enzymes in saliva also help break down solids and further release aromas that are carried by the saliva and delivered to these olfactory receptors.[2]

Digestion

As previously mentioned, enzymes in our saliva are present to help break down starches and starch-containing food. The enzyme most cited in the literature is alpha-amylase (1,4,-glucan 4-glucanohydrolase).[2]

Protection

Saliva also acts as a buffer against very acidic foods and environments. The buffering properties come from the presence of bicarbonate and carbonic anhydrase VI. When acidic foods are introduced, salivary flow increases, and the hydrogen ions from acidic foods interact with bicarbonate to form carbonic acid. The carbonic anhydrase VI then springs into action to convert carbonic acid into water and gas.[2] As you can imagine, vomiting can also be very harmful to the oral mucosa. The hydrochloric acid from the stomach also increases salivary flow, and the bicarbonate in the oral cavity will also work to buffer the gastric contents entering the mouth. As previously mentioned, saliva lubricates the esophagus and oral cavity, which softens and lubricates the foods we consume. The esophagus is lined by 600 to 700 mucous glands that secrete bicarbonate and mucus that help form a protective surface layer 95 μm thick.[2]

Teeth

Saliva has a very prominent role in the acquired enamel pellicle that surrounds teeth. Salivary proteins are found in bulk within this pellicle, which provides multiple protective factors. The pellicle decreases the friction from opposing teeth and provides protection against attrition, abrasion, and foreign trauma. Our enamel and dentin are composed of hydroxyapatite ($Ca_{10}(PO_4)_6(OH)_2$) crystals; the main components are calcium, phosphate, and hydroxide ions. Saliva is supersaturated with both calcium and phosphate ions. These ions can diffuse through the enamel pellicle to assist in remineralizing the enamel.[2] Patients who have a decreased salivary flow or composition have an increased risk of caries formation because they have lost that protective component provided by saliva.

When the oral cavity is subjected to an acidic environment, there is an increase in the concentration of H+ ions and a decrease in the pH. In this environment, the H+ ions act to displace the phosphate from hydroxyapatite, which manifests as erosion. Saliva, being supersaturated with phosphate, helps buffer the acidic environment. In patients who have a decreased salivary function, there will be a concurrent decreased buffering capacity, and you will begin observing erosion and dental caries precipitated by acidogenic organisms in plaque.[2] Saliva is also rich in urea. Microorganisms in plaque release urease, which converts urea into ammonia and carbon dioxide. Ammonia is a strong base that neutralizes carbon dioxide and increases the pH.[2]

WHAT ARE THE OTHER PROTECTIVE PROPERTIES OF SALIVA?

Along with the aforementioned properties, saliva also contains antibacterial, antifungal, and antiviral properties that keep the oral microbiota population stabilized. During dental training, the authors had a professor who described the oral microbiota as a "see-saw." There was a balance of protective proteins living in conjunction with healthy and harmful microorganisms. Whenever you had an altered balance from external factors, the see-saw would turn and disrupt the balance, manifesting as the oral health problems we see today. The saliva is also home to multiple growth factors such as endothelia growth factor and vascular endothelial growth factor, which assist in angiogenesis and allow reepithelialization and regulation of the extracellular matrix.[2]

HOW IS IT MEASURED?

As previously described, xerostomia is the subjective feeling of dry mouth, whereas hyposalivation is the measured decrease in salivary outflow. Various measures are present to quantify the decrease in the measured outflow.

1. The most commonly and conveniently used technique is "the spitting and drooling" method. This measures the unstimulated salivary flow. A patient will allow for saliva to accumulate in the mouth for 5 minutes and spit into a collection tube, and this is repeated for a fixed time period. The stimulated flow can be measured by the patient chewing or using a sialogogue (a medication that promotes the secretion of saliva).
2. The modified Schirmer test (MST) uses paper strips that are placed in a blue dye that mark the amount of flow.
3. In sialography, a radiopaque contrast medium is introduced in the major duct of a major salivary gland, followed by routine radiographs, and the image is called a sialogram. In Sjogren syndrome, areas of destruction are seen in the radiographs. MRI sialography is more accurate than conventional sialography.[3]

MEDICATIONS WITH THE STRONGEST EVIDENCE OF INTERFERENCE WITH SALIVARY GLAND FUNCTION

The authors are using the compiled list from Dr Wolff's systematic review "Guide to medications inducing salivary gland dysfunction, xerostomia and subjective sialorrhea." This review compiled a list of medications with documented effects on salivary gland function or symptoms. The reviewers performed an in-depth analysis in literature that found links between medications and salivary gland dysfunction. They also stratified these studies with a degree of relevance and strength. They provided a list of 56 medications with strong evidence of interference with salivary gland function. Later, the authors describe the highest cited medications commonly used that are linked to xerostomia and salivary gland dysfunction. They also include a table with the other medications that present with high evidence.[4]

Alendronate (Fosamax)

The oral specialist should be very familiar with alendronic acid and its fellow bisphosphonate derivatives. This medication is among many others to be cited in the literature for increased risk of medication-related osteonecrosis to the jaw (MRONJ) along with links causing salivary gland hypofunction.[5]

Mechanism of action
Alendronate is a nitrogen containing bisphosphonate that attaches to hydroxyapatite crystals in the bone. When osteoclasts begin their function

to resorb bone, it releases and inhibits further function by decreasing binding, resorptive activity, and inducing apoptosis.[6]

Uses
Alendronate is most commonly used in conditions that cause excessive bone resorption such as osteoporosis, Paget disease, and metastatic bone diseases.[6]

Adverse affects
According to the AAOMS position paper on MRONJ, there is a derived incidence of 0.004% (4 cases per 10,000) patient-years of exposure to alendronate.[5]

Amitriptyline

Imipramine (Tofranil) was the first drug in the tricyclic antidepressant family, although initially used to treat bed wetting (enuresis) in children during the 1950s. Increased observations at this time revealed increased evidence that in 1958, imipramine (Tofranil) was successful in the treatment of depression. Amitriptyline is among many tricyclic antidepressants that were synthesized in 1960 after the success of imipramine. These tricyclic antidepressants (TCAs) had become the first line of treatment for 30 years in the treatment of depression before the development of serotonin reuptake inhibitors.[7]

Mechanism of action
Amitriptyline (tertiary amine), as other TCAs, are named based on their structure and side chain functions. They are divided into 2 classes: tertiary amines and secondary amines. Tertiary amines have 2 methyl groups, whereas secondary amines have one methyl group at the end of their side chain.[8] They act primarily by increasing serotonergic and noradrenergic neurons by inhibiting central serotonin and noradrenaline reuptake at the synapse.[7] Tertiary amines are more potent at blocking reuptake of serotonin, whereas secondary amines are more potent in blocking norepinephrine.[8]

Uses
Amitriptyline is approved by Food and Drug Administration (FDA) for the treatment of depression. Its off-label use includes treatment of anxiety, chronic pain syndromes, migraines, sialorrhea, and posttraumatic stress disorder among others.[9]

Metabolism
They are metabolized by first pass hepatic metabolism in the liver by cytochrome p450 enzymes CYP2D6 and CYP2C19 to nortriptyline.[7]

Adverse effects
The use of amitriptyline has decreased after the introduction of selective serotonin reuptake inhibitors (SSRIs). This decrease can be attributed to its adverse side effects, which includes its potential for cardiac toxicity, serotonin syndrome (confusion, agitation, dilated pupils, headache, nausea, vomiting diarrhea, tachycardia, twitching diaphoresis, and shivering), and antimuscarinic effect.

Cardiac effects: alone or when administered with other medications, TCAs such as amitriptyline can cause prolongation of the QT interval, which increases risk of ventricular arrhythmias.

Antimuscarinic effects include dry eyes, hyposalivary gland function, xerostomia, and sedation.[7] As discussed previously, hyposalivation and xerostomia can increase the incidence of dental caries and other oral detriment.

Seizures: all tricyclic antidepressants decrease the seizure threshold and thus increase likeliness to increase seizures. Amitriptyline has a seizure rate of 1% to 4% at doses 250 mg/d to 450 mg/d.[8]

Aripiprazole (Abilify)

Aripiprazole was cited 5 times with a high evidence of inducing xerostomia according to the world workshop oral medicine systematic review. It is classified as an atypical antipsychotic indicated for treatment of mania associated with bipolar I disorder.[10]

Mechanism of action
Aripiprazole acts as a partial agonist of dopamine D2 and D3 and serotonin 5-HT1A receptors and also antagonizes the 5-HT2A receptor. It is hypothesized that dopamine hyperactivity contributes to mania, thus when aripiprazole binds to the receptor, it stimulates the receptor to 25% to 30% of maximal dopamine activity.[10] Aripiprazole has moderate alpha-1 adrenergic and H1 receptor activity and mild muscarinic receptor activity.[10]

Adverse reactions
Because of the mild alpha-1 adrenergic antagonism, there is possibility for antihypertensive when coadministered with central acting drugs or alcohol.[10]

Metabolism
Abilify is extensively metabolized by the liver via dehydrogenation and hydroxylation by P450 (CYP) 3A4 and CYP2D6 enzymes and N-dealkylation by the CYP3A4 enzyme.[10]

Atropine

Atropine (Atropen) is a commonly used anticholinergic agent primarily indicated for the treatment of symptomatic bradycardia. Other uses include use as an inhibitor of salivation and secretions.[11]

Atropine is given intravenously or intramuscularly, 0.5 to 1 mg, every 3 to 5 minutes to a maximum total dose of 3 mg for the treatment of symptomatic bradycardia.

Mechanism of action

Atropine works by inhibiting acetylcholine at parasympathetic sites in smooth muscles and secretory glands, innervated by the central nervous system, and this will cause an increase in cardiac output and inhibit secretions. It also works to reverse cholinergic poisoning.

Adverse reactions

Cardiovascular: lethal arrhythmias, asystole, atrial fibrillation, aches pain, decreased blood pressure, electrocardiogram changes, ectopic beats, ventricular fibrillation, and ventricular flutter.

Ophthalmic: abnormal eye movements, dry eyes, and decreased secretions.

Bupropion (Wellbutrin)

Bupropion is a monocyclic aminoketone and classified as an atypical antidepressant, a different class when compared with SSRIs and TCAs. It is commonly used in patients with major depression or in situations where the other classes are not effective or are creating undesirable side effect.[12]

Mechanism of action

Bupropion inhibits reuptake of dopamine and norepinephrine in the presynaptic terminal. It has a larger effect on dopamine than norepinephrine.[13]

Black box warning

Bupropion has a potential effect of suicide ideation, which must be discussed with the patient.

Adverse reactions

Patients taking bupropion also are at an increased risk of seizures, dry mouth, nausea, insomnia, dizziness, anxiety, sinusitis, and tremor.[14]

Twenty-one percent of patients on bupropion complain of dry mouth, and it is one of the most highly cited drugs in connection with xerostomia.[14]

Clozapine (Clozaril)

Similar to bupropion, clozapine is characterized as an atypical antipsychotic (second generation). It is most commonly used in the treatment of schizophrenia, especially those who fail to respond to classic antipsychotic treatment. Clozapine is also used to reduce suicidal behavior in patients with schizophrenia.

Off-label uses

Clozapine is used for bipolar disorder, especially when standard treatment is not effective, and for psychosis/agitation and psychosis in Parkinson disease.

Mechanism of action

Clozapine is an antagonist to the dopamine type 2 (D2) and serotonin type 2A receptors. It also acts as an antagonist to histamine, cholinergic, and alpha-adrenergic receptors.

Black box warning

Clozapine can cause severe neutropenia. Because of the risks associated with clozapine, clozapine is only available through the REMS program (Clozapine Risk Evaluation and Mitigation Strategy Program). It will not be dispensed without both your doctor and pharmacist being registered in REMS. Other warnings include orthostatic hypotension, bradycardia, syncope, secures, and myocarditis. Clozapine has anticholinergic effects and is highly associated with development of xerostomia, constipation, and urinary retention.

Adverse reactions

Clozaril can cause hypertension, hypotension, tachycardia, constipation, nausea, sialorrhea, vomiting, dizziness, and drowsiness.

Duloxetine (Cymbalta) and Venlafaxine (Effexor)

Duloxetine and venlafaxine are serotonin-norepinephrine reuptake inhibitors (SNRIs) that are prescribed for depressive conditions such as unipolar major depression, persistent depressive disorder, and anxiety disorder.[15] Duloxetine is also used for chronic pain syndromes and fibromyalgia.[15]

Mechanism of action

SNRIs treat depression by blocking presynaptic serotonin and norepinephrine transporter proteins that cause an increase in postsynaptic stimulation. Duloxetine is also a more potent inhibitor of serotonin reuptake.[16,17]

Black box warning

In young adults and pediatric patients, duloxetine and venlafaxine have been associated with an increased risk of suicidal ideation and suicidal behavior.[15]

Adverse effects

Clinical studies performed by Hudson showed adverse effects of duloxetine, which included nausea, xerostomia, constipation, insomnia, dizziness, fatigue, diarrhea, somnolence, diaphoresis, and anorexia.[18]

Olanzapine (Zyprexa) and Quetiapine (Seroquel)

Quetiapine is a commonly used second-generation antipsychotic for bipolar I or II major depression disorders. The American Psychiatric Association's diagnostic and statistical manual of mental disorders (DSM-5 th edition) defines major depressive disorder (unipolar major depression) as a period lasting at least 2 weeks, with 5 or more of the following symptoms: depressed mood, loss of interest or pleasure in most activities, insomnia or hypersonic, change in appetite or weight, psychomotor retardation or agitation, decreased energy, poor concentration, thoughts of worthlessness or guilt, and recurrent thoughts about death or suicide.[19] Bipolar disorder is marked by episodes of mania, hypomania, and nearly includes episodes of major depression. For patients with bipolar major depression, olanzapine is frequently used as a monotherapy.[20]

Black box warning
Increased mortality in elderly patients with dementia-related psychosis.

Mechanism of action
As previously described, olanzapine and quetiapine are second-generation antipsychotics and work as antagonist to the serotonin 5-HT2A and 5-HT2C, dopamine, histamine H1, and alpha-1 adrenergic receptors.

Adverse effects
According to a systematic review and meta-analysis, quetiapine has been found to cause major adverse effects such as sedation, weight gain, *xerostomia,* headache, dizziness, nausea, constipation, and extrapyramidal symptoms.[20] That same systematic analysis has found olanzapine to cause sedation, weight gain, increased appetite, xerostomia and possible hypo salivary gland function, weakness, headache, hypercholesterolemia, hypertriglyceridemia, hyperglycemia, and neutropenia.

Oxybutynin (Oxytrol and Ditropan), Solifenacin (VESIcare), and Tolterodine (Detrol)

The primary therapy involved in urinary incontinence involves conservative therapy. These include changes to lifestyle/obesity factors, kegel exercises, and bladder training.[21] If primary measures do not improve symptoms, pharmacologic therapies are available. The 2 types of therapies include antimuscarinic agents and beta-adrenergic therapy.

Oxybutynin, solifenacin, and tolterodine are 3 of 6 commonly prescribed muscarinics for treatment of urinary incontinence.

Mechanism of action
Oxybutynin has a direct antispasmodic effect on smooth muscle and also is an acetylcholine inhibitor on smooth muscle.[21]

Solifenacin inhibits muscarinic receptors that decrease contraction of the urinary bladder, increase residual urine volume, and decrease detrusor muscle pressure.[21]

Tolterodine is a competitive antagonist of muscarinic receptors and very selective for receptors in the bladder.

Adverse reactions
Because of their anticholinergic activity, all 3 of these medications cause xerostomia and salivary gland dysfunction (**Table 1**).

TREATMENT

Numerous treatments are available for xerostomia. The patient should be advised to increase hydration. There are over-the-counter medications consisting of saliva substitutes, and mouth rinses are available to improve daily quality of life. Saliva Orthana is a mucin-based product that stimulates release of the lubricant and stimulates salivation. The oral gel, Biotene is another saliva substitute that has an antimicrobial action as well as decreases the sensation of dryness.[3] Sugar-free sour candy is also a simple method to stimulate salivary flow.

There are 2 prescription medications approved by the FDA for treatment of xerostomia: pilocarpine (Isopto Carpine and Salagen) and cevimeline (Evoxac). Both of these medications act as cholinergic agonists that increase serous secretions. Cevimeline is used to treat dry mouth associated with Sjogren syndrome as a cholinergic stimulant to increase salivary production. Common side effects of Evoxac include sweating, excessive salivation, nausea, loss of appetite, runny or stuffy nose, frequent urge to urinate, dizziness, weakness, and diarrhea. Pilocarpine is only approved for patients undergoing head and neck radiation and patients with Sjogren syndrome.[1] Pilocarpine is contraindicated in patients with uncontrolled asthma, closed angle/narrow angle glaucoma, and liver disease.[1]

BURNING MOUTH SYNDROME

Burning mouth syndrome (BMS) has been referred to with different names based on the location and

Table 1
Medications that cause xerostomia or salivary gland hypofunction with high level of evidence

Drug Name	Drug Category	Mechanism of Action	Xerostomia or SGH
Baclofen	Central acting skeletal muscle relaxant	GABA agonist: reduces release of excitatory glutamate	Xerostomia
Bendroflumethiazide	Weak diuretic	Inhibits reabsorption of NaCl in distal tubule of nephron	SGH
Bevacizumab	Antineoplastic	Monoclonal antibody: inhibits vascular proliferation and tumor growth	Xerostomia
Brimonidine	Antiglaucoma	Alpha-2 adrenergic agonist	Xerostomia
Buprenorphine	Opioid analgesic	Mixed receptor actions; kappa-opioid antagonist and partial mu-opioid agonist	Xerostomia
Butorphanol	Opioid analgesic	Mixed receptor actions; kappa-agonist and mu-antagonist	Xerostomia
Chlorpromazine	Antipsychotic	Antagonist to dopamine, 5-HT, histamine (H1), muscarinic and alpha(1,2) adrenergic receptors	Xerostomia
Citalopram	Antidepressant	Selective 5-HT reuptake inhibitor	Xerostomia
Clonidine	Antihypertensive/ antimigraine	Alpha-2 adrenergic agonist	SGH
Clozapine	Atypical antipsychotic	Dopamine antagonist, partial 5-HT and partial muscarinic(M1) agonist muscarinic (M3) antagonist, and alpha1 adrenergic antagonist	Xerostomia
Cyclobenzaprine	Centrally acting skeletal muscle relaxant	Histamine (H1) and muscarinic antagonist	Xerostomia
Dexmethylphenidate	Psychostimulant—ADHD	Indirect sympathomimetic and NE/dopamine reuptake inhibitor	Xerostomia
Dimebon	Antidementia	Unknown—proposed histamine (H1) and 5-HT antagonist	Xerostomia
Doxylamine	Hypnotic	Antihistamine, histamine (H1), and muscarinic antagonist	Xerostomia
Duloxetine	Antidepressant	5-HT/NE reuptake inhibitor	Xerostomia

(continued on next page)

Table 1
(continued)

Drug Name	Drug Category	Mechanism of Action	Xerostomia or SGH
Escitalopram	Antidepressant	Selective 5-HT reuptake inhibitor	Xerostomia
Fluoxetine	Antidepressant	Selective 5-HT reuptake inhibitor	Xerostomia and SGH
Furosemide	Diuretic	Inhibits reabsorption of NaCl in thick ascending loop of Henle	Xerostomia and SGH
Gabapentin	Anticonvulsant	Stimulates GABA synthesis and GABA release	Xerostomia
Imidafenacin	Reduces bladder activity	Antimuscarinic	Xerostomia
Imipramine	Anti-depressant	5-HT/NE reuptake inhibitor, inhibitor to histamine, 5-HT, muscarinic, and alpha 1 adrenergic receptors	Xerostomia
Lisdexamfetamine	Psychostimulant—ADHD	5-HT/NE reuptake inhibitor	Xerostomia
Lithium	Antipsychotic	Mood stabilizer; inhibits dopamine/NE release and intracellular $Ca2+$ mobilization	Xerostomia
Loxapine	Antipsychotic	Dopamine/5-HT antagonist	Xerostomia
Methylphenidate	Psychostimulant—ADHD	Indirect sympathomimetic release of dopamine and NE/5-HT reuptake inhibitor	Xerostomia
Nortriptyline	Antidepressant	NE reuptake inhibitor, antagonist to histamine (H1), 5-HT, alpha-1 adrenergic, and muscarinics	Xerostomia
Paliperidone	Atypical antipsychotic	Antagonist to dopamine, 5-HT, alpha(1,2)-adrenergics, and histamine	Xerostomia
Paroxetine	Antidepressant	5-HT reuptake inhibitor	Xerostomia and SGH
Perphenazine	Antipsychotic	Antagonist to 5-HT, dopamine, histamine (H1), muscarinic, and alpha-1 adrenergic receptors	Xerostomia
Phentermine	Appetite suppressant	Releases NE and to a lesser degree dopamine and 5-HT	Xerostomia
Propantheline	Antiperistaltic/spasmolytic	Antimuscarinic	Xerostomia and SGH

(continued on next page)

Table 1
(continued)

Drug Name	Drug Category	Mechanism of Action	Xerostomia or SGH
Propiverine	Urological—reduces bladder activity	Antimuscarinic	Xerostomia and SGH
Reboxetine	Antidepressant	NE Reuptake inhibitor, antimuscarinic	Xerostomia
Ziprasidone	Atypical antipsychotic	5-HT, dopamine, and alpha-adrenergic antagonist	Xerostomia
Zolpidem	Hypnotic/sedative	Agonist of GABAa receptor	Xerostomia

Abbreviations: ADHD, attention-deficit hyperactivity disorder; GABA, gamma aminobutyric acid; HT, hydroxytryptamine; NE, norepinephrine; SGH, salivary gland hypofunction.

Data from Wolff A, Joshi RK, Ekström J, Aframian D, Pedersen AM, Proctor G, Narayana N, Villa A, Sia YW, Aliko A, McGowan R, Kerr AR, Jensen SB, Vissink A, Dawes C. A Guide to Medications Inducing Salivary Gland Dysfunction, Xerostomia, and Subjective Sialorrhea: A Systematic Review Sponsored by the World Workshop on Oral Medicine VI. Drugs R D. 2017 Mar;17(1):1-28.

quality of pain: burning mouth condition, burning lips syndrome, scalded mouth syndrome, stomatodynia, oral dysesthesia, glossopyrosis, and stomatopyrosis. BMS is defined by the International Association for the Study of Pain as burning in the tongue or other oral mucous membrane associated with normal laboratory findings that lasts 4 to 6 months. The International classification of Headache Disorders describes it as an intraoral burning sensation for which there are no medical- or dental-related causes.[22]

Epidemiology

The incidence that women experience BMS is 3 to 16x more likely than men: highest incidence in postmenopausal women aged 50 to 89 years with maximal incidence in women aged 70 to 79 years.[22]

Clinical Findings

The most common affected areas are the anterior two-thirds, tip, the dorsum, and the anterior lateral margins of the tongue. Other areas include the anterior hard palate, mucosal aspect of the lip, and mandibular alveolar regions. BMS is typically bilateral and symmetric. Most patients with BMS will subjectively report xerostomia, dyspepsia, sialorrhea, halitosis and dysphaigia.[22]

Clinical signs of BMS include the following:

1. Frothy saliva (indicative of parotid hypofunction and dominance of mucoid-type submandibular gland saliva)
2. Dryness of the lower lip
3. Scalloping of the lateral lingual marginals due to habitual pressure against the adjacent teeth

4. Buccal mucosal irregularity with leukoedema, translucent keratosis, and a prominent linea alba
5. Low-grade erythema of the anterior dorsum of the tongue to traumatic abrasion of the filiform papillae and exposure of the sensitive fungiform papillae
6. Low-grade erythema of the coincident anterior hard palate
7. Low-grade linear erythema of the inner aspect of the lip

Causes

1. Hormonal: studies found that among menopausal women with BMS, follicle-stimulating hormones were higher, whereas estradiol was significantly lower.[22]
2. Smoking: there is a significant link between cigarette smoking and patients with BMS.
3. Medications: as noted in the previous sections, many medications can alter salivary flow; these medications have also been found in patients with BMS.[22]
4. Xerostomia and salivary gland hypofunction: it is multifactorial, comprising both physiologic and psychological reasons. Please refer to previous section.
5. Nutritional deficiencies: BMS has links to nutritional deficiencies including vitamins and minerals, more specifically those associated with anemia: iron and vitamin B12 deficiency. Others include zinc and vitamin B complexes.
6. Candidiasis: candidiasis has been linked to BMS very closely due to similar predisposing factors such as nutritional deficiency, diabetes, and change in salivary function.[23]

Burning Mouth Syndrome Classification

Type 1: characterize day burning sensation that is not present on waking but develops late in the morning and progresses throughout the day with greatest discomfort in the evening (**Fig. 1**).

Type 2: a burning sensation that remains constant throughout the day and prevents the patient from falling asleep.

Type 3: characterize day intermittent symptoms and symptom-free periods with variable presence between days and may experience the symptoms at unusual sites (floor of mouth and buccal mucosa).

Primary BMS: when no clinical or laboratory test abnormalities are present.

Secondary BMS: there is an identifiable underlying cause for BMS.

Pathophysiology

Neuropathic: dysfunction in the trigeminal nerve and chorda tympani induces an alteration of the sensitivity threshold and reflection in the trigeminal area. Neural alterations reduce the threshold of pain transmission and transmit an ascending nociceptive signal that is not transmitted under healthy conditions. In BMS, alteration of gray matter is recognized in the prefrontal cortex, anterior cingulate gyrus, and hippocampus. Thus, it is proposed that central sensitization is one of the many entities that plays a role in BMS.[22]

Endocrine: decreased synthesis of ovarian steroids after menopause induces deficiency or dysfunction in adrenal steroids, which abolishes the neuroprotective effects of steroids on neural tissues.[22]

Psychological: several studies suggest link between anxiety and depressive disorders in unexplained somatic symptoms. The patients with BMS have self-reported poorer health and complain of more illnesses, gastrointestinal problems, chronic fatigue, disturbed sleep patterns, and headaches; are anxious; and have low self-esteem. BMS have higher levels of neuroticism in all facets: anxiety, anger, hostility, depression, self-consciousness, impulsiveness, and vulnerability. To support this somatoform pain disorder model of BMS anxiolytic drugs, such as SSRI and amisulpride, can cause an improvement in BMS symptoms.[22]

Treatment

There are no standard treatment protocols. However, physiologic and psychological aspects of this disease can be managed and addressed through various means (**Table 2**).

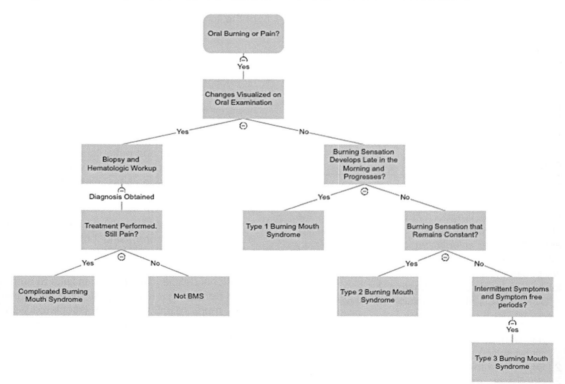

Fig. 1. Burning mouth syndrome classification.

Table 2
Treatment of burning mouth syndrome

Drug Name	Drug Category	Mechanism	Topical or Systemic
Clonazepam	Benzodiazepine	Agonist of GABA receptor	Topical and systemic
Capsaicin	Topical analgesic	TRPV1 agonist	Topical
Alpha-lipoic acid	Antioxidant	Debated in literature	Systemic
Gabapentin	Anticonvulsant	GABA agonist	Systemic
Nystatin	Antifungal	Binds to ergosterol	Topical
Vitamin B complex	Multivitamin	Cofactor	Systemic
Magic mouthwash	Combination therapy	Multiple mechanisms	Topical

CLINICS CARE POINTS

- Xerostomia is the subjective feeling of dry mouth or sensation of oral dryness, whereas hyposalivation is the actual decrease in measured salivary outflow.

- Mean unstimulated salivary outflow of healthy persons ranges from 0.3 to 0.4 mL/min. An unstimulated flow of less than 0.1 mL/min is considered evidence of salivary hypofunction.

- Lubrication, moistening, and protection of the oral mucosa and esophagus, as well as assisting in both taste and smell. Saliva also provides enzymes that aid in digestion.

- The acquired enamel pellicle that surrounds teeth are composed of salivary proteins that act to protect teeth. They decrease friction from opposing teeth and protect against attrition, abrasion, and foreign trauma.

- The MST uses paper strips that are placed in a blue dye that mark the amount of salivary flow.

- The 2 prescription medications approved by the FDA for xerostomia are pilocarpine and cevimeline.

REFERENCES

1. Rayman S, Dincer E, Almas K. Xerostomia. Diagnosis and management in dental practice. N Y State Dent J 2010;76(2):24–7.
2. Dawes C, et al. The functions of human saliva: a review sponsored by the World Workshop on Oral Medicine VI. Arch Oral Biol 2015;60(6):863–74.
3. Eveson JW. Xerostomia. Periodontology 2000;48(1):85–91.
4. Wolff A, et al. A guide to medications inducing salivary gland dysfunction, xerostomia, and subjective sialorrhea: a systematic review sponsored by the world workshop on oral medicine VI. Drugs R D 2017;17(1):1–28.
5. Ruggiero SL, et al. American Association of Oral and Maxillofacial Surgeons position paper on medication-related osteonecrosis of the jaw—2014 update. J Oral Maxill Surg 2014;72(10):1938–56.
6. Drake MT, Clarke BL, Khosla S. Bisphosphonates: mechanism of action and role in clinical practice. Mayo Clinic Proc 2008;83(9):1032–45.
7. Devine K. Amitriptyline. Pract Diabetes 2016;33(1):34–5.
8. Nelson JC. Tricyclic and tetracyclic drugs. In: Schatzberg AF, Nemeroff CB, editors. The American psychiatric association publishing textbook of psychopharmacology. Fifth edition. Arlington, VA: American Psychiatric Association Publishing; 2017. p. 305.
9. Radley DC, Finkelstein SN, Stafford RS. Off-label prescribing among office-based physicians. Arch Intern Med 2006;166(9):1021–6.
10. Dhillon S. Aripiprazole. Drugs 2012;72(1):133–62.
11. Peterson LJ. Peterson's principles of oral and maxillofacial surgery, vol. 1. PMPH-USA; 2012.
12. Rush AJ, et al. Bupropion-SR, sertraline, or venlafaxine-XR after failure of SSRIs for depression. N Engl J Med 2006;354(12):1231–42.
13. Horst WD, Preskorn SH. Mechanisms of action and clinical characteristics of three atypical antidepressants: venlafaxine, nefazodone, bupropion. J Affect Disord 1998;51(3):237–54.
14. Clayton AH, Gillespie EH. Bupropion 2009.
15. Norris S, Blier P. Duloxetine, milnacipran, and levomilnacipran. In: Schatzberg AF, Nemeroff CB, editors. The American psychiatric association publishing textbook of psychopharmacology. 2017. p. 529–47.
16. Thase ME, Sloan DM. Venlafaxine and desvenlafaxine. In: The American psychiatric publishing textbook of psychopharmacology. 4th edition. Arlington, VA: American Psychiatric Publishing; 2009. p. 439–52.
17. Tyrer P. Drug treatment of psychiatric patients in general practice. Br Med J 1978;2(6143):1008–10.

18. Hudson JI, et al. Safety and tolerability of duloxetine in the treatment of major depressive disorder: analysis of pooled data from eight placebo-controlled clinical trials. Hum Psychopharmacol Clin Exp 2005;20(5):327–41.

19. Edition F. Diagnostic and statistical manual of mental disorders. Am Psychiatr Assoc 2013;21.

20. De Fruyt J, et al. Second generation antipsychotics in the treatment of bipolar depression: a systematic review and meta-analysis. J Psychopharmacol 2012;26(5):603–17.

21. Wood LN, Anger JT. Urinary incontinence in women. BMJ 2014;349.

22. Dym H, Lin S, Thakkar J. Neuropathic pain and burning mouth syndrome: an overview and current update. Dent Clin 2020;64(2):379–99.

23. Terai H, Shimahara M. Glossodynia from Candida-associated lesions, burning mouth syndrome, or mixed causes. Pain Med 2010;11(6):856–60.

Updates on Topical and Local Anesthesia Agents

Junaid Mundiya, DMD*, Edward Woodbine, DDS

KEYWORDS

- Topical anesthesia • Local anesthesia • Local anesthesia delivery
- Local anesthesia potency and toxicity

KEY POINTS

- The goal for topical anesthesia is to blunt the effect of administration of local anesthesia.
- Local anesthetics are divided into esters and amides, amides being commonly used.
- Local anesthesia is dose dependent. Maximum dosage should be calculated to prevent toxicity in pediatrics and adult patients.
- Amide local anesthesia is safe for breastfeeding women.
- Advances in local anesthesia administration can make the experience more tolerable for the patients.

INTRODUCTION

Use of topical and local anesthesia (LA) is the workhorse of all aspects of dentistry.[1] There was a time in the past when dentistry was performed without any local pain control. Owing to this there are patients with dental anxiety and fear of a dental office. The media portraying dentistry as being painful, or showing a dentist with needles, enlists fear and distrust of dentists. In contrast, pain is what brings the patient to the dental office and with local pain control measures a dentist is able to alleviate the patient's cause of pain.[1]

TOPICAL ANESTHETICS

The role of topical anesthetic is to minimize painful stimuli or dull the effect of the procedure. A painful stimulus can be a procedure, injections, or to blunt gag reflexes. LA can be administered as gels, cream, ointment, liquid, sprays, or lotions.

Benzocaine is one of the most common topical anesthetics; it can be purchased over the counter or prescription based. Benzocaine is an ester derivative topical anesthetic.[2] The pharmacophysiology of benzocaine is that it binds selectively to the intracellular surface of sodium channels to block influx of sodium into axons.[2] The role of benzocaine in dentistry is to provide relief from dental pain or to lessen the painful experience of injection of LA. There are different formulations, combinations, and brands of topical anesthesia. Cetacaine is a combination of benzocaine, tetracaine, butyl aminobenzoate, and benzalkonium chloride.[1] Cetacaine is available as a spray, and it is commonly used before dental impressions to control the gag reflex.

Tetracaine is an ester-type local anesthetic. Ester is metabolized in the plasma and in the liver by plasma pseudocholinesterase. Tetracaine should not be used in patients with liver disease.[3] Tetracaine is commonly used in medicine for spinal anesthesia, and LA to the eye and nose for diagnostic examinations; it is not commonly used in dentistry.[4]

Flurori-methane is a topical local anesthetic spray that aids in myofascial pain in patients with temporomandibular dysfunction. The goal of the local anesthetic spray is to assist in stretch therapy after application of the spray. The spray should be 12 in away from the muscle, and care should be taken to cover the patient's eyes before application.[2]

Department of Dentistry and Oral and Maxillofacial Surgery, The Brooklyn Hospital Center, 121 DeKalb Avenue, Brooklyn, NY 11201, USA
* Corresponding author.
E-mail address: Junaidmundiya@gmail.com

Oral Maxillofacial Surg Clin N Am 34 (2022) 147–155
https://doi.org/10.1016/j.coms.2021.08.003
1042-3699/22/© 2021 Elsevier Inc. All rights reserved.

Lidocaine is probably the most common topical and local anesthetic; it is classified as an amide. Topical lidocaine is available as 5% base and 2% water soluble. When lidocaine is used in its viscous state (0.5%, 1.0%, and 2.0%) form, the goal is to help patients with pain in mucositis secondary to chemotherapy and radiation therapy. The topical application also helps patients suffering from autoimmune blistering disease such as pemphigus and pemphigoid of the oral cavity. Most obstetricians and gynecologists prefer lidocaine applications in their patients because it is classified as a category B drug.[1] In the pediatric population the clinician must be aware of the maximum dosage of lidocaine that should be considered, which is 4 mg/kg without epinephrine.[1]

LOCAL ANESTHETICS

The goal for LA is to provide loss of sensation at the area of the body by depression of excitation in nerve endings and inhibition of the conduction process in peripheral nerves. LA takes its effect by decreasing the permeability of the ion channels to sodium therefore decreasing the rate of depolarization.[5] All the local anesthetics have an aromatic ring that gives them lipid solubility. Adequate LA has been found to reduce the need for inhalation anesthetics for patients undergoing general anesthesia Local anesthetics are divided into amides and ester.[5]

Ideal properties for local anesthetics are they should not be an irritant, and they should not be neurotoxic, which can lead to permanent alteration of nerve structures. The systemic toxicity should be low. Their efficacy is comparable when injected into deep tissue as well as mucous membranes. The duration of onset is short. The duration of LA is based on the drug selected, which is based on the length of the procedure. There is potency for anesthesia without the use of harmful concentration. One should also choose a local anesthetic that does not cause an allergic reaction. The drug is able to undergo biotransformation in the body.

Amide local anesthetics are metabolized in the liver and no *para*-aminobenzoic acid (PABA) is formed. The amine terminal end gives these local anesthetics their water solubility. Common amide local anesthetics include lidocaine, mepivacaine, prilocaine, articaine, etidocaine, and bupivacaine. The dosage of amide local anesthetic should be adjusted for patients with medical comorbidities[5] (**Table 1**).

Ester local anesthetics are hydrolyzed in the plasma by pseudocholinesterase, and they form PABA as their by-product from metabolism.

PABA is known to cause allergic reactions including tissue sloughing and dermatitis. Ester local anesthetics are also potent vasodilators, therefore increasing the rate of absorption of local anesthetic and decreasing its duration of action.[5] Ester local anesthetics are not used commonly in dentistry because of their allergic potential and decreased efficacy compared with amides (**Table 2**).

There are a few factors that affect local anesthetic transformation and distribution in the body. These factors for amide local anesthetic include liver function. If the liver function is not in its normal limits, the half-life of amides is increased. LA plasma protein binding capacity and blood volume also contribute to biotransformation and distribution.[4] Generally speaking, the primary excretory organ for local anesthetics is the kidneys. In patients with renal pathology, the maximum calculated drug dose should be decreased.[4]

When selecting local anesthetic for a procedure the length of the procedure and the duration of the local anesthetic should be considered.[6] The duration of LA depends on individual variation of the drug, which is depicted by a normal distribution, and the accuracy of administration. A drug administered close to a targeted nerve will lead to a longer duration and greater depth of anesthesia. In contrast, when the LA is administered away from the targeted nerve the efficacy and duration will be decreased. When administering LA in an infected site, the vascularity and pH of the tissue should be considered.[6] The LA duration and efficacy is usually decreased in infected tissue.

The central nervous system (CNS) and the cardiovascular system are most susceptible to the increased level of plasma levels of local anesthetic. Blood levels of local anesthetic depend on biotransformation, distribution, and rate of uptake. CNS effects of LA can be seen as CNS depression.[1] Local anesthetics can easily cross the blood-brain barrier and cause biphasic reactions and seizures. CNS depression can also lead to respiratory arrest. In the cardiovascular system, local anesthesia can decrease electrical excitability of the myocardium, which results in decrease in the rate of conduction, and hence a decrease in the force of contraction.[1] Vasodilation is seen initially as the plasma level of local anesthetic increases; it is followed by myocardium depression and decrease in blood pressure. CNS depression is seen before cardiovascular system depression. Clinical signs and symptoms of LA overdose are blurred vision, dizziness, headache, ringing in ears, disorientation, flushing, numbness of tongue, perioral numbness, and possibly loss of consciousness.[1]

Table 1
Amide local anesthesia

Drug	Facts[1,6]	Comments
Lidocaine	• Classification = Amide • Metabolism = Liver • Excretion = Kidneys (>80% metabolites, <10% unchanged) • pH (with epi) = 3.5 • pKa = 7.9 • Onset = 3–5 min • Half-life = 1.6 h	• Introduced in 1948 • First amide to be marketed • Commonly used as a 2% solution with 1: 100,000 epi in dentistry • Toxicity may present as initial mild sedation instead of excitatory symptoms • Less vasodilation compared with procaine • More vasodilation compared with prilocaine or bupivacaine • Topical anesthetic is available • Compared with procaine, rapid onset of action, longer duration, and greater potency • epi-sensitive patients are limited to 2 carpules of 1: 100,000 epi • Use 1: 50,000 epi for hemostasis
Mepivacaine	• Classification = Amide • Metabolism = Liver • Excretion = Kidney (<16% excreted unchanged) • pKa = 7.6 • pH = 5.5–6.0 • Onset = 3–5 min • Half- life = 1.9 h	• Introduced in 1960 • Produce slight vasoconstriction. Therefore, longer duration of anesthesia relative to others without vasoconstrictors • Use 3% without epi in patient in whom a vasoconstrictor is not indicated
Prilocaine	• Classification = Amide • Metabolism = In the liver, kidney, and lung • Excretion = Kidneys • pKa = 7.9 • pH (with epi) = 3.0–4.0 • Onset = 2–4 min • Half-life = 1.6 h	• Introduced in 1960 • Not available as a topical • Renal clearance • Metabolism in the liver produces carbon dioxide, orthotolidine, and N-propyl alanine • In larger doses, orthotolidine can lead to methemoglobinemia. This will reduce the blood oxygen-carrying capacity • Less toxic due to plasma levels decreasing more rapidly compared with lidocaine • Less vasodilation effect, therefore can be used as a plain solution • CNS toxicity signs are brief and less severe than lidocaine • Cardiac patients can receive a maximum of 4 carpules of prilocaine with 1:200,000 epi • Indicated for epi-sensitive patients • Relative contraindication in patients with methemoglobinemia, sickle cell anemia, or symptoms of hypoxia

(continued on next page)

Table 1
(continued)

Drug	Facts[1,6]	Comments
Articaine	• Classification = Amide • Metabolism = Plasma and liver producing free carboxylic acid. • Excretion = Via kidney (<10% unchanged, >90% metabolites) • pKa = 7.8 • pH (with epi) = 3.5–4.0 • Onset = 1–3 min • Half-life = 1.25 h	• Introduced in 1976 • Faster onset of action compared with other amides • An analogue to prilocaine in which benzene rings found in all other amides have been replaced with thiophene rings • Vasodilatory properties similar to lidocaine • Methemoglobinemia is a potential side effect • Contraindicated in patients with sulfa allergies because it contains methylparaben
Bupivacaine	• Classification = Amide • Metabolism = Liver • Excretion = Kidney • pKa = 8.1 • pH (with epi) = 3.0–4.5 • Onset = 6–10 min • Half-life = 2.7 h	• Introduced in 1983 • The carbons added to mepivacaine molecules increase potency and duration of action • Greater vasodilation than lidocaine but less than procaine • Indicated for management of postoperative pain • Longer onset compared with lidocaine or mepivacaine
Etidocaine	• Classification = Amide • Metabolism = N- dealkylation in the liver. • Excretion = Kidney • pKa = 7.7 • pH (with epi) = 3.0–3.5 • Onset = 1.5–3.0 min • Half- life = 2.6 h	• Carbons are added to the lidocaine molecule, which increases potency and duration of action • No longer in the market • Greater vasodilation than lidocaine • Longer acting and has similar indications to bupivacaine

Abbreviation: epi, epinephrine.
Adapted from Boyce RA, Kirpalani T, Mohan N. Updates of topical and local anesthesia agents. Dent Clin North Am. 2016 Apr;60(2):445-71.

The role of vasoconstrictors in LA is to constrict the blood vessels in the area of injection. Vasoconstrictor plays a role in lowering the rate of absorption of local anesthetic in the bloodstream. In result, there is a prolonged effect of LA and lower risk of toxicity. Epinephrine is a common vasoconstrictor injected with local anesthetic.[7] The advantages of epinephrine are reduction of blood level of the local anesthetic being administered, longer pulpal anesthesia, and reduction of blood loss. The maximum dose of epinephrine is 0.2 mg for healthy patients and 0.04 mg for cardiac patients.[7] If local anesthetic with epinephrine is administered greater than the maximum dose, elevated systolic blood pressure, increased heart rate, abnormal cardigan rhythm, and conduction can be seen; this can result in dysrhythmias, and cardiac arrest. Bisulfite preservatives are added to local anesthetic containing epinephrine. If there is an allergic reaction in patients, it can be attributed to bisulfites. In patients with reported history of local anesthetic allergies, consideration should be made to administer local anesthetic without epinephrine. Levonordefrin is a substitute for epinephrine; it is an isomer and purely synthetic. The intensity of hemostasis is inferior to epinephrine. Levonordefrin is also less likely to produce cardiac side effects compared with epinephrine.[1]

Table 2
Ester local anesthesia

Drug	Facts[1,6]	Comments
Procaine	• Classification = Ester • Metabolism = Hydrolyzed in plasma by plasma pseudocholinesterase • Excretion = 90% as *para*-aminobenzoic acid, 8% as diethylaminoethanol, 2% unchanged in the urine • pKa = 9.1 • pH (with epi) = 3.5–5.5 • Onset = 6–10 min (slow) • Half-life = 30 min	• It is the first injectable local anesthesia to be synthesized • It has the greatest vasodilation properties • There is increased bleeding at the surgical site • Slow onset • Not available as topical • If there is an allergy to *para*-aminobenzoic acid, it can be used • Toxicity may present initial mild sedation instead of excitatory symptoms
Propoxycaine	• Classification = Ester • Metabolism = Hydrolyzed in plasma and liver • Excretion = Kidney • Onset = 2–3 min	• It is combined with procaine for rapid onset and longer duration • It is highly toxic • Not available as a topical
Cocaine HCL	• Metabolism = Liver • Excretion = Urine • Onset (topical) = 1 min	• First LA to be widely used in dentistry • Highly soluble in water • Known for its vasoconstriction ability • Absorbed rapidly • Eliminated slowly • Blocks reuptake and enhances release of norepinephrine • Crosses the blood-brain barrier • Repetitive administration can cause beta receptors in the heart and dopamine receptors in the brain to be sensitized • Epinephrine can cause cardiac arrhythmias and hypertensive crisis • Not recommended as topical due to potential of abuse • Short duration of action

Abbreviation: epi, epinephrine.

Adapted from Boyce RA, Kirpalani T, Mohan N. Updates of topical and local anesthesia agents. Dent Clin North Am. 2016 Apr;60(2):445-71.

Lidocaine

Lidocaine is the gold standard to evaluate the safety and effectiveness of other local anesthetics. About 90% lidocaine is metabolized by the liver. The remaining 10% is excreted in the original form.[8] The dissociation constant (pKa) of lidocaine is 7.85, and it can be decomposed into numerous recharged local anesthetic molecules that act on myelin sheath to produce nerve block. Lidocaine is a vasodilator and absorbed by the body in a short time. Therefore a local constrictor is added to delay drug absorption. Lidocaine is the most commonly used local anesthetic in dentistry and is commonly used in acute myocardial infarction and various rapid ventricular arrhythmias.[9]

Articaine

Articaine contains a thiophene ring, which results in stronger lipid solubility of articaine compared with lidocaine, which contains a benzene ring.[10,11] Articaine is also able to form hydrogen bonds, which improves lipid solubility of articaine. Articaine is able to fold its molecules into tissues and better able to penetrate nerve sheath. Articaine is metabolized in the liver, and in the blood it is broken down into nontoxic and inactive metabolite, articainic acid. Articaine is commonly locally infiltrated in the maxilla and mandible in dentistry. The use of articaine for mandibular block is a controversial topic because of the high risk of nerve injury.[9]

Prilocaine

Prilocaine is an amide local anesthetic. Prilocaine contains a benzene ring similar to lidocaine.[12] Prilocaine is the weakest vasodilator among other amide local anesthetics. Prilocaine can be used in patients who have contraindications to adrenaline.[13] The pKa of prilocaine is 7.7 indicating more uncharged base molecules in the body to accelerate the anesthetic process. Prilocaine is metabolized in the liver, kidney, and lungs. The first stage of metabolism occurs in the kidney and lungs. The metabolites from the first stage can be decomposed in the liver.[14] Therefore prilocaine is metabolized faster and is less likely to reach toxic levels. While using prilocaine there is a potential risk of developing methemoglobin in susceptible patients.[15]

Mepivacaine

The pKa of mepivacaine is lower than that of lidocaine hence mepivacaine has quick action and long-term effect.[16] Mepivacaine is a weak vasodilator, therefore it promotes longer anesthesia. Mepivacaine is completely metabolized in the liver. Mepivacaine has been considered a preferred local anesthetic for patients with cardiovascular disease.[16]

TOPICAL AND LOCAL ANESTHESIA IN BREASTFEEDING PATIENTS

Topical anesthesia generally does not cause a serious concern in breastfeeding patients as long as it is not directly applied to breast, nipples, or other parts of the body with direct contact to infants.[17] If topical anesthetic is ingested, it is known to cause gastrointestinal symptoms, seizures, arrhythmias, and death in an infant.[18,19]

Local ester anesthetics that are administered are rapidly inactivated by plasma pseudocholinesterase and are unlikely to be found in breast milk. Consideration should be taken when administering prilocaine.[17] Owing to prilocaine's ability to cause methemoglobinemia it should not be used

in nursing mothers.[17] Lidocaine and bupivacaine have extensive documented use in nursing mothers and are preferred local anesthetics during breastfeeding.[17]

DOSE CALCULATION

The maximum dose of local anesthetic is limited by the maximum dose of epinephrine, or vasoconstrictor. After the maximum dosage is calculated, the maximum number of carpules that can be administered should be considered. One dental carpule contains 1.8 mL local anesthetic.

MAXIMUM DOSES OF LOCAL ANESTHETIC[1]

- X% = (1000X) mg/100 mL
- MRD = Y mg/kg
- Weight of individual = Z kg
- Volume of 1 carpule = 1.8 mL
- Total amount of anesthetic that can be given to patients = (Z*Y) mg
- Total amount of anesthetic in 1 carpule = [(1.8/100)*(1000X)] mg/carpule = (18X) mg/carpule
- Maximum number of carpules that can be given to patients = [(Z*Y)/18X] carpules

MAXIMUM DOSES OF VASOCONSTRICTOR

- Dosage equivalence of epinephrine (epi) = A mg/mL[1] (Table 3)
- Amount of epi in 1 carpule = (A mg/mL)*(1.8 mL/carpule) = 1.8 A mg/carpule
- Maximum dose of epinephrine for patients = B mg
- Maximum number of carpules that can be given to patients = [(B/1.8 A)] carpules

PEDIATRIC CONSIDERATION

Clark's rule for pediatric dosage of local anesthetic for children is based on the weight of the patient and not the age.[20] The American Academy of Pediatric Dentistry (2015) suggests using body mass index for calculation.[20]

- Dose = (Child weight/adult weight) * (Adult dose)
- The maximum number of dental cartridges to be administered is [(Z * Y)/18X].
- The Z value represents the patient's weight, Y for maximum dose and X for the percentage concentration.

ROLE OF pKa AND pH

Understanding acid-base equilibrium is important to understand the physiology of local anesthetic. When local anesthetic interacts with tissue at

Table 3	
Maximum doses of vasoconstrictor	
Concentration	**Dose Equivalence (mg/mL)**
1:1000	1.0
1:10,000	0.1
1:100,000	0.01
1:200,000	0.005

Adapted from Boyce RA, Kirpalani T, Mohan N. Updates of topical and local anesthesia agents. Dent Clin North Am. 2016 Apr;60(2):445-71.

physiologic pH, the anesthetic dissociates. The uncharged basic form is an active form of the local anesthetic. In the uncharged basic form, the local anesthetic has the ability to diffuse through the membrane of the neuronal tissue. The pKa of the anesthetic describes the amount of uncharged form compared with the charged form[1]; this can be calculated using the Henderson- Hasselbalch equation:

$$pKa = pH - log [base]/[acid]$$

An equilibrium is established when pH of surrounding tissue equals pKa. Local anesthetics are typically manufactured with pH from 3.5 to 6.0 and pKa typically ranging from 7.7 to 8.9.[21] The pKa determines the onset time of local anesthesia. The local anesthetic with lower pKa will have faster onset compared with that with higher pKa, which has slower onset times (**Table 4**).

LIPID SOLUBILITY

Lipid solubility of local anesthetic determines how potent it is. A potent local anesthetic will require a lower dose of drug to have similar effect compared with a less potent local anesthetic. Highly potent local anesthetics are highly lipid soluble. The ability to penetrate neuronal tissue is also affected by lipid solubility[21] (**Table 5**).

ADVANCES IN LOCAL ANESTHETIC DELIVERY DEVICES

The goal of newer technologies for delivery of local anesthetic is to reduce pain during their administration.[22] There are vibrotactile devices, computer-controlled local anesthetic delivery systems, jet injectors, and safety dental syringes that can be used.[22]

Vibrotactile devices use simultaneous activation of nerve fiber through the use of vibration.[23] The pain reduction from vibration results from tactile induced pain inhibition within the cerebral cortex. The inhibition occurs without any contribution at

the spinal level. VibraJect is a battery-operated attachment that attaches to a dental syringe.[24] The goal of VibraJect is to deliver high-frequency vibration to the needle that is strong enough for the patient to feel. DentalVibe (BING Innovations LLC, Crystal Lake, IL, USA) is a wireless, rechargeable handheld device that delivers soothing, pulsed, percussive micro-oscillation to the injection site.[22] Accupal (ACCUPAL, Inc., Hot Springs, AR, USA) is another wireless device that uses vibration and pressure to precondition the oral mucosa.[22] The goal of these vibrotactile devices is to reduce pain at the injection site, which also can be achieved with manual manipulation of soft tissue at the time of administration of local anesthetic.

Computer-controlled local anesthetic delivery system controls the rate of flow of the local anesthetic.[22] The Wand (Milestone Scientific, Inc, Livingston, NJ, USA) is a lightweight handpiece that provides users with tactile sensation and control over a traditional syringe. The rate of delivery of local anesthetic is controlled by a computer, therefore it is consistent. Competitive to The Wand is Comfort Control Syringe (Dentsply International, York, PA, USA). With the Comfort Control Syringe there is no foot pedal and there are 5 preset speeds for the delivery of local anesthetic. However, Comfort Control Syringe is bulky and therefore more difficult to use.[25]

Jet infectors use mechanical energy sources to create sufficient pressure to deliver the local anesthetic.[24,26] There is no needle involved. There is enough force to deliver a small dose through the soft tissue into subcutaneous tissue. Jet injectors are said to offer fast and easy use, with little or no pain, less tissue damage, and faster drug absorption. There are 2 brands Syrijet Mark II (Keystone Industries [aka Mizzy], Cherry Hill, NJ, USA) and MED-JET (Medical International

Table 4		
Characteristics of commonly used local anesthetics at physiologic pH		
Medication	**pKa**	**Free Base (%)**
Mepivacaine	7.7	33
Lidocaine	7.8	29
Articaine	7.8	29
Bupivacaine	8.1	17
Procaine	8.9	3

Adapted from Boyce RA, Kirpalani T, Mohan N. Updates of topical and local anesthesia agents. Dent Clin North Am. 2016 Apr;60(2):445-71.

Table 5	
Lipid solubility of commonly used anesthetics	
Anesthetic Drug	**Lipid Solubility**
Articaine	40
Mepivacaine	42
Lidocaine	110
Bupivacaine	560

Adapted from Boyce RA, Kirpalani T, Mohan N. Updates of topical and local anesthesia agents. Dent Clin North Am. 2016 Apr;60(2):445-71.

Technologies, Montreal, QC, Canada) that are currently available.

As the Occupational Safety and Health Administration and the Centers for Disease Control and Prevention are recommending health care personnel safety and advocating using medical devices with safety features, there is development of a safe dental syringe to minimize needle stick injury in the work environment. These syringes possess a sheath that locks over the needle when it is removed from patients' tissue preventing accidental needle stick.[22]

CLINICS CARE POINTS

- Topical anesthesia is adjunct to pain control, and to assist in delivery of local anesthetics.
- There are 2 groups of local anesthetics, ester and amide. Amide local anesthetics are more commonly used.
- Local anesthetic such as lidocaine is safe for breastfeeding females.
- Maximum dosage of local anesthetic should be calculated before administrating LA especially in pediatric patients.
- There are many adjunct devices to assist in delivery of local anesthetic to make the experience more tolerable.

DISCLOSURE

The authors have nothing to disclose.

REFERENCES

1. Boyce RA, Kirpalani T, Mohan N. Updates of topical and local anesthesia agents. Dent Clin North Am 2016;60(2):445–71. Erratum in: Dent Clin North Am. 2017 Apr;61(2):xiii. PMID: 27040295.
2. Wynn RL, Meiller TF, Crossley HL. Drug information handbook for dentistry: oral medicine for medically-compromised patients & specific oral conditions. 7th edition. Hudson (OH): Lexi-Comp Inc; 2002. p. 352.
3. Nasri-Heir C, Khan J, Heir GM. Topical medications as treatment of neuropathic orofacial pain. Dent Clin North Am 2013;57:541.
4. Malamed SF. Handbook of local anesthesia by Malamed. 6th edition. St. Louis (MO): Elsevier; 2013.
5. Hersh EV. "Local anesthetics" lecture. Philadelphia: UPenn SDM; 2010.
6. Malamed SF. Clinical actions of specific agents. In: Handbook of local anesthesia by Malamed. 6th edition. St. Louis (MO): Elsevier; 2013. p. 52–75.
7. Turk DC. Assess the person, not just the pain. Pain 2013;1:1–4.
8. Klimitz JMI, editor. Handbook of LA, vol. 102, 5th edition. Maryland Heights: Alpha Omegan; 2009. p. 161–2.
9. Wang YH, Wang DR, Liu JY, et al. Local anesthesia in oral and maxillofacial surgery: a review of current opinion. J Dental Sci 2021;16(4):1055–65.
10. Gazal G. Is articaine more potent than mepivacaine for use in oral surgery? J Oral Maxillofac Res 2018;9:e5.
11. Singla M, Subbiah A, Aggarwal V, et al. Comparison of the anaesthetic efficacy of different volumes of 4% articaine (1.8 and 3.6 mL) as supplemental buccal infiltration after failed inferior alveolar nerve block. Int Endod J 2015;48:103–8.
12. Alsharif A, Omar E, Alolayan AB, et al. Gazal "2% lidocaine versus 3% prilocaine for oral and maxillofacial surgerySaudi. J Anaesth 2018;12:571–7.
13. Gazal G. Does articaine, rather than prilocaine, increase the success rate of anaesthesia for the extraction of maxillary teeth Saudi. J Anaesth 2020;14:297–301.
14. Torres-Lagares D, Serrera-Figallo MÁ, Machuca-Portillo G, et al. Cardiovascular effect of dental anesthesia with articaine (40 mg with epinephrine 0,5 mg % and 40 mg with epinephrine 1 mg%) versus mepivacaine (30 mg and 20 mg with epinephrine 1 mg%) in medically compromised cardiac patients: a cross-over, randomized, single blinded study. Med Oral Patol Oral Cir Bucal 2012;17:e655–60.
15. Kreutz RW, Kinni ME. Life-threatening toxic methemoglobinemia induced by prilocaine. Oral Surg Oral Med Oral Pathol 1983;56:480–2.
16. Visconti RP, Tortamano IP, Buscariolo IA. Comparison of the anesthetic efficacy of mepivacaine and lidocaine in patients with irreversible pulpitis: a double-blind randomized clinical trial. J Endod 2016;42:1314–9.

17. Anderson PO. Local anesthesia and breastfeeding. Breastfeed Med 2021;16(3):173–4.

18. Dayan PS, Litovitz TL, Crouch BI, et al. Fatal accidental dibucaine poisoning in children. Ann Emerg Med 1996;28:442–5.

19. Nelsen J, Holland M, Dougherty M, et al. Severe central nervous system and cardiovascular toxicity in a pediatric patient after ingestion of an over-the-counter local anesthetic. Pediatr Emerg Care 2009; 25:670–3.

20. DAA Khan S, et al. Updates of local anesthesia in pediatric dentistry: a review. Annals of clinical and analytical medicine. ACAM 2020;9(3):331–4.

21. Drasner K. Local anesthetics. In: Miller R, Pardo M, editors. Basics of anesthesia. 6th edition. Philadelphia: Elsevier Saunders; 2011. p. 130–42.

22. Saxena P, Gupta SK, Newaskar V, et al. Advances in dental local anesthesia techniques and devices: An update. Natl J Maxillofac Surg 2013;4(1):19–24.

23. Melzack R, Wall PD. Pain mechanisms: a new theory. Science 1965;150:971–9.

24. Ogle OE, Mahjoubi G. Advances in local anesthesia in dentistry. Dent Clin North Am 2011;55:481–99.

25. Clark TM, Yagiela JA. Advanced techniques and armamentarium for dental local anesthesia. Dent Clin North Am 2010;54:757–68.

26. Massoomi N. Local anesthetics. In: Fonseca RJ, editor. Oral and maxillofacial sur[1]gery, vol. I, 2nd edition. St Louis (MO): Saunders Elsevier; 2009. p. 35–56.

Current Concepts in Prophylactic Antibiotics in Oral and Maxillofacial Surgery

Chad Dammling, DDS, MD[a],*, Shelly Abramowicz, DMD, MPH[b],
Brian Kinard, DMD, MD[a]

KEYWORDS

- Antibiotic • Prophylaxis • Maxillofacial surgery

KEY POINTS

- Antibiotic prophylaxis use should be limited to established guidelines and standardized protocols to avoid risk of antimicrobial resistance, toxicity, and excess cost.
- In addition to sterile surgical technique, proper perioperative administration and antibiotic selection are imperative to prevent surgical site infections.
- Surgical procedures are classified as class I to IV based on the presence of active infection and their involvement of the respiratory, alimentary, gastrointestinal, or urinary tract lining.
- Most dentoalveolar procedures do not require antibiotic prophylaxis, although special considerations exist for infective endocarditis prevention and foreign body placement.
- Use of perioperative prophylactic antibiotics for other maxillofacial procedures depends on the surgical classification and exposure to oral or pharyngeal mucosa.

INTRODUCTION

When performing any surgical procedure, the prevention of infection at local and distant sites is always a concomitant goal.[1] There are a variety of factors that influence the rate of surgical site and distant infections that must be taken into consideration. Foreign bodies (eg, dental implants, reconstructive hardware) have the potential to increase infection rates.[1] Patient-related risk factors include the age of the patient, immune status, medical comorbidities (eg, diabetes), tobacco use, and nutritional status. Surgical factors are wound closure, contamination level, duration of operation, and tissue quality.[2] Further, there are critical steps during all operations that decrease the likelihood of infection, such as adequate irrigation, clean incisions, removal of debris, hemostasis, and properly placed mucoperiosteal flaps.[3]

Antimicrobial prophylaxis is the use of antibiotics in the perioperative period in order to prevent infection at the surgical site or at distant locations.[4] This can be directly contrasted with therapeutic antibiotics which treat and eradicate active infections often for an extended period of time.[5] Surgical wounds can be classified as class I-IV based upon their degree of contamination and involvement of respiratory, alimentary, gastrointestinal, or urinary tract lining (**Table 1**). For each of these classifications, specific guidelines and recommendations exist for antimicrobial prophylaxis prior to surgery.

Class I surgery (clean surgery) occurs when there are no breaks in the respiratory, gastrointestinal, or urinary tract barriers and there is no preoperative inflammation at the surgical site.[1] Examples of these surgeries include extraoral lymph node excisions and parotidectomies. Class I surgery has an infection rate of approximately 2%

[a] Department of Oral and Maxillofacial Surgery, School of Dentistry, University of Alabama at Birmingham, 1919 7th Avenue South, Room 406, Birmingham, AL 35233, USA; [b] Division of Oral and Maxillofacial Surgery, Department of Surgery, Emory University School of Medicine, Oral and Maxillofacial Surgery, Children's Healthcare of Atlanta, 1365 Clifton Road, Building B, Suite 2300, Atlanta, GA 30322, USA
* Corresponding author.
E-mail address: Dammling@uab.edu

Oral Maxillofacial Surg Clin N Am 34 (2022) 157–167
https://doi.org/10.1016/j.coms.2021.08.015
1042-3699/22/

Table 1
Surgical classification system

Classification	Criteria and Examples	Risk of Infection (%)
Clean	Parotidectomy, lymph node excision Elective: nonemergent, nontraumatic. No acute inflammation. No break in respiratory, gastrointestinal, biliary, or genitourinary tracts	<2
Clean-contaminated	Cleft lip or palate surgery. Orthognathic surgery. Cyst enucleation Urgent or emergency care that is otherwise clean, or elective opening of respiratory, gastrointestinal, biliary, or genitourinary tract with minimal spillage	<10
Contaminated	Mandibular fractures Nonpurulent inflammation. Gross spillage from gastrointestinal or genitourinary tract. Penetrating trauma <4 h old. Chronic open wounds	Approximately 20
Dirty	Odontogenic abscess Purulent inflammation with preoperative perforation of respiratory, gastrointestinal, or genitourinary tract. Penetrating trauma >4 h old	Approximately 40

Adapted from Halpern LR, Adams DR. The Dentoalveolar Surgical Patient: Perioperative Principles Based on Contemporary Controversies. *Oral Maxillofac Surg Clin North Am.* 2020;32(4):495-510.

when prophylactic antibiotics are not given. In contrast, procedures that disrupt the mucosa or respiratory epithelium (class II or clean-contaminated surgery) have been reported to have an infection risk rate of approximately 10% to 15% when prophylactic antibiotics are not provided.[1,3] All intraoral procedures are considered class II and can cause a transient bacteremia requiring antimicrobial prophylaxis.[6,7] When prophylactic antibiotics are given and combined with good surgical technique, these rates can be decreased to as low as 1%.[2,3]

Salivary flora introduces a multitude of bacteria (ie, gram-positive aerobes and anaerobic bacteria) into the surgical site. Gram-negative aerobes are generally not part of the head and neck but often colonize the oropharynx in patients with upper aerodigestive tract cancers or poor oral health.[8]

When performing class III procedures (contaminated surgery; eg, open mandibular fractures) or class IV procedures (dirty surgery; eg, odontogenic abscesses), therapeutic antibiotics may be indicated in addition to preoperative prophylactic therapy.[4]

The overall goal of prophylactic antibiotic therapy is to provide adequate blood levels of an antibiotic during the procedure to reduce contamination from transient bacteremia caused by physiologic flora.[5] These optimal levels of prophylactic antibiotics should occur before incision, and therefore proper timing and dosage are crucial.[9] For operations that last more than 2 hours,

repeat intraoperative dosing may be necessary to maintain adequate serum levels.[9,10] The patient's weight (especially in obese or pediatric patients) must be taken into consideration to achieve adequate steady-state levels.

Antibiotic prophylaxis use should be limited to established guidelines and standardized indications to avoid risk of antimicrobial resistance, toxicity, and excess cost.[11] In the past several years, guidelines have greatly narrowed the indications for use because of increased risk to benefit ratios.[12] These potential risks include life-threatening anaphylaxis and specific antibiotic-associated side effects, such as *Clostridium difficile* colitis and tendon injury associated with clindamycin and fluoroquinolones, respectively.[11] Judicious use of antibiotics is also critical to prevent multiple drug-resistant strains of bacteria that have already evolved because of excessive overprescribing and overuse.[4] Even short-term use through prophylaxis with a single dose has been shown to select for resistant viridans streptococci.[13]

According to the American Society of Health-System Pharmacists (ASHP) guidelines, the goals of an antimicrobial agent for prophylaxis should be to prevent surgical site infections, prevent surgical site infection morbidity and mortality, reduce the duration and cost of health care, produce no adverse effects, and have no adverse consequences to the flora of the hospital or of the patient.[9] Further, whichever agent is chosen should be active against most pathogens at the surgical site and administered for the shortest time frame possible.[9] Cefazolin is the most frequently chosen regimen because it has proven efficacy against skin flora, including *Staphylococcus aureus* and coagulase-negative staphylococci. These guidelines for antimicrobial prophylaxis also correlate with recommendations by the Surgical Care Improvement Project (SCIP).[14] Seven of these guidelines apply directly to the perioperative period: (1) antibiotics provided 1 hour before incision, (2) antibiotic coverage for the most probable contaminant, (3) antibiotics discontinued with 24 hours after surgery, (4) euglycemia throughout surgery and through the first 2 postoperative days, (5) hair clipped at the surgical site, (6) Foley catheters removed within the first 2 postoperative days, and (7) normothermia throughout the surgical procedure (**Table 2**). The establishment of these protocols has further standardized perioperative care and reduced the incidence of surgical site infections since their introduction in 2006.

This article discusses indications for antibiotic prophylaxis use during oral and maxillofacial surgery procedures. For most dentoalveolar procedures, prophylactic antibiotics are not indicated unless foreign bodies are to be placed, such as dental implants.[4] Perioperative prophylactic antibiotics for other maxillofacial procedures depend on the surgical classification and exposure to oral or pharyngeal mucosa. When prophylactic antibiotics are indicated, published guidelines and dosages are further reviewed here.

Dentoalveolar Procedures and Cardiac Conditions

Infective endocarditis (IE) is a rare but lethal disease.[12] Despite advancements in the management and treatment of IE, patients still have high morbidity and mortality.[12,15] The most common organisms isolated in IE are *S aureus*, viridans streptococci, and enterococci species. Other, although rarer, bacteria include *Haemophilus* species, *Aggregatibacter* species, *Cardiobacterium hominis*, *Eikenella corrodens*, and *Kingella*.[17]

The American Heart Association (AHA) published guidelines for IE in 1955 and most recently in 2021.[15,16] These guidelines have been thoroughly studied and revised after analysis and risk stratification. Antibiotic premedication is indicated for patients with risk factors for complications from IE and for select dental procedures that pierce the oral mucosa or manipulate gingival tissue/periapical region of teeth (**Boxes 1 and 2**). For this reason, routine anesthetic injections (through healthy tissue), radiographs, prosthodontic or orthodontic work, and exfoliation of deciduous teeth do not require a prophylactic antibiotic.

Overall, the AHA found that the cumulative bacteremia risk from daily activity (eg, chewing, brushing of teeth) is higher than those caused by dental, genitourinary, or gastrointestinal procedures.[11,15] For most patients, the risk of adverse events from antibiotic use exceeds the benefit of prophylactic therapy unless they have risk factors for serious IE complications.[11] As a result of the findings discussed earlier, the AHA promotes the maintenance of oral health and hygiene as more important than prophylactic antibiotics in the prevention of IE in most patients.[17]

If a preoperative antibiotic is indicated, a single dose 30 to 60 minutes before the procedure should be provided to cover for the transient bacteremia caused by oral bacterial flora (**Table 3**). If this dose is inadvertently missed preoperatively, the medication can be administered up to 2 hours following the procedure.[15,18] Further, if a patient is already taking an antibiotic for another condition (eg, amoxicillin for sinusitis), it is recommended that a medication from a different class be chosen for prophylactic coverage.[6] Alternatively, treatment can be delayed for 10 days following the completion of the antibiotic course to allow for reestablishment of oral flora.[18] Then the oral and maxillofacial surgeon (OMS) may proceed with routine IE prophylaxis.

Dentoalveolar Procedures and Prosthetic Joints

Based on current evidence, prophylactic antibiotics for dentoalveolar procedures are not indicated for patients with prosthetic joints.[18,19] A panel of experts selected by the American Dental Association (ADA) in 2014 evaluated current evidence of prosthetic joint infections (PJIs) and found no relationship between infections and dental procedures. Similar to antibiotic use for prevention of IE, the risk of adverse drug reactions, costs, and antibiotic resistance outweighed the benefit of prescribing antibiotics for PJI prophylaxis (**Box 3**).

Of note, some patients have conditions causing an immunocompromised state (eg, rheumatoid arthritis) and the OMS should discuss need for a prophylactic regimen with the orthopedic surgeon or primary care physician. If this occurs, it is most appropriate to have the orthopedic surgeon or primary care doctor prescribe the appropriate therapy.[18]

Perioperative prophylactic antibiotics for temporomandibular joint (TMJ) replacement surgery are discussed later in this article. For patients

Table 2
Surgical Care Improvement Project criteria in the immediate postoperative period

SCIP Measure Designator	Performance Measure Title
INF-1	Prophylactic antibiotic received within 1 h before incision
INF-2	Prophylactic antibiotic selection for surgical patient applicable to flora
INF -3	Prophylactic antibiotics discontinued within 24 h after surgery end time
INF-4	Cardiac surgery patients with controlled 6 AM and postoperative blood glucose
INF-6	Surgery patients with appropriate hair removal
INF-9	Urinary catheter removal on postoperative day 1 or postoperative day 2
INF-10	Surgery patients with perioperative temperature management

INF, infection measure designators.
Adapted from Dua A, Desai SS, Seabrook GR, Brown KR, Lewis BD, Rossi PJ, Edmiston CE, Lee CJ. The effect of Surgical Care Improvement Project measures on national trends on surgical site infections in open vascular procedures. J Vasc Surg. 2014 Dec;60(6):1635–9.

already with a TMJ prosthesis, it is recommended that they are treated with prophylactic antibiotics to cover for oral flora if they are to receive an inferior alveolar nerve injection during the procedure. During the administration of local anesthesia, the tip of the needle can potentially come in close contact with or touch the condylar component fixation screws as they are positioned in the pterygomandibular space.[20]

Dental Implants and Bone Grafting

Infections around dental implants can be extremely difficult to eradicate and often warrant removal of the implant.[21] Antibiotic prophylaxis for dental implant procedures has been shown to be beneficial in reducing implant failure and postoperative infection rates.[21,22] A Cochrane Review summarized these findings and recommended 2 or 3 g of amoxicillin 1 hour preoperatively to significantly reduce the failure rate of implants caused by infection. In a separate retrospective analysis, no differences were noted between clindamycin, amoxicillin, or cephalosporins when given preoperatively.[4] For both autogenous and allogeneic

Box 1
AP for a dental procedure: underlying conditions for which AP is suggested

Prosthetic cardiac valve or material

  Presence of cardiac prosthetic valve

  Transcatheter implantation of prosthetic valves

  Cardiac valve repair with devices, including annuloplasty, rings, or clips

  Left ventricular assist devices or implantable heart

Previous, relapse, or recurrent IE

CHD

  Unrepaired cyanotic congenital CHD, including palliative shunts and conduits.

  Completely repaired congenital heart defect with prosthetic material or device, whether placed by surgery or by transcatheter during the first 6 mo after the procedure

  Repaired CHD with residual defects at the site of or adjacent to the site of a prosthetic patch or prosthetic device

  Surgical or transcatheter pulmonary artery valve or conduit placement such as Melody valve and Contegra conduit

Cardiac transplant recipients who develop cardiac valvulopathy

AP for a dental procedure not suggested

  Implantable electronic devices such as a pacemaker or similar devices

  Septal defect closure devices when complete closure is achieved

  Peripheral vascular grafts and patches, including those used for hemodialysis

  Coronary artery stents or other vascular stents

  CNS ventriculoatrial shunts

  Vena cava filters

  Pledgets

AP indicates antibiotic prophylaxis; CHD, congenital heart disease; CNS, central nervous system; and IE, infective endocarditis.

From Wilson WR, Gewitz M, Lockhart PB, Bolger AF, DeSimone DC, Kazi DS, Couper DJ, Beaton A, Kilmartin C, Miro JM, Sable C, Jackson MA, Baddour LM; American Heart Association Young Hearts Rheumatic Fever, Endocarditis and Kawasaki Disease Committee of the Council on Lifelong Congenital Heart Disease and Heart Health in the Young; Council on Cardiovascular and Stroke Nursing; and the Council on Quality of Care and Outcomes Research. Prevention of Viridans Group Streptococcal Infective Endocarditis: A Scientific Statement From the American Heart Association. Circulation. 2021 May 18;143(20):e963-e978.

bone grafting, a meta-analysis by Khouly and colleagues[23] found that there are insufficient data to support the use of prophylactic antibiotics for bone grafting when performed without implant placement. An additional review by Klinge and colleagues[24] found a similar lack of evidence in the literature. There still remains a need for an adequate randomized controlled trial to evaluate prophylaxis when bone grafts are placed independent of dental implants.

Postoperatively, antibiotics have not been shown to be beneficial to prevent infections of dental implants. Because of increased risk of adverse events and antibiotic resistance, postoperative antibiotics are not indicated following placement of dental implants.[25] Despite this lack of evidence or standardized guidelines, many dentists empirically provide a postoperative course of therapy ranging from 1 to 5 days.[23] The Misch International Institute recommends both prophylactic and postoperative antibiotic therapy based on the patient's health status and the procedural intervention (**Table 4**).[26] Although there are no long-term randomized controls validating these protocols, their guidelines have been successfully implemented by the many doctors that have completed training through their institutions.[23,26]

Table 3
Antibiotic regimens for a dental procedure regimen: single dose 30 to 60 minutes before procedure

Situation	Agent	Adults	Children
Oral	Amoxicillin	2g	50 mg/kg
Unable to take oral medication	Ampicillin OR Cefazolin or ceftriaxone	2 g IM or IV 1 g IM or IV	50 mg/kg IM or IV 50 mg/kg IM or IV
Allergic to penicillin or ampicillin—oral	Cephalexin[a] OR Azithromycin or clarithromycin OR Doxycydine	2g 500 mg 100 mg	50 mg/kg 15 mg/kg <45 kg, 2.2 mg/kg >45 kg, 100 mg
Allergic to penicillin or ampicillin and unable to take oral medication	Cefazolin or ceftriaxone[b]	1 g IM or IV	50 mg/kg IM or IV

Clindamycin is no longer recommended for antibiotic prophylaxis for a dental procedure.
IM indicates intramuscular; and IV, intravenous.
[a] Or other first- or second-generation oral cephalosporin in equivalent adult or pediatric dosing.
[b] Cephalosporins should not be used in an individual with a history of anaphylaxis, angioedema, or urticarial with penicillin or ampicillin.
From Wilson WR, Gewitz M, Lockhart PB, Bolger AF, DeSimone DC, Kazi DS, Couper DJ, Beaton A, Kilmartin C, Miro JM, Sable C, Jackson MA, Baddour LM; American Heart Association Young Hearts Rheumatic Fever, Endocarditis and Kawasaki Disease Committee of the Council on Lifelong Congenital Heart Disease and Heart Health in the Young; Council on Cardiovascular and Stroke Nursing; and the Council on Quality of Care and Outcomes Research. Prevention of Viridans Group Streptococcal Infective Endocarditis: A Scientific Statement From the American Heart Association. Circulation. 2021 May 18;143(20):e963-e978.

Box 3
Management of patients with prosthetic joints undergoing dental procedures

Clinical recommendations:

In general, for patients with prosthetic joint implants, prophylactic antibiotics are not recommended before dental procedures to prevent PJI.

For patients with a history of complications associated with their joint replacement surgery who are undergoing dental procedures that include gingival manipulation or mucosal incision, prophylactic antibiotics should only be considered after consultation with the patient and orthopedic surgeon. To assess a patient's medical status, a complete health history is always recommended when making final decisions regarding the need for antibiotic prophylaxis.

Clinical reasoning for the recommendation:

- There is evidence that dental procedures are not associated with prosthetic joint implant infections.
- There is evidence that antibiotics provided before oral care do not prevent prosthetic joint implant infections.
- There are potential harms of antibiotics, including risk for anaphylaxis, antibiotic resistance, and opportunistic infections such as *C difficile*.
- The benefits of antibiotic prophylaxis may not exceed the harms for most patients.
- The individual patient's circumstances and preference should be considered when deciding whether to prescribe prophylactic antibiotics before dental procedures.

Adapted from Sollecito TP, Abt E, Lockhart PB, et al. The use of prophylactic antibiotics prior to Dental procedures in patients with prosthetic joints: Evidence-based clinical practice guideline for dental practitioners-a report of the American Dental Association Council on Scientific Affairs. *J Am Dent Assoc.* 2015;146(1):11-16.e8.

Other Maxillofacial Procedures

Aside from the dentoalveolar procedures discussed earlier, other maxillofacial procedures often require antibiotic prophylaxis based on their involvement of respiratory or alimentary tracts (ie, oral, nasal, pharyngeal mucosa). Examples of clean procedures include thyroidectomy, extraoral lymph node excisions, and blepharoplasties, whereas clean-contaminated surgeries include orthognathic procedures, rhinoplasty, and cleft palate repair.[9]

Infection rates for clean procedures are extremely low, even without antibiotic prophylaxis, and are estimated at less than 2%. Systemic antibiotics have not been proved effective in reducing surgical site infections and generally a single dose to cover for skin flora is indicated.[9] If placement of a prosthetic material such as hardware or an implant is planned, a similar perioperative dose of a cephalosporin or clindamycin is indicated.[9] Routine sterile preparation and draping remain recommended for all procedures.

Compared with class I procedures, the current literature recommends prophylactic antibiotics for any incisions through oral, nasal, or pharyngeal mucosa.[9] This recommendation includes coverage for *S aureus*, oropharyngeal anaerobes, and enteric gram-negative bacilli with cefazolin plus metronidazole, ampicillin/sulbactam, clindamycin, or cefuroxime plus metronidazole.[11] It has been shown that a short course of antimicrobial therapy (<24 hours) has improved outcomes compared with an extended course (>72 hours) for both oral surgery and ear, nose, and throat procedures. The administration of antibiotics for more than 72 hours was associated with more adverse effects than the short-term dose even in just the perioperative period.[27,28]

Head and neck oncology

Head and neck oncologic procedures are at an increased risk of infection because of the presence of multiple wound locations, including the primary tumor site, neck dissection, free flap donor sites, and tracheostomy. The diverse flora present within these locations and exposure to the oral cavity contribute to persistently high rates of infection despite perioperative and postoperative antibiotic therapy[29] (**Table 5**). Free flap reconstruction increases the risk of surgical site infection by 2.2 to 2.8 times and tracheotomy increases infection risk 3-fold.[8] A total laryngectomy caries the highest risk of postoperative surgical site infection out of all head and neck procedures.

Surgical site infections in these patient populations are increasingly problematic because of potential delays in adjuvant therapy and prolonged tracheostomy status.[29] For these reasons, the modifiable risk factors discussed earlier are imperative to address preoperatively, including malnutrition and tobacco use. Proper assessment of nutritional status is critical given that many of these disorders can severely limit adequate oral intake.

Surgical site infections in head and neck oncologic procedures are estimated at 24% to 87% if prophylactic antibiotics are not provided.[9] For patients treated with perioperative prophylactic antibiotics, infection rates are decreased to 5.8% to

Table 4
Misch International Implant Institute prophylaxis protocol

Type	Patient Selection	Procedure	Antibiotic	Antimicrobial
Type 1	ASA 1 or 2	• Simple extraction of uninfected teeth • Single-tooth implant • Second-stage surgery • Limited soft tissue reflection surgery	None	Chlorhexidine 14.8 mL (0.5 oz) BID for 2 wk
Type 2	ASA 1 or 2	• Multiple simple extractions • Traumatic extractions • Multiple implants/limited reflection • Socket grafting • Immediate implants/no disorder	Amoxicillin 1 g 1 h before surgery and 500 mg 6 h later	Chlorhexidine 14.8 mL (0.5 oz) BID for 2 wk
Type 3	ASA 1 or 2	• Membrane bone grafting (allograft, xenograft, or alloplast) • Multiple implants/extensive reflection • Multiple immediate implants	Amoxicillin 1 g 1 h before surgery and 500 mg TID for 3 d	Chlorhexidine 14.8 mL (0.5 oz) BID for 2 wk
Type 4	ASA>2 • Long-duration surgery • Less experienced surgeon • Immunocompromised • Active periodontal disease	• Full-arch implants • Sinus lift • Autogenous bone graft	Amoxicillin 1 g 1 h before surgery and 500 mg TID for 5 d	Chlorhexidine 14.8 mL (0.5 oz) BID for 2 wk
Type 4 Sinus	Sinus augmentation patients	• Sinus patients	Augmentin 875/125 mg BID starting 1 d before and 5 d after	Chlorhexidine 14.8 mL (0.5 oz) BID for 2 wk

Abbreviation: ASA, American Society of Anesthesiologists; BID, twice a day; TID, 3 times a day.
Adapted from Resnik RR, Misch C. Prophylactic antibiotic regimens in oral implantology: Rationale and protocol. *Implant Dent.* 2008;17(2):142-150.

Table 5
Risk factors for infection complications in head and neck surgery

Type of surgery	Upper aerodigestive tract, clean-contaminated surgery, tracheostomy, and osteocutaneous flap reconstruction
Surgical factors	Duration of surgery, operative blood loss, flap failure, operative takebacks, and microsurgical revision
Medical factors	ASA classification, advanced age, diabetes, increased BMI
Factors that affect wound healing	Nutrition status, hypoalbuminemia, hypothyroidism, smoking, tobacco use, MRSA colonization
Previous therapies	Previous radiation and previous surgery
Antibiotic selection	Clindamycin

Abbreviations: BMI, body mass index; MRSA, methicillin-resistant *S aureus*.
From Cannon RB, Houlton JJ, Mendez E, Futran ND. Methods to reduce postoperative surgical site infections after head and neck oncology surgery. Lancet Oncol. 2017;18(7):e405-e413. Reprinted with permission of Elsevier, Inc.

38%.[9] Existing evidence recommends broad-spectrum antibiotics that cover gram-positive, gram-negative, and anaerobic bacteria with cefazolin plus metronidazole, or ampicillin/sulbactam. For patients with a severe β-lactam allergy, the combination of clindamycin and an aminoglycoside (generally gentamycin), ciprofloxacin, or aztreonam should be used.[8,29] Clindamycin monotherapy should be avoided because there are increased risks of surgical site infections caused by the presence of increased gram-negative organisms and increased resistance in the head and neck.[8,29,30] Clindamycin monotherapy was also found to increase the length of hospital stay to 18 versus 11.4 days because of both medical and surgical infections.[31] It is recommended that clinicians still consider the use of cefazolin plus metronidazole if mild allergies are noted given low cross-reactivity rates between penicillin and cephalosporins (~2%).[8,29]

Postoperatively, no difference in efficacy has been reported in regimens of 24 hours of antibiotics versus longer therapies for 7 days.[9,29]

Despite this research, institutional protocols following free flap reconstructive procedures generally include 2 to 5 days of antibiotic coverage because of the increased infectious risk discussed earlier.

Orthognathic surgery
For orthognathic surgery, there is a general lack of consensus for the preferred duration of prophylactic antibiotic therapy.[13] Without any antibiotic prophylaxis, the rate of infection can vary between 10% and 25% and, given the procedure is classified as clean-contaminated, prophylactic antibiotics are always indicated immediately before incision.[22,32–34] Systematic reviews by Naimi-Akbar and colleagues[13] and Oomens and colleagues[32] found that there is a high amount of bias in previous orthognathic studies that discuss the use of postoperative prophylactic antibiotic regimens.[22] There is no evidence regarding the effectiveness of a postoperative regimen and both investigators conclude that a single preoperative dose for bacterial coverage as discussed earlier for clean-contaminated surgery is sufficient.[35]

Temporomandibular joint replacement
Surgical site infections following alloplastic joint replacement can be a devastating complication and often require removal of the entire joint. The use of clean operating rooms, stringent protocols, and appropriate antibiotic therapy has decreased orthopedic infection rates to approximately 1% during primary joint replacements.[9] When infections occur, they present as early (within 3 months of surgery), delayed (3–12 months), or late (after 12 months). A major contributing factor to the development of late infections is bacterial formation of a biofilm on the prosthesis, which also must be carefully monitored during TMJ replacements.

There is a significant amount of data from the orthopedic literature supporting the use of prophylactic antibiotic therapy to cover for skin flora in any joint replacement even though there is no break in the respiratory or gastrointestinal epithelium.[9] Further, for patients that are colonized with methicillin-resistant *S aureus* (MRSA) preoperatively or at hospitals with high rates of MRSA infections, vancomycin is often given in addition to cefazolin. Nasal mupirocin should also be administered preoperatively to patients that are colonized with MRSA.

TMJ replacement infections have been estimated to occur 1.5% to 2.7% of the time.[20] The use of prophylactic antibiotics with correct timing and dose remains the most important factor in preventing PJI.[20] Comparable with the orthopedic literature, cephalosporins are used for prophylaxis (clindamycin if allergic) and vancomycin is indicated if the patient is a carrier for MRSA. It also has been recommended that TMJ prostheses are soaked in a vancomycin solution before implantation into the patient. All TMJ replacement instrumentation and devices should strictly be kept separate from contamination from the oral cavity.[36] Following the procedure, a total of 7 to 10 days of continued oral antibiotic prophylaxis are recommended to prevent contamination by the parotid gland, ear canal, or oral cavity.[20]

SUMMARY

Aside from a few exceptions, most dentoalveolar procedures performed by OMSs do not require antibiotic prophylaxis. If a patient meets criteria for risk of IE, then premedication with the appropriate antibiotic coverage 30 to 60 minutes before the procedure should occur. For nondentoalveolar head and neck procedures, the decision to provide prophylactic antibiotics is based on the disturbance of the oral, nasal, or pharyngeal barrier. If these areas are violated or involved in the surgery, then the procedure is considered a clean-contaminated procedure (assuming no active infection is already present). The transient bacteremia initiated by this involvement incurs a 10% risk of infection without treatment and prophylactic antibiotics are indicated. In contrast, clean procedures do not require antibiotics unless a foreign body or implant is to be placed. As with all procedures, clinical judgment and evaluation of the patient's medical status must be taken into consideration to stratify the risk of infection and need for prophylactic and/or postoperative antibiotics.

CLINICS CARE POINTS

- The goals of antimicrobial prophylaxis are to: prevent surgical site infections, prevent surgical site infection morbidity and mortality; reduce the duration and cost of healthcare; produce no adverse effects; and have no adverse consequences to the flora of a hospital or of the patient.
- The Surgical Care Improvement Project (SCIP) has laid out specific guidelines on how to reduce surgical site infections. Seven of these guidelines apply directly to the perioperative period: 1) antibiotics provided one hour prior to incision; 2) antibiotic coverage for the most probable contaminant; 3) antibiotics

discontinued with 24 hours after surgery; 4) euglycemia throughout surgery and through the first two post-operative days; 5) hair clipped at the surgical site; 6) foley catheters removed within the first two post-operative days; and 7) normothermia throughout the surgical case.
- Prophylactic antibiotics are generally not indicated for most routine dentoalveolar procedures.
- Infective endocarditis (IE) prophylaxis is indicated in patients with the presence of a cardiac valves, previous or recurrent infective endocarditis, unrepaired congenital heart defects or repaired defects with residual deficits, and cardiac transplant recipients who develop cardiac valvulopathies.
- IE prophylaxis is not indicated in patients with pacemakers, peripheral vascular grafts, stents, CNS shunts, vena cava filters or cardiac pledgets.
- Compared to the previous 2007 AHA guidelines regarding antibiotic prophylaxis, clindamycin is no longer recommended for patients that are penicillin allergic.
- Class I surgery (clean surgery) occurs when there are no breaks in the respiratory, gastrointestinal, or urinary tract barriers and there is no preoperative inflammation at the surgical site. Generally, a single dose to cover for normal skin flora is indicated in addition to routine sterile prep and drape.
- Class II procedures include any incision through oral, nasal, or pharyngeal mucosa. Prophylactic antibiotics are indicated for coverage of Staphylococcus aureus, oropharyngeal anaerobes, and enteric gram-negative bacilli with cefazolin plus metronidazole, ampicillin/sulbactam, clindamycin, or cefuroxime plus metronidazole.
- When performing class III procedures (contaminated surgery i.e. an open mandibular fractures) or class IV procedures (dirty surgery i.e. odontogenic abscesses), therapeutic antibiotics may be indicated in addition to preoperative prophylactic therapy.
- Head and neck oncologic procedures are at an increased risk of infection due to the presence of diverse flora and multiple wound locations including the primary tumor site, neck dissection, free flap donor sites, and tracheostomy.

DISCLOSURE

The authors have nothing to disclose.

REFERENCES

1. Peterson LJ. Antibiotic prophylaxis against wound infections in oral and maxillofacial surgery. J Oral Maxillofac Surg 1990;48(6):617–20.
2. Posnick JC, Choi E, Chavda A. Surgical site infections following bimaxillary orthognathic, osseous genioplasty, and intranasal surgery: a retrospective cohort study. J Oral Maxillofac Surg 2017;75(3):584–95.
3. Salmerón-Escobar JI, del Amo-Fernández de Velasco A. Antibiotic prophylaxis in Oral and Maxillofacial Surgery. Med Oral Patol Oral Cir Bucal 2006;11(3):292–6.
4. Blatt S, Al-Nawas B. A systematic review of latest evidence for antibiotic prophylaxis and therapy in oral and maxillofacial surgery, vol. 47. Germany: Springer Berlin Heidelberg; 2019.
5. Sancho-Puchades M, Herráez-Vilas JM, Berini-Aytés L, et al. Antibiotic prophylaxis to prevent local infection in oral surgery: use or abuse? Med Oral Patol Oral Cir Bucal 2009;14(1):E28–33.
6. Halpern LR, Adams DR. The dentoalveolar surgical patient: perioperative principles based on contemporary controversies. Oral Maxillofac Surg Clin North Am 2020;32(4):495–510.
7. Ariyan S, Martin J, Lal A, et al. Antibiotic prophylaxis for preventing surgical-site infection in plastic surgery: an evidence-based consensus conference statement from the American Association of Plastic Surgeons. Plast Reconstr Surg 2015;135(6):1723–39.
8. Vander Poorten V, Uyttebroek S, Robbins KT, et al. Perioperative antibiotics in clean-contaminated head and neck surgery: a systematic review and meta-analysis. Adv Ther 2020;37(4):1360–80.
9. Bratzler DW, Dellinger EP, Olsen KM, et al. Clinical practice guidelines for antimicrobial prophylaxis in surgery. Surg Infect (Larchmt) 2013;14(1):73–156.
10. Orzechowska-Wylęgała B, Wylęgała A, Buliński M, et al. Antibiotic therapies in maxillofacial surgery in the context of prophylaxis. Biomed Res Int 2015;2015:819086.
11. Enzler MJ, Berbari E, Osmon DR. Antimicrobial prophylaxis in adults. Mayo Clin Proc 2011;86(7):686–701.
12. Hafner S, Albittar M, Abdel-Kahaar E, et al. Antibiotic prophylaxis of infective endocarditis in oral and maxillofacial surgery: incomplete implementation of guidelines in everyday clinical practice. Int J Oral Maxillofac Surg 2020;49(4):522–8.
13. Naimi-Akbar A, Hultin M, Klinge A, et al. Antibiotic prophylaxis in orthognathic surgery: a complex systematic review. PLoS One 2018;13(1):1–16.
14. Rosenberger LH, Politano AD, Sawyer RG. The surgical care improvement project and prevention of post-operative infection, including surgical site infection. Surg Infect (Larchmt) 2011;12(3):163–8.
15. Wilson W, Taubert KA, Gewitz M, et al. Prevention of infective endocarditis: guidelines from the American Heart Association. Circulation 2007;116(15):1736–54.
16. Wilson WR, Gewitz M, Lockhart PB. Prevention of Viridans GRoup Streptococcal Infective Endocarditis. A scientific statement from the American Heart Association. Circulation 2021;142:e963–78.
17. Revision L. Antibiotic prophylaxis for dental patients at risk for infection - Best practices: antibiotic prophylaxis the reference manual of pediatric dentistry 2019. p. 417–21. Available at: http://circ.ahajournals.org/.
18. American Association of Endodontists. Antibiotic prophylaxis 2017 update. Supplement 2017. p. 1–3. Available at: https://www.aae.org/specialty/wp-content/uploads/sites/2/2017/06/aae_antibiotic-prophylaxis-2017update.pdf.
19. Sollecito TP, Abt E, Lockhart PB, et al. The use of prophylactic antibiotics prior to dental procedures in patients with prosthetic joints: evidence-based clinical practice guideline for dental practitioners-a report of the American Dental Association Council on Scientific Affairs. J Am Dent Assoc 2015;146(1):11–6.e8.
20. Mercuri LG. Prevention and detection of prosthetic temporomandibular joint infections—update. Int J Oral Maxillofac Surg 2019;48(2):217–24.
21. Esposito M, Grusovin MG, Worthington HV. Interventions for replacing missing teeth: antibiotics at dental implant placement to prevent complications. Cochrane Database of Systematic Reviews 2013;7:CD004152.
22. Lund B, Hultin M, Tranæus S, et al. Complex systematic review - perioperative antibiotics in conjunction with dental implant placement. Clin Oral Implants Res 2015;26:1–14.
23. Khouly I, Braun RS, Silvestre T, et al. Efficacy of antibiotic prophylaxis in intraoral bone grafting procedures: a systematic review and meta-analysis. Int J Oral Maxillofac Surg 2020;49(2):250–63.
24. Klinge A, Khalil D, Klinge B, et al. Prophylactic antibiotics for staged bone augmentation in implant dentistry. Acta Odontol Scand 2020;78(1):64–73.
25. Romandini M, De Tullio I, Congedi F, et al. PGA prophylaxis at dental implant placement: W is the best protocol? A systematic review and network meta-analysis. J Clin Periodontol 2019;46(3):382–95.
26. Resnik RR, Misch C. Prophylactic antibiotic regimens in oral implantology: rationale and protocol. Implant Dent 2008;17(2):142–50.
27. Oppelaar MC, Zijtveld C, Kuipers S, et al. Evaluation of prolonged vs short courses of antibiotic prophylaxis following ear, nose, throat, and oral and maxillofacial surgery: a systematic review and meta-

analysis. JAMA Otolaryngol Head Neck Surg 2019; 145:610–6.

28. Bartella AK, Lemmen S, Burnic A, et al. Influence of a strictly perioperative antibiotic prophylaxis vs a prolonged postoperative prophylaxis on surgical site infections in maxillofacial surgery. Infection 2018;46(2):225–30.

29. Veve MP, Davis SL, Williams AM, et al. Considerations for antibiotic prophylaxis in head and neck cancer surgery. Oral Oncol 2017;74(August):181–7.

30. Cannon RB, Houlton JJ, Mendez E, et al. Methods to reduce postoperative surgical site infections after head and neck oncology surgery. Lancet Oncol 2017;18(7):e405–13.

31. Saunders S, Reese S, Lam J, et al. Extended use of perioperative antibiotics in head and neck microvascular reconstruction. Am J Otolaryngol Head Neck Med Surg 2017;38(2):204–7.

32. Oomens MA, Verlinden CRA, Goey Y, et al. Prescribing antibiotic prophylaxis in orthognathic surgery: a systematic review. Int J Oral Maxillofac Surg 2014; 43(6):725–31.

33. Zijderveld SA, Smeele LE, Kostense PJ, et al. Preoperative antibiotic prophylaxis in orthognathic surgery: a randomized, double-blind, and placebo-controlled clinical study. J Oral Maxillofac Surg 1999;57(12):1403–6.

34. Danda AK, Wahab A, Narayanan V, et al. Single-dose versus single-day antibiotic prophylaxis for orthognathic surgery: a prospective, randomized, double-blind clinical study. J Oral Maxillofac Surg 2010;68(2):344–6.

35. Tan SK, Lo J, Zwahlen RA. Perioperative antibiotic prophylaxis in orthognathic surgery: A systematic review and meta-analysis of clinical trials. Oral Surg Oral Med Oral Pathol Oral Radiol Endod 2011;112(1):19–27.

36. Mercuri LG. Avoiding and managing temporomandibular joint total joint replacement surgical site infections. J Oral Maxillofac Surg 2012;70(10):2280–9.

Update on Antimicrobial Therapy in Management of Acute Odontogenic Infection in Oral and Maxillofacial Surgery

Check for updates

Sam R. Caruso, DMD[a],*, Elena Yamaguchi, MD[b],
Jason E. Portnof, DMD, MD, FACD, FICD[c,d]

KEYWORDS

- Odontogenic infections • Antibiotics • Caries • Head & neck infections • Antimicrobial therapy
- Oral flora • Incision and drainage

KEY POINTS

- Odontogenic infections have many presentations and contribute primarily to health disorders seen in both inpatient and outpatient settings across the United States and worldwide.
- There are varying antimicrobial therapies that can be used for patients with odontogenic infections. Each case should be assessed in full before concluding the antibiotic of choice for the patient's therapy; this is a continually evolving scenario that requires close follow-up with the possibility for change.
- Pharmacotherapy is an adjuvant therapy, not the definitive treatment for odontogenic infections.

INTRODUCTION

This article focuses on the antimicrobial therapy of head and neck infections from odontogenic origin. It will not discuss the antimicrobial treatment of uncomplicated dental caries and periodontal disease. This discussion is limited to adult immunocompetent patients; pediatrics, pregnant patients, patients with renal, hepatic, and cardiac problems are excluded, and management of these patients should be addressed on a case-by-case basis by the provider.

Odontogenic infections are among the most common infections of the oral cavity. They are sourced primarily from dental caries and periodontal disease (gingivitis and periodontitis). Many odontogenic infections are self-limiting and may drain spontaneously. However, these infections may drain into the

anatomic spaces adjacent to the oral cavity and spread along the contiguous facial planes, leading to more serious infections.[1] Holmes and Pellecchia[1] divide facial infections by primary and secondary spaces. Primary spaces include buccal, canine, sublingual, submandibular, submental, and vestibular spaces. After a direct primary infection, secondary infection can take place. These spaces include pterygomandibular, infratemporal, masseteric, lateral pharyngeal, superficial, and deep temporal, masticator, and retropharyngeal.

Infections in the head and neck have an array of presentations. However, they most often demonstrate classic signs and symptoms of infection in the early stages, including inflammation, edema, redness, and pain (calor [heat], rubor [redness], dolor [pain], tumor [swelling]). As the infection persists, systemic symptoms may result, including

[a] Department of Oral & Maxillofacial Surgery, Broward Health Medical Center, Nova Southeastern University College of Dental Medicine, 1600 S. Andrews Avenue, Fort Lauderdale, FL 33301, USA; [b] Private Practice, Infectious Diseases, 13550 South Jog Rd, Suite 202A, Delray, FL 33446, USA; [c] Department of Oral & Maxillofacial Surgery, Nova Southeastern University College of Dental Medicine, 3200 S. University Dr., Davie, FL 33314, USA; [d] Private Practice, Oral & Maxillofacial Surgery, Surgical Arts of Boca Raton, 9980 North Central Park Bvld, Suite #113, Boca Raton, FL 33428, USA
* Corresponding author.
E-mail address: scaruso@browardhealth.org

Oral Maxillofacial Surg Clin N Am 34 (2022) 169–177
https://doi.org/10.1016/j.coms.2021.08.005
1042-3699/22/© 2021 Elsevier Inc. All rights reserved.

more significant generalized or pronounced edema, trismus, tachycardia, dysphagia fever, fatigue, and malaise.[2]

These infections pose many threats, including patient mortality. Primary concern of the disease is that of airway security. In the past, the major cause of mortality was due to airway obstruction. Modern treatment guidelines for early airway security and surgical intervention have reduced this airway-related mortality. A 2015 study by Bali and colleagues[3] demonstrated that embarrassment of the airway was a tertiary cause of mortality accounting for only 5% of 18 deaths among 2790 patients. The 2 most common causes of mortalities in these patients were sepsis and preexisting organ failure. In addition, there are morbidities related to the course of spread to critical structures, which can include the orbit, brain, and spine.[1] Risks of odontogenic infection also include progression to sepsis, bacteremia, endocarditis, and acute respiratory distress syndrome.[4–7]

For the modern oral and maxillofacial surgeon or surgical trainee, these infections are commonly seen in an emergent setting, whether in office or in the local emergency department. In 2007, the Nationwide Emergency Department Sample database included 302,507 Emergency Department visits for facial cellulitis in the United States.[8] These patient encounters led to a significant financial expense. Kim and colleagues[9] showed many factors associated with increased length of stay in odontogenic infections with a mean cost of $24,290 per patient.

Abramowicz and colleagues[10] explored the nationwide inpatient sample from 2012 and 2013 showing that facial cellulitis accounted for 74,480 hospitalizations. Demographic results from the study show a greater number of women than men and mean age of 47.5 years.[10] In the retrospective analysis of the nationwide inpatient sample, 86.1% of the patients were routinely discharged and 0.2% of the patients died inthe hospital.[10] Of note, this study did not distinguish between odontogenic and other causes of facial cellulitis. It is inferred that many of these infections are odontogenic in nature. Other sources for head and neck infections could include peritonsillar, intravenous (IV) drug abuse, and foreign bodies.[11]

MICROBIOLOGY OF ODONTOGENIC INFECTIONS

Odontogenic infections are usually attributed to the endogenous flora of the mouth and not the introduction of nonresident bacteria.[12] It is important to emphasize that suppurative odontogenic infections are typically polymicrobial in nature, with mixed aerobic and anaerobic bacteria present.[13–15] However, the anaerobes generally outnumber the aerobic bacteria by a factor of 3- to 4fold.[16,17]

Knowledge of the usual microbial flora of the mouth and dental surfaces will help in the selection of empiric antimicrobial therapy while awaiting final culture results. In general, it is recommended to use antibiotics that cover these organisms, including anaerobic bacteria, as these may not necessarily grow with the usual available techniques or because of delays in getting samples to the microbiology laboratory. When "normal oropharyngeal flora" results are obtained from culture, practitioners should choose broad-spectrum antibiotics and not consider these results true negative cultures.

Actinomycosis is a rare subacute to chronic bacterial infection caused by *Actinomyces* spp, a bacterium that normally colonizes the human mouth. One of the common presentations includes cervicofacial actinomycosis.[18] It is characterized by contiguous spread, suppurative and granulomatous inflammation, and formation of multiple abscesses and sinus tracts that may discharge sulfur granules.[18] It is important to consider Actinomycosis in the differential diagnosis of orofacial and head and neck infections, as treatment with antimicrobial therapy is quite different from the treatment of other odontogenic infections. The preferred treatment for Actinomycosis is penicillin G 18 to 24 million units IV daily in divided doses for 2 to 6 weeks and then amoxicillin 500 to 750 mg orally 3 to 4 times a day for 6 to 12 months.[18]

DIAGNOSTICS OF ODONTOGENIC INFECTIONS
Imaging

A careful history and physical examination are important in the diagnosis of odontogenic infections. Clinical symptoms, vital signs, microbiological evaluation, and diagnostic imaging are all crucial in identifying the cause of infection and to help guide the course of treatment.

Modern imaging techniques provide the surgeon excellent topography of the spreading infection, but not all active infections warrant computed tomography (CT) imaging for definitive treatment.[19,20] There are "red-flag" clinical symptoms to consider CT imaging and likely inpatient stay. These "red-flag" clinical symptoms include but are not limited to trismus, fever, dysphagia, odynophagia, pain, and dyspnea.[1,19,20]

Weyh and colleagues[19] suggested "red-flag" clinical signs that warrant the use of CT imaging and include fever, pain, voice change, elevated floor of mouth, signs of inflammation of deep fascial spaces, periorbital edema, nonpalpable inferior border of the mandible, dyspnea, dysphagia or odynophagia, and trismus. The study found 56.6% of CT imaging was unnecessary. Christensen and colleagues[20] performed a study that determined emergency medicine physicians conducted CT imaging on 61.7% of patients who did not require CT imaging by study standards. Recommendations were made to increase education to providers to avoid unnecessary imaging.[20]

There is a wide array of clinical imaging that can be used to assess head and neck infections in the emergency setting, but the most common is CT imaging with IV contrast in a hospital setting and cone beam CT or panoramic film if the patient is being evaluated in an outpatient clinic. CT is particularly sensitive for soft tissue with IV contrast and remains the imaging modality of choice for assessment of most odontogenic infections (Fig. 1).[21]

CT 3-dimensional imaging will show ring enhancing loculations of well-formed abscesses, gas formation or entrapment, and finally, the soft tissue edema associated with these infections. Using IV contrast-enhanced CT for emergency diagnosis of head and neck infections is currently routine because it is fast, readily available, and relatively inexpensive.[22,23] However, limited soft tissue contrast and artifacts from bone and dental implants may compromise accurate delineation of neck disease.[21]

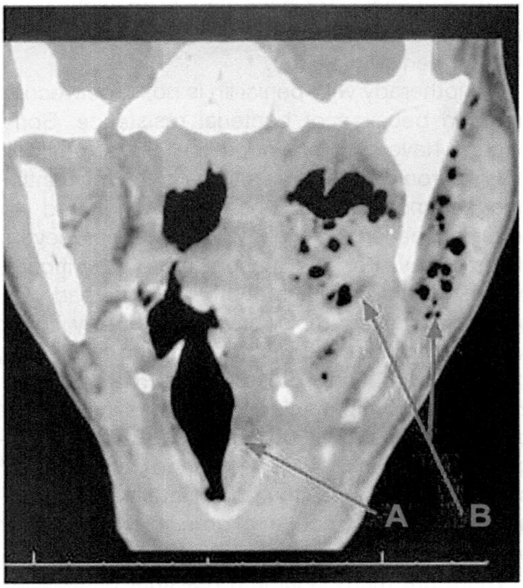

Although in-office panoramic imaging may be readily available, it is only beneficial in identifying a possible odontogenic source of the infection, as the soft tissue is not adequately visualized. Panoramic imaging can be reserved for an outpatient setting or should medical CT be unavailable.[19]

In patients with persistent odontogenic infections that are not clearly diagnosed by CT imaging with IV contrast and/or MRI, nuclear medicine studies, such as triple-phase bone scan or indium-labeled scans, can be used especially in cases of osteomyelitis of the jaw, but they are not typically used because they can be difficult to interpret.[24]

Microbiology

Obtaining appropriate material for culture and processing is important in the diagnosis of odontogenic infections. One of the difficulties in defining etiologic agents for odontogenic infections is the presence of normal resident flora. For closed space infections, it is very important that the normal oral flora be excluded during the specimen collection. Needle aspiration of loculated pus by an extraoral approach is desirable, and specimens should be transported immediately to the laboratory under anaerobic conditions. **Figs. 2** and **3** show a clinical specimen of an odontogenic abscess.

Contamination by the resident oral flora is inevitable for intraoral infections. In this setting, direct microscopic examination of stained smears,

Fig. 1. Gross airway deviation, infection, and gas formation in the deep spaces. (A) The gross deviation of the airway of the patient (arrow). (B) The gas formation from infection in the pterygomandibular and inferior temporal deep spaces (arrows).

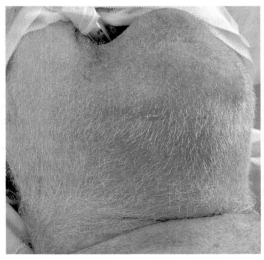

Fig. 2. A submandibular space abscess of odontogenic origin.

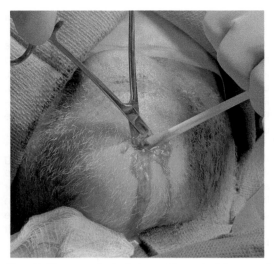

Fig. 3. The surgical intervention, incision and drainage, of the submandibular abscess and culture of purulent material.

such as Gram stain, often provides more useful information than culture results from surface swabs.

The gram-stain step is implemented to provide basic information about the culture sample and to provide some information to the clinician while awaiting culture results. If the sample shows excess epithelial cells, the laboratory can conclude that the sample was poorly obtained and includes skin or oral mucous membrane flora. If the presence of white blood cells is predominant, it can be assumed that the clinician gathered a good collection of purulent material.

Gram stains can also be helpful if they show a mixture of gram-positive and gram-negative bacteria and the aerobic culture is negative. This should raise the suspicion of anaerobic involvement. This information is useful especially if only aerobic cultures are sent.

Cultures will be specifically plated for both aerobic and anaerobic growth. The plates are monitored based on hospital protocol, with a minimum of daily evaluation. Aerobic growth assessment begins at 24 hours, and anaerobic growth assessment begins at 48 hours (**Fig. 4**).

In addition to cultures from abscesses or drainage, tissue biopsies should be routinely examined for histopathological evidence of acute or chronic inflammation and infection. Tissue biopsies should also be sent for aerobic and anaerobic cultures and if suspected for acid fast and fungal cultures before they are sent to the pathology laboratory. Specific microbial agents can sometimes be detected by immunofluorescence or polymerase chain reaction.

OUTPATIENT MANAGEMENT OF ODONTOGENIC INFECTIONS

Most outpatient odontogenic infections are treated with β-lactam antibiotics. The β-lactam ring is crucial to the bactericidal activity of the medication because of their inhibition of bacterial cell wall biosynthesis. β-Lactam antibiotics include penicillin derivatives, cephalosporins, cephamycins, monobactams, carbapenems and cabacephems.

The first-generation penicillins include penicillin V, which is orally administered, and penicillin G, which is administered parenterally. The usual adult dose for penicillin is 250 to 500 mg orally 4 times a day.

Third-generation penicillins (aminopenicillins) are effective against a wider spectrum of bacteria than first-generation penicillins and are generally used as a first-line agent against odontogenic infections. Amoxicillin is a third-generation penicillin that is commonly prescribed for adults as 500 mg orally 3 times a day or 500 to 875 mg orally 2 times a day. As β-lactamase production among oral anaerobes, such as *Prevotella* and *Fusobacterium* spp, is increasing, monotherapy treatment with standard penicillin has been found to be less effective. For this reason, it is not recommended.[25] Also, the need to take the oral penicillin 3 to 4 times a day on an empty stomach, because gastric acid inactivates the drug with the result that only 30% of the oral dose is absorbed, makes amoxicillin the drug of choice for initial empiric antibiotic treatment of mild odontogenic infections in patients without penicillin allergy.

Monotherapy with penicillin is no longer recommended because of bacterial resistance. Some experts have recommended the use of penicillin plus metronidazole as an alternative. A multiantibiotic regimen is less commonly adhered to, requiring patients to take 2 medications several times a day. For this reason, more practitioners are using amoxicillin monotherapy instead. The authors of this article have anecdotally found more compliance with patients taking twice-daily dosing and routinely prescribe 875 mg amoxicillin 2 times a day in patients for 7 days as the first-line outpatient treatment of dental and mild odontogenic infections. Al-Belasy and colleagues[26] showed that along with appropriate surgical management, a 3-day course of amoxicillin has shown similar clinical outcomes to a 7-day course.

There are many β-lactam-resistant bacteria inside the oral cavity. These bacteria produce β-lactamase, thereby inactivating the β-lactam ring. Bacteria that produce β-lactamase enzymes will be resistant to β-lactam antibiotics. β-Lactamase

A

B

C

D

E

F

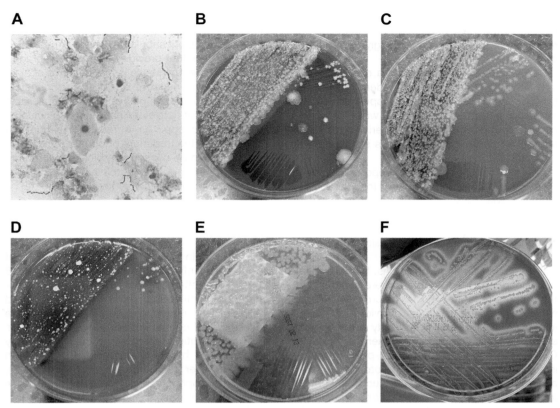

Fig. 4. In vitro microbiological evaluation of odontogenic abscesses and some regularly studied samples. (*A*) Gram stain showing gram-positive cocci in chains throughout, a large epithelial cell in the center, and several white blood cells throughout. (*B*) Blood agar plate from culture of oral flora. (*C*) Chocolate agar plate highlighting *Haemophilus*. (*D*) Columbia CNA plate highlighting alpha streptococcus and coagulase-negative *Staphylococcus*. (*E*) MacConkey agar growing enteric gram-negative bacilli. These same colonies can also be pictured in panels *D* and *E*. (*F*). Beta-hemolysis of blood agar.

enzymes are generally secreted by gram-negative bacteria. The β-lactamase inhibitor, clavulanic acid (clavulanate), is a β-lactam, structurally similar to the penicillins, and is often coformulated with the β-lactam antibiotics amoxicillin or ticarcillin. The combination of amoxicillin with clavulanate potassium is generally prescribed as 875 mg orally 2 times a day. The authors recommend switching to amoxicillin-clavulanic acid when there is not an adequate response to amoxicillin in 48 hours or use amoxicillin-clavulanic acid from the beginning when the infection is moderate or if there is involvement of the maxillary sinuses.

Clindamycin has excellent activity against gram-positive organisms, such as *Staphylococcus aureus*, *Streptococcus* spp, and most anaerobes above the diaphragm and β-lactamase-producing strains, and is used primarily in patients with odontogenic infections that are allergic to penicillin. Clindamycin binds to the 50S ribosomal subunit of susceptible bacteria and interferes with protein synthesis.[27]

More than 90% of clindamycin is absorbed following oral administration. Absorption is delayed but not decreased with the ingestion of food. Clindamycin's broad-spectrum coverage and excellent clinical efficacy, coupled with the increase in both penicillin resistance and the reports of treatment failures with penicillin, has prompted some experts to recommend clindamycin to be the drug of choice in treating odontogenic infections.[28]

The principal side effect associated with clindamycin is diarrhea, with a reported incidence ranging from 0.1% to 17%.[12] Clindamycin has also been associated with pseudomembranous colitis. This concern may be exaggerated, however, and the risk is probably no greater than with other broad-spectrum antimicrobials, including broad-spectrum penicillins and cephalosporins.[29]

The usual dose of clindamycin for odontogenic infections is 300 to 450 mg orally every 6 hours.[27] Knowledge of the local susceptibilities pattern is important, as in some areas *Streptococcus anginosus*, a prominent pathogen in odontogenic infections, is becoming increasingly resistant to clindamycin.[27]

Cephalosporin antibiotics are a class of β-lactam family antibiotics, originally derived from the fungus, *Acremonium*. Cephalosporins act by inhibiting enzymes in the cell walls of gram-positive and gram-negative bacteria in the same fashion as penicillins but are less susceptible to β-lactamases.

Cephalosporins have been reported to have cross-sensitivity with penicillins. However, cross-reactivity with penicillins and other classes of β-lactams, including other cephalosporins, is less common than previously thought, especially among patients who have had mild (nonanaphylactic) reactions to penicillins.

In patients allergic to penicillins, but tolerant to cephalosporins, and unable to take clindamycin, the authors recommend oral cefuroxime 500 mg twice daily for the treatment of mild odontogenic infections. Cefuroxime is the only oral cephalosporin that has coverage for anaerobic bacteria. Cefuroxime covers aerobic gram-positive organisms, such as *S aureus*, *Streptococcus* spp, anaerobic gram-positive cocci such as *Peptostreptococcus* spp, and *Viridans streptococci*. For more serious cases, metronidazole 500 mg orally every 8 hours is recommended in addition to cefuroxime. The other cephalosporins do not provide adequate anaerobic coverage, and they must be used in combination with either clindamycin or metronidazole.

As bactericidal antibiotics, quinolones inhibit the bacterial enzyme DNA gyrase and topoisomerase IV. They are not used as first-line oral agents in the treatment of odontogenic infections. Use should be limited to patients with positive cultures with Gram negatives that are not covered by amoxicillin or amoxicillin-clavulanic acid. Quinolones should be used in combination with amoxicillin or amoxicillin-clavulanic acid, clindamycin or metronidazole, as many quinolones do not have excellent activity against gram-positive cocci, and they do not cover anaerobes.

The FDA recommends avoiding unnecessary treatment of patients with quinolones unless the patient lacks alternatives. Quinolones can cause disabling and potential irreversible reactions, including tendonitis/tendon rupture, peripheral neuropathy, central nervous system effects, and worsening of myasthenia gravis symptoms, including muscle weakness.

Macrolide antibiotics include azithromycin, clarithromycin, and erythromycin. Al-Belasy and Hairam[26] described azithromycin and erythromycin as effective adjunctive treatments in the treatment of relatively mild odontogenic orofacial infections but should be used in combination with antibiotics that provide anaerobic coverage.

Although metronidazole is highly active against anaerobic gram-negative bacilli and spirochetes, it is only moderately active against anaerobic cocci and is not active against aerobes, including *Streptococcus* spp. As a result, it cannot be used alone in the treatment of odontogenic infections. It should be used in combination with penicillins, cephalosporins, macrolides, or quinolones in the appropriate clinical setting.

INPATIENT MANAGEMENT OF COMPLICATED ODONTOGENIC INFECTIONS

For patients in which signs and symptoms of odontogenic infection do not improve within 48 to 72 hours after surgical drainage and appropriate oral antibiotics, referral to an oral and maxillofacial surgeon and an infectious disease specialist is recommended. Severe infections must be identified promptly, as they can rapidly progress and be life threatening. Patients with persistent fever (temperature $\geq 38°C$ or 100.4 F), stridor, odynophagia, rapid progression and the involvement of multiple spaces, and secondary anatomic spaces should be treated in an inpatient hospital setting.

When evaluating antimicrobial options for inpatient management of odontogenic infections, ampicillin-sulbactam (Unasyn) remains the first choice for empiric coverage of most inpatients without penicillin allergy. This is formally an "off-label" use for odontogenic infections. The recommended dose is IV 3 g every 6 to 8 hours; duration is 7 to 14 days (including oral step-down therapy).[30] Unasyn provides broad extended coverage, including those that produce β-lactamases. Unasyn is the treatment of choice in immunocompetent patients. Penicillin G in combination with metronidazole can also be considered. This combination would be delivered as penicillin G, 2 to 4 million units IV every 4 to 6 hours along with 500 mg of metronidazole IV or orally every 8 hours. For penicillin-allergic patients, the current standard of care is clindamycin 600 mg IV every 8 hours plus levofloxacin 500 to 750 mg IV or PO every 24 hours.

Some experts advise against isolated clindamycin for initial therapy because of resistant *S anginosus* (millergi group) in 20-30% of isolates. Equally Prevotella can be resistant to clindamycin in about 20-30% of isolates.[27] This susceptibility is dependent on local patterns of resistance. Information for local resistance patterns should be available within the local hospital microbiology department.

If the penicillin allergy is confirmed as nonsevere, one could prescribe ceftriaxone (a third-generation cephalosporin 1 to 2 g IV every 24 hours) plus metronidazole (500 mg IV every 8 hours) or ceftriaxone 1-2 g IV every 24 hours and Clindamycin 600-900 mg IV every 6 to 8 hours. If available, cefoxitin 2 g every 6 hours or cefotetan 2 g IV every 12 hours is also an option. The above antibiotic combinations are not exhaustive and are the antibiotic combinations preferred by the authors, but different antibiotic regimens can be selected taking in consideration the presence or absence of antibiotic allergies, drug interactions and local susceptibility patterns of antibiotic resistance.

CHLORHEXIDINE GLUCONATE

Oral suspension of 0.12% chlorhexidine gluconate mouth rinse is a regular part of the oral infection and postoperative regimen of many oral and maxillofacial surgeons and dentists. In light of the abundance of use of the suspension, there appears to be a relative lack of recent data on the use of chlorhexidine gluconate suspension in the prevention and treatment of odontogenic infections. Much of its use in modern oral and maxillofacial surgery and dentistry is based on anecdotal practices.

Halabi and colleagues[31] showed that chlorhexidine gluconate mouth rinse was a safe and effective way to reduce alveolar osteitis postoperatively in patients with tooth extraction. Chlorhexidine gluconate has also been shown to significantly reduce plaque and gingival bleeding sores over placebos in periodontal studies.[32] A review by Daly and colleagues[33] suggested there were benefits to chlorhexidine gluconate (both 0.12% and 0.2%) rinse after tooth extraction in the prevention of alveolar osteitis, but also identified incidents of patient adverse reactions to the solution. Given the high frequency that this medication is prescribed, the authors recommend further study of this topic, and evidence-based prescribing practices.

STEROIDS

The use of steroids in acute odontogenic infection has been the source of some controversy. Synthetic glucocorticoids tend to be much more potent than their natural corticosteroid counterparts. Methylprednisolone is about 5 times as potent, and betamethasone and dexamethasone are 20 to 30 times as potent as natural corticosteroids.[34] There are contraindications for the use of steroids. For example, a common contraindication includes a medical history significant for diabetes mellitus

due to the risk of worsening hyperglycemia.[35–37] A survey of maxillofacial specialists in the United Kingdom in 2017 showed that 15% of practitioners used steroids to combat odontogenic infections.[38] This number increased to 60% when the infection threatened airway compromise.[38] The use of corticosteroids in treating odontogenic infections is quite debated with evidence supporting both arguments for and against.[39]

SUMMARY

Antibiotics are an important aspect of care of the patient with an acute odontogenic infection. Antibiotics are not a substitute for definitive surgical management. Incision and drainage and the elimination of the infection source are the main factors in a favorable outcome.[26]

Some minor odontogenic infections can be treated effectively with surgery alone, and without additional antimicrobial drugs.[26] However, these patients should be monitored closely for progression or resolution of the infection. Medical management, including antibiotic medications, combined with surgery for removal of the infective source will provide ultimate treatment for the infection.

CLINICS CARE POINTS

- Appropriate management of odontogenic infections has a major effect on total health care dollars and overall patient outcomes.

- Outpatient vs inpatient management of odontogenic infections varies dramatically in both surgical intervention and medication selection.

- Working closely with a microbiology laboratory could improve outcomes by providing clinicians more data about the source and delivering guidance for specific antibiotic therapy.

- Chlorhexidine gluconate is used regularly for these infections, but further studies should be conducted to support its use.

- The use of steroids in odontogenic infections is a debated topic with strong literature both for and against. Steroids should be used on a case-by-case basis.

- Surgical intervention is the gold-standard treatment for odontogenic infections, but pharmacotherapy is an important adjuvant in successful outcomes.

DISCLOSURES

All authors of this article have no conflicts of interests to disclose.

ACKNOWLEDGMENTS

The authors would like to provide a special thanks to Elizabeth George, Assistant Chief Medical Technologist of Microbiology at Memorial Healthcare System, Hollywood, FL, and her team for their assistance with this article.

REFERENCES

1. Holmes CJ, Pellecchia R. Antimicrobial therapy in management of odontogenic infections in general dentistry. Dent Clin North Am 2016;60(2):497–507.
2. Martins JR, Chagas OL, Velasques BD, et al. The use of antibiotics in odontogenic infections: what is the best choice? A systematic review. J Oral Maxillofac Surg 2017;75(12):2606.e1–11.
3. Bali RK, Sharma P, Gaba S, et al. A review of complications of odontogenic infections. Natl J Maxillofac Surg 2015;6(2):136–43.
4. Haggerty CJ, Tender GC. Actinomycotic brain abscess and subdural empyema of odontogenic origin: case report and review of the literature. J Oral Maxillofac Surg 2012;70(3):e210–3.
5. Rajab B, Laskin DM, Abubaker AO. Odontogenic infection leading to adult respiratory distress syndrome. J Oral Maxillofac Surg 2013;71(2):302–4.
6. Roberts GJ, Holzel HS, Sury MR, et al. Dental bacteremia in children. Pediatr Cardiol 1997;18(1):24–7.
7. Parahitiyawa NB, Jin LJ, Leung WK, et al. Microbiology of odontogenic bacteremia: beyond endocarditis. Clin Microbiol Rev 2009;22(1):46–64.
8. Kim MK, Allareddy V, Nalliah RP, et al. Burden of facial cellulitis: estimates from the nationwide emergency department sample. Oral Surg Oral Med Oral Pathol Oral Radiol 2012;114(3):312–7.
9. Kim MK, Nalliah RP, Lee MK, et al. Factors associated with length of stay and hospital charges for patients hospitalized with mouth cellulitis. Oral Surg Oral Med Oral Pathol Oral Radiol 2012;113(1):21–8.
10. Abramowicz S, Rampa S, Allareddy V, et al. The burden of facial cellulitis leading to inpatient hospitalization. J Oral Maxillofac Surg 2017;75(8):1656–67.
11. Ridder GJ, Technau-Ihling K, Sander A, et al. Spectrum and management of deep neck space infections: an 8-year experience of 234 cases. Otolaryngol Head Neck Surg 2005;133(5):709–14.
12. Sandor GK, Low DE, Judd PL, et al. Antimicrobial treatment options in the management of odontogenic infections. J Can Dent Assoc 1998;64(7):508–14.
13. Greenberg RN, James RB, Marier RL, et al. Microbiologic and antibiotic aspects of infections in the oral and maxillofacial region. J Oral Surg 1979;37(12):873–84.
14. Kannangara DW, Thadepalli H, McQuirter JL. Bacteriology and treatment of dental infections. Oral Surg Oral Med Oral Pathol 1980;50(2):103–9.
15. von Konow L, Nord CE, Nordenram A. Anaerobic bacteria in dentoalveolar infections. Int J Oral Surg 1981;10(5):313–22.
16. Baker KA, Fotos PG. The management of odontogenic infections. A rationale for appropriate chemotherapy. Dent Clin North Am 1994;38(4):689–706.
17. Sands T, Pynn BR, Katsikeris N. Odontogenic infections: part two. Microbiology, antibiotics and management. Oral Health 1995;85(6):11–4, 17–21, 23 passim.
18. Valour F, Sénéchal A, Dupieux C, et al. Actinomycosis: etiology, clinical features, diagnosis, treatment, and management. Infect Drug Resist 2014;7:183–97.
19. Weyh A, Busby E, Smotherman C, et al. Overutilization of computed tomography for odontogenic infections. J Oral Maxillofac Surg 2019;77(3):528–35.
20. Christensen BJ, Park EP, Nelson S, et al. Are emergency medicine physicians able to determine the need for computed tomography and specialist consultation in odontogenic maxillofacial infections? J Oral Maxillofac Surg 2018;76(12):2559–63.
21. Hurley MC, Heran MKS. Imaging studies for head and neck infections. Infect Dis Clin North Am 2007;21(2):305–53, v–vi.
22. Kamalian S, Avery L, Lev MH, et al. Nontraumatic head and neck emergencies. Radiogr Rev Publ Radiol Soc N Am Inc 2019;39(6):1808–23.
23. Maroldi R, Farina D, Ravanelli M, et al. Emergency imaging assessment of deep neck space infections. Semin Ultrasound CT MR 2012;33(5):432–42.
24. Boronat-Ferrater M, Simó-Perdigó M, Cuberas-Borrós G, et al. Bone scintigraphy and radiolabeled white blood cell scintigraphy for the diagnosis of mandibular osteomyelitis. Clin Nucl Med 2011;36(4):273–6.
25. Brook I. Antibiotic resistance of oral anaerobic bacteria and their effect on the management of upper respiratory tract and head and neck infections. Semin Respir Infect 2002;17(3):195–203.
26. Al-Belasy FA, Hairam AR. The efficacy of azithromycin in the treatment of acute infraorbital space infection. J Oral Maxillofac Surg 2003;61(3):310–6.
27. Guidelines for treatment of odontogenic infections in hospitalized adults. 2018. Available at: https://www.med.umich.edu/asp/pdf/adult_guidelines/Odontogenic_ADULT.pdf. Accessed April 21, 2021.

28. Gilbert DN, Chambers HF, Eliopoulos GM, et al. The Sanford guide to antimicrobial therapy 2019. 49th edition. Antimibrobial Therapy, Inc; 2019.

29. Devenyi AG. Antibiotic-induced colitis. Semin Pediatr Surg 1995;4(4):215–20.

30. Chow AW. Complications, diagnosis, and treatment of odontogenic infections. Available at: http://www.uptodate.com. Accessed March 29, 2019.

31. Halabi D, Escobar J, Alvarado C, et al. Chlorhexidine for prevention of alveolar osteitis: a randomised clinical trial. J Appl Oral Sci Rev 2018;26:e20170245.

32. Sanz M, Newman MG, Anderson L, et al. Clinical enhancement of post-periodontal surgical therapy by a 0.12% chlorhexidine gluconate mouthrinse. J Periodontol 1989;60(10):570–6.

33. Daly TE, Drane JB, MacComb WS. Management of problems of the teeth and jaw in patients undergoing irradiation. Am J Surg 1972;124(4):539–42.

34. Bodnar J. Corticosteroids and oral surgery. Anesth Prog 2001;48(4):130–2.

35. Ko H-H, Chien W-C, Lin Y-H, et al. Examining the correlation between diabetes and odontogenic infection: a nationwide, retrospective, matched-cohort study in Taiwan. PLoS One 2017;12(6):e0178941.

36. Weise H, Naros A, Weise C, et al. Severe odontogenic infections with septic progress - a constant and increasing challenge: a retrospective analysis. BMC Oral Health 2019;19(1):173.

37. Juncar M, Popa AR, Baciuț MF, et al. Evolution assessment of head and neck infections in diabetic patients–a case control study. J Craniomaxillofac Surg 2014;42(5):498–502.

38. McDonald C, Hennedige A, Henry A, et al. Management of cervicofacial infections: a survey of current practice in maxillofacial units in the UK. Br J Oral Maxillofac Surg 2017;55(9):940–5.

39. Tami A, Othman S, Sudhakar A, et al. Ludwig's angina and steroid use: a narrative review. Am J Otolaryngol 2020;41(3):102411.

Medication Management of Selected Pathological Jaw Lesions

Yijiao Fan, DDS[a],*, Allen Glied, DDS[b]

KEYWORDS

- Jaw lesions • Nonsurgical • Oral surgery • ABC • CGCG • Fibrous dysplasia
- Paget's disease of bone • MRONJ

KEY POINTS

- Most jaw lesions are treated surgically, but there is evidence for treating select jaw lesions pharmaceutically.
- Most jaw lesions are osteolytic, so drugs that target the physiology of bone turnover are effective.
- Bisphosphonates and denosumab are a common group of drugs that can be used to treat select bone lesions, but they can also cause medication-related osteonecrosis of the jaw.
- Necrosis of the jaw either owing to medications or radiation can also be treated pharmaceutically.

INTRODUCTION

Most jaw lesions are treated by surgical removal. Minimizing or eliminating surgical trauma is beneficial to patients whenever possible. Interest is growing in nonsurgical treatment alternatives, especially in pharmaceutical therapy, for surgery refractory or surgery contraindicated patients. Some of the evidence is taken from orthopedic literature studying extragnathic lesions that also occur in the jaw. Some drugs work by targeting a cellular mechanism antithetical to the pathophysiology of a specific lesion. Other drugs work by promoting bone fill through global mechanisms because jaw lesions are predominantly osteolytic. Drugs that target the osteoblast–osteoclast relationship to build bone or prevent bone resorption are especially common. Select jaw lesions with well-studied pharmaceutical treatments are presented.

CENTRAL GIANT CELL GRANULOMA

Nonsurgical treatments for central giant cell granulomas (CGCG) are the most studied in jaw lesions. CGCGs are benign, locally destructive intraosseous lesions predominantly found in the anterior mandible but can occur anywhere in the jaw bones.[1,2] First described by Jaffe in 1953 as a reparative non-neoplastic lesion, it has a female predilection and occurs most commonly in young people between 10 and 25 years of age.[3] It is characterized microscopically by proliferating giant cells in a stroma of oval and spindle mesenchymal cells, especially around areas of hemorrhage.[2,4] Radiographically, CGCGs are osteolytic or radiolucent, with the ability to displace teeth and expand or perforate gnathic contours, and may be unilocular or multilocular. In 1986, Chuong distinguished between 2 types of CGCGs, namely, nonaggressive and aggressive.[5] The former describes an indolent lesion that usually presents with painless asymptomatic swelling of the jaw but aggressive lesions were described as showing more neoplastic characteristics including presence of pain, paresthesia, root resorption, rapid growth, cortical perforation, and high recurrence after curettage. Histologically, however, the 2 types of CGCGs were indistinguishable.[2,4] Multiple lesions are rare but possible, and have bene associated

[a] Department of Oral and Maxillofacial Surgery, The Brooklyn Hospital Center, 121 Dekalb Avenue, Brooklyn, NY 11201, USA; [b] Department of Dentistry, St. Barnabas Hospital, 4422 Third Avenue, Bronx, NY 10457, USA
* Corresponding author.
E-mail address: yfan@tbh.org

Oral Maxillofacial Surg Clin N Am 34 (2022) 179–187
https://doi.org/10.1016/j.coms.2021.08.004
1042-3699/22/© 2021 Elsevier Inc. All rights reserved.

with genetic syndromes especially Noonan syndrome, which is associated with growth deformities, cardiac problems, and coagulopathies.[6] The recognition of the aggressive variant and syndromic links call into question if CGCGs are entirely reparative in nature. Although the exact etiology of CGCG is unclear, it is hypothesized that the actual proliferating cells in CGCGs are spindle cells in the stroma, which act to recruit giant cells from adjacent vasculature. Although abundant, giant cells seem to be histologically non-neoplastic under a microscope. Nevertheless, the abundant giant cells are reactive to RANKL, and when activated promote osteoclastogenesis, thereby producing a lysis of regional bone.[2]

The most common treatment modality is surgery. Enucleation alone has been shown to exhibit up to 72% recurrence.[4] Resection had much high long-term success, but still can have recurrence.[7] Nonsurgical treatment modalities are well studied for CGCGs.

Intralesional Steroid Injections in Central Giant Cell Granulomas

In 1988, Jacoway was the first to report treatment of CGCG with corticosteroids. Since then, numerous investigators have reported success with intralesional steroid injections as monotherapy or in combination with surgery.[2] Osterne and associates[8] reviewed 41 cases of CGCG treated with intralesional steroid between 1994 and 2011. The patients were split 20:21 male:female, with an average age of 15.9 years. There were 12 lesions in the maxilla and 29 lesions in the mandible. On follow-up (range, 7 months to 7 years), 32 (78%) were considered good responses, 6 (15%) were considered moderate responses, and 3 (7%) were considered negative responses. Seventeen patients (41%) did require additional surgical treatment; 9 (22%) underwent further osteoplasty, 5 (12%) underwent further curettage, and 3 (7%) required resection. Additionally, 3 patients (7%) received additional steroid injections on follow-up, although they did not require surgery. Predictably, when the data were stratified, nonaggressive lesions (18 [44%]) were more responsive to steroid injections. No cases had negative responses. Sixteen patients (89%) reported good response to therapy versus 2 (11%) who reported moderate response to therapy. Four patients (22%) required additional osteoplasty, 3 (17%) required additional curettage, and 2 cases required additional injections; no cases resulted in resection. Aggressive lesions (23 [56%]) showed less overall but significant response to steroid injections. Sixteen patients

(70%) reported a good response, 4 (17%) reported a moderate response, and 3 (13%) reported a negative response. Four patients (17%) required additional osteoplasty, 2 (9%) required additional curettage, and 3 (13%) ultimately needed resection, but it is useful to note that 14 (61%) did not require surgical treatment after corticosteroid therapy.[8] From these data, it can be inferred that there may be a clinical benefit to use of corticosteroid intralesional injections in both aggressive and nonaggressive lesions.

The mechanism of corticosteroids' therapeutic effect is not well-understood. All CGCG lesions seem to express receptors for glucocorticoids to some degree.[9] On one hand, dexamethasone was shown in vitro to stimulate osteoclast precursor differentiation and proliferation.[10] On the other hand, it seems like corticosteroids induce apoptosis of osteoclastlike cells.[11] The net effect clinically sees to be the inhibition of bone resorption.[1,2,11]

Most commonly, the steroid used for injection was triamcinolone acetonide (10 mg/mL) or triamcinolone hexacetonide (20 mg/mL), diluted with equal parts lidocaine or marcaine, and injected weekly or biweekly for 6 weeks. Two milliliters of injection fluid was generally injected for every 2 cm of radiolucency, with 1 mL of fluid for every 1 cm^3 of lesion was used reported. Common side effects include injection site pain, bleeding, bruising, infection, contact dermatitis (generally only if there is a preservative), and impaired wound healing. Systemic side effects are unlikely due to the localized route of delivery, but can potentially include allergic reactions, glucose intolerance, Cushing syndrome, hirsutism, osteoporosis, muscle weakness, tendon rupture, and cardiac and neurologic problems.[1,12]

Calcitonin in Central Giant Cell Granulomas

Calcitonin is a peptide hormone produced primarily by the thyroid parafollicular cells that regulate blood calcium levels by directly inhibiting the activity of osteoclasts and decreasing the activity of calcium resorption in the kidneys.[13] Calcitonin has also been demonstrated to interfere with osteoclast precursor differentiation. Calcitonin receptors are found in osteoclast cells and the giant cells in CGCG have been shown to be osteoclasts.[2,14] Therefore, calcitonin should have a direct inhibitive effect in decreasing bone resorptive activity of CGCG giant cells. Both human and salmon calcitonin have been implicated in CGCG therapy, with the latter being approximately 1.5× as potent, but with the former being potentially less immunogenic. In vitro studies showed no difference in bone-resorptive effects between human and salmon calcitonin.[15] Calcitonin can be injected subcutaneously 50 to 100 IU/d or sprayed nasally 100 to 200 IU/d. There is no consensus regarding the efficacy injection versus nasal spray, but bioavailability is estimated to be approximately 70% for injections and 3% to 25% for nasal spray.[2] Harris[16] was the first to suggest the use of human and salmon calcitonin via injection (100 IU/d) and nasal spray (200 IU/d) in 4 patients with CGCG. He claimed complete remission, but 2 patients had to undergo additional surgery. Studies following Harris generally showed partial to complete remission with varying calcitonin regimen.[2] However, in the largest of such studies by De Lange,[2] 14 patients with CGCG treated by salmon nasal spray 200 IU/d showed no response to only partial remission. The inconsistency in the clinical efficacy of calcitonin therapy for CGCG may be related to varying expressions of calcitonin receptors in CGCG lesions. Vered and coworkers[9] observed that only 23 of 41 CGCG lesions stained positive for calcitonin receptors, and of the lesions that were positive, the intensity of staining varied. Side effects can be inferred from the use of calcitonin subcutaneous injections for osteoporosis, which include nausea, abdominal pain, diarrhea, vomiting, flushing, injection site swelling or redness, salty taste in the mouth, increased urination, or loss of appetite.[17]

Interferon in Central Giant Cell Granulomas

Interferon (IFN) is a cellular mediator that has antiviral and antiangiogenic effects.[2] Some investigators have observed that CGCG are associated with high vascularity and have speculated that decreasing vascular growth to the lesions may act to suppress lesion proliferation. An in vitro study with porcine mesenchymal stem cells also showed that IFN stimulated differentiation of precursors to osteoblasts. The efficacy of IFN in literature is promising. De Lange[2] and associates presented 6 studies totaling 32 patients in 2006. All showed arrest or slowing of lesion growth; however, only 2 of 6 studies claimed complete remission. Three of the 6 studies had patients undergo additional surgery after IFN therapy. It is hypothesized that IFN's antiangiogenic and bone-forming effects can terminate rapid growth in CGCG, but because there are no direct effects on the proliferating cells, complete remission is unlikely in most cases. IFN is given as a subcutaneous injection 1×10^6 to 9×10^6 IU per day for 2 to 14 months.

The use of IFN is also limited by its well-known side effects, including headache, fatigue, diarrhea, upset stomach, appetite loss, dizziness, xerostomia, dysgeusia, nausea/vomiting, and, most important, pancytopenia. Blood counts should be monitored regularly during therapy. Liver damage has also been reported. IFN is contraindicated in patients with autoimmune or decompensated liver disease, pregnancy, and known hypersensitivity reactions.[1] Therefore, surgery is preferred over or used in combination with IFN. IFN has rarely been used as monotherapy.

Bisphosphonates and Denosumab in Central Giant Cell Granulomas

Antiresorptives are medications that prevent bone resorption and include bisphosphonates (eg, zoledronate) and monoclonal antibodies that inhibit the osteoclast activator RANKL (eg, denosumab). It is intuitively sound that lytic lesions such as CGCG should respond to antiresorptive therapy, and in fact bisphosphonates will be making multiple appearances throughout this write up. Bisphosphonates being the older of the 2 are also used to strengthen bone in a myriad of destructive bone diseases such as osteoporosis and metastatic bone disease. Bisphosphonates are small molecules with a structure similar to inorganic phosphate and they work in 2 main ways. First, bisphosphonates bind strongly to the mineral component of bone thereby disrupting the normal process of conversion between amorphous calcium and phosphate molecules and crystal hydroxyapatite. Second, they disrupt osteoclasts intracellularly, eventually inducing programmed cell death. There is also evidence to suggest that they downregulate osteoclast precursors. Their strong binding affinity to bone allows them to stay embedded in bone, being effective years after administration.[18] Denosumab on the other hand was created after discovery of the RANK/RANKL system between stromal cells and osteoclast precursors to activate osteoclasts. Denosumab is a monoclonal antibody that disrupts this interaction, thereby downregulating the availability of activated osteoclasts. The effect of denosumab is much shorter and also stronger compared with bisphosphonates.[18]

Landesberg and colleagues[19] reported 3 cases of use of intravenous bisphosphonate therapy with varying degree of success. One patient was treated with a single treatment of 4 mg zoledronic acid and lesion showed complete regression after 6 months. The second patient was treated by 2 treatments of 90 mg pamidronate at 6 months intervals, which resulted in a 30% decrease in lesion size on a computed tomography scan. The patient was then lost to follow-up. The third patient received 3 doses of 4 mg zoledronic acid at yearly intervals. The lesion stabilized but did not regress. The patient ended up requiring surgical excision. In the pediatric population, alternatives to surgery are preferred when possible; however, antiresorptives are not often used owing to concerns of skeletal growth disruption. However, in cases where the initial surgery failed to achieve adequate resolution, Chien and associates[20] were able to describe 4 pediatric patients with CGCG treated with zoledronic acid, 3 of whom had resolution of lesions without need for additional therapy. Chien and associates reported that there were instances of flulike symptoms and phosphate depletion after treatment, but the therapy was generally well-tolerated without evidence of long term effects on projected anthropometric growth parameters. Choe and coworkers[21] also reported that CGCG in children can be treated by denosumab. Choe and coworkers described 2 cases where denosumab was used successfully to achieve a positive response in lesions, indicated by bone fill on CBCT and histopathologic evaluation showing viable in lieu of giant cells. One of the 2 cases also received intralesoinal corticosteroid injections. Facial deformity was also reduced for each patient. Denosumab was given monthly by 120 mg subcutaneous injections.

The most common side effects of antiresorptives include extremity pain, back pain, and headache. More serious side effects include hypocalcemia, hypophosphatemia, anemia, and osteonecrosis of the jaw. There is also concern of disruption of linear growth when used in pediatric patients. However, this is difficult to study owing to long-term follow-up and we have found no reports in literature.

In this author's opinion, the role of antiresorptives in the treatment of CGCG is supported by case studies, albeit with limited evidence. Surgery remains the first-line treatment, and in surgery-refractory cases or pediatric cases indicated for a more conservative approach, there are other pharmaceutical treatments such as intralesional steroid injections that do not have the potential to cause stunted growth or osteonecrosis of the jaw. Medication related osteonecrosis of the jaw in the dental and oral surgery community has been an active topic and its relationship to antiresorptive use before trauma to the jaw bones is well-documented. Osteonecrosis of the jaw is a rare but chronic complication that can cause prolonged morbidity to the patient, sometimes requiring extensive invasive surgery. In fact, many of the cases in literature supporting use of antiresorptives were in patients with other prior or concurrent non–antiresorptive pharmaceutical therapy.

ANEURYSMAL BONE CYST

The aneurysmal bone cyst (ABC) is, despite its name, a pseudocyst of the skeleton that occurs in the jaw in approximately 2% of cases. It is a non-neoplastic bony lytic lesion filled with blood.[22] ABCs occur mostly in the pediatric population. The etiology is unclear. Some investigators have hypothesized that ABCs are secondary lesions arising from other primary lesions of the jaw because microcysts and cysts filled with blood are also found in many other jaw lesions such as the aforementioned CGCG, Paget's disease of bone (PDOB), fibrous dysplasia (FD), and so on.[23] ABCs occur more in the mandible compared with the maxilla, with the condyle and ramus being the most common areas of occurrence.[24] In literature, the majority of cases were treated by surgical curettage or resection. Successful cryotherapy and spontaneous healing have also been observed.[24] Estimated recurrence ranges from 13.3% to 59.0% and, owing to its vascular nature and increased risk of perioperative hemorrhage, nonsurgical pharmaceutical agents have been proposed as surgical alternatives or adjuncts.[24,25]

Sclerosing Agents (Percutaneous Embolization) in Aneurysmal Bone Cysts

Sclerosing agents disable a vascular source or lesion, traditionally endovascularly. Percutaneous embolization of an ABC introduces the sclerosing agent directly into the bony cavity of the ABC. Alcoholic zein (Ethibloc) is one of the most widely used sclerosing agents. Zein is a storage protein found in corn and is thrombogenic. Dissolved in alcohol as Ethibloc, the zein component causes a local inflammatory reaction.[25] Harvey George studied patients with ABCs treated with 4.0 to 7.5 mL of alcoholic zein via direct intralesional injections. He found that 58% of patients exhibited complete resolution and 35% exhibited partial healing (with asymptomatic residual nonprogressive lytic areas) at 22 to 90 months follow-ups on a postprocedural computed tomography scan. Harvey's review did not, however, include cases of ABC in the jaw. Baldo and colleagues[26] reported a case of a 7 year old with ABC in the left mandible being treated with histoacryl. Histoacryl is n-butyl-2-cyanoacrylate, a resin based sclerosing agent that polymerizes upon contact with blood thereby sealing the area of the bleed. Histoacryl is used 1:1 with a lipiodol carrier to prevent premature polymerization. In the case that Baldo and associates treated, the lesion showed no sign of recurrence and the patient also underwent successful orthodontic treatment involving movement of teeth in the area of the lesion with preservation of teeth vitality. The biggest risk of using sclerosing agents is venous drainage. Contrast or dye is injected before introducing the sclerosing agent to the control risk of unwanted sclerosing of the downstream vasculature or the creation of an embolus. Other complications reported included aseptic fistulation, infection of the bone and soft tissue, and systemic immune reactions such as fever.

Aqueous Calcium Sulfate in Aneurysmal Bone Cyst

Some consider ABCs as not only secondary lesions, but reparative lesions. Delloye and associates[27] reported healing of ABCs treated with nothing but demineralized bone and bone marrow to facilitate the reparative process. Ossification was seen in the within 3 months postoperatively. However, this procedure required surgical access that was not so different from a curettage procedure. Clayer[28] advanced this concept by injecting aqueous calcium sulfate directly into the cyst, which he hypothesized has the same osteoconductive properties within the lesion without the surgical trauma. In his pool of 15 patients, Clayer noted a 90% response rate in increased ossification of lesions by 8 weeks without surgical morbidity. He also reported a decrease in preoperative pain around the lesions in all but 1 patient. The report had a recurrence rate of 2 patients among 15 and pathologic fracture despite radiographic signs of healing. On a spectrum of treatment options, aqueous calcium sulfate is one of the more conservative treatment options.

PAGET'S DISEASE OF BONE AND CRANIOFACIAL FIBROUS DYSPLASIA

PDOB and craniofacial FD are 2 fibro-osseous conditions that have similar skeletal phenotypic presentations and have similar treatments. PDOB was first described by James Paget in 1877 and is predominantly polyostotic and predominantly in people over the age of 30.[29] It is a rare disease of bone turnover characterized by 3 distinct phases. Phase I (early) is a period of osteolysis. It is the most aggressive time of the PDOB and appears and behaves like other lytic lesions of the jaw. It is thought of as an imbalance of osteoclastic to osteoblastic activity. Phase II (intermediate) is a period of disordered bone growth. It is the most dominant phase in PDOB, where diseased phase I bone is interspersed with immature woven bone resulting in a net gain but weaker stock of bone. In phase III (late), the disease burns out. Previously late immature bone is remodeled to sclerotic hard bone, clinically presenting as multiple abnormal bone overgrowths. The etiology is not clear, with possible genetic and/or environmental factors such as bony reactions or low-grade viral infections. FD also compromises the integrity of the skeleton, but tends to be mono-ostotic rather than polyostotic. It has a well-characterized genetic basis in mutations involving the GNAS1 gene, a component of the ubiquitous G protein involved in intracellular secondary messaging. This factor explains that FD is associated with McCune–Albright syndrome, a multisystem syndromic condition with endocrine dysfunction, somatic lesions, and polyostotic FD. Similar to PDOB, normal bone architecture is disrupted by proliferation of GNAS1 mutated osteoblasts creating soft spongy bone that is predisposed to fractures. All of these patients have weakened and sometimes abnormally shaped bone, which can lead to facial deformities, pathologic fractures, and impingement of nearby nerves. Surgery is not always indicated, except for severe cases; for example, if the bony expansion is invading nearby vital structures such as the first and seventh cranial nerves, possibly leading to blindness or deafness, surgery is indicated. Without surgery, these patients are treated pharmacologically when needed.[29]

Bisphosphonates in Paget's Disease of Bone

Bisphosphonates are commonly used in conditions that weaken the skeleton such as osteoporosis and metastatic bone disease. PDOB and FD both have clinically weakened bone prone to fracture. Bisphosphonates are the mainstay for treatment of PDOB before surgery. Ralston and associates[30] conducted a systematic review of the literature on the diagnosis and treatments of Paget's disease, including the use of bisphosphonates. One meta-analysis of 418 patients showed that predominately bisphosphonate-treated patients achieved a decrease in bone pain at 45% versus 23% in placebo. Intravenous zoledronate was inferred to be the preferred agent for bone pain. Zoledronic acid (4 mg) for bone pain was found to be superior to 30 mg IV pamidronate when given on 2 consecutive days every 3 months. One other study also found that 5 mg zoledronic acid provided more pain relief than 30 mg risedronate given orally. The same study found that bone pain relapsed a lot more (10 times more with zoledronic acid and 25% more with risedronate) than biochemical relapse, suggesting there are separate mechanisms dictating the 2 entities. Ralston and coworker's review also showed that quality of life (as surrogated by the Short Form 36 physical summary score) consistently was slightly elevated when using zoledronic acid. However, the effect was not statistically significant in any of the included articles that studied this parameter. On the effect of bisphosphonates on the incidence of pathologic fractures, Ralston and colleagues reported that there was insufficient evidence to recommend bisphosphonates for fracture prophylaxis. Similarly, insufficient evidence was found to recommend bisphosphonates for limiting the progression of osteoarthritis or for limiting progression of hearing loss. One study in Ralston and associate's data reported that 7 of 8 patients treated with etidronate or clodronate for between 1 and 6 years developed less facial deformity, as measured by facial or skull volume. For limiting neurologic symptoms, Ralston and colleagues stated that bisphosphonates may be considered, but there was no conclusive evidence. Work that studied this parameter studied bisphosphonates in conjunction with calcitonin, which has been shown independently to improve neurologic symptoms in patients with PDOB. Last, Ralston and colleagues reported that bisphosphonates are highly effective in reducing metabolic activity in PDOB, as evidenced by decreased serum alkaline phosphatase (ALP) levels. In a Cochrane review, bisphosphonates achieved a 50% greater decrease in ALP versus placebo. The same review showed that nitrogen containing bisphosphonates such as zoledronic acid was more effective than non-nitrogen–containing bisphosphonates. One study showed that the healing of lytic lesions was achieved in 47.8% of patients treated with alendronic acid. Histopathology showed lower turnover in these patients versus placebo.[30]

Adverse events for bisphosphonate use for PDOB is similar to those reported for bisphosphonate use for CGCG in the previous section, and includes atypical femoral fractures, uveitis, osteonecrosis of the jaw, hypocalcemia, and kidney damage. The estimated medication-related osteonecrosis of the jaw (MRONJ) incidence rate is estimated to be 0.06%, lower than in osteoporosis. The risk of adverse events was not found to be lower after discontinuation of bisphosphonates. This finding is consistent with the long functional half-life of bisphosphonates from embedding in bone matrices. Zoledronic acid being the most efficacious for control of PDOB symptoms also was reported as having an increased risk of adverse effects versus placebo. The most common adverse event reported with zoledronic acid was flulike symptoms.[30]

Commonly, zoledronic acid is given as a single dose 5 mg intravenously. Pamidronate is given 30 mg intravenously for 3 consecutive days. Alendronate is given 40 mg orally daily for 6 months. Risedronate is give 30 mg orally once daily for 2 months.[29]

Calcitonin in Paget's Disease of Bone

Similar to its use for CGCG described elsewhere in this article, calcitonin is used in PDOB for its inhibitory effects on osteoclast activity. Ralston and associates[30] reported on a case series of 38 patients with active PDOB who received porcine calcitonin therapy (80 units/d). Bone pain improved in 82% of the patients. The serum ALP decreased from 899 to 579 in the pretreatment and post-treatment groups. Six patients developed side effects such as nausea and diarrhea. Calcitonin, when used in combination with etidronate, was more effective at decreasing ALP than etidronate alone. In 2 independent studies, calcitonin was found to have improved neurologic dysfunction in 20 of 21 patients.[30] A common regimen for calcitonin for PDOB is 100 IU subcutaneous or intramuscular once daily for 6 to 18 months.[30]

Denosumab in Paget's Disease of Bone

Denosumab, as discussed elsewhere in this article. is an antiresorptive that has a similar effect on bone integrity as bisphosphonates but a shorter clinical half-life. Two case reports using 60 mg by subcutaneous injection every 6 months in PDOB patients resulted in decreased ALP serum concentrations.[30] Although intuitively the use of denosumab is logical, there is a scarcity of evidence in literature to support the use of denosumab for PDOB at this time.

FIBROUS DYSPLASIA
Bisphosphonates in Fibrous Dysplasia

The rationale for bisphosphonate therapy in FDOB is similar to the rationale for bisphosphonate therapy in Paget's disease in that the end goal of therapy is the same, namely, to strengthen pathologically weakened bone through inhibition of osteoclasts. Numerous reports of bisphosphonates used in FDOB can be found. Liens and coworkers[31] reported 9 patients with FDOB with 60 mg pamidronate infusions every 6 months. At 4 years of follow-up, bone density increased, although serum ALP and bone pain decreased. Chapurlat and colleagues[32] also treated 20 patients with the same pamidronate regimen ,except the subjects were also given calcium and vitamin D supplements. Again, lesions resolved in approximately one-half of the patients. Kos and colleagues[33] treated 6 children with progressive cranial facial monostotic FD with 1 mg/kg IV pamidronate every 4 to 6 months because they believed the children could ill tolerate major surgery. Pain relief was achieved in all cases. Increases in bone density and a decrease in lesion size was also noted. The only side effects reported were flulike symptoms in a report by Egner-Höbarth and coworkers.[34] However, given what we know about bisphosphonates, MRONJ and increased bone brittleness is expected.

Denosumab in Fibrous Dysplasia

Raborn and colleagues[35] presented a case of a 13-year-old female patient, who developed a biopsy confirmed FD of the left maxilla at 6 years of age. Owing to progressive increases in lesion size, including encroachment on the nasal cavity, she underwent surgical debulking. However, 1 year later, her symptoms returned. She would continue to undergo 3 more debulking surgeries and was treated with both pamidronate and zoledronate. These treatments relieved her symptoms temporarily each time, with bisphosphonates especially effective for her bone pain, but her lesion remained active. Raborn and associates treated her with 1 mg/kg denosumab every 4 weeks for 18 months followed by 70 mg every 4 weeks for 3.5 years. She reported resolution of pain. She was noted to have progressive an increase in bone density and stabilization of her lesion. Her therapy was discontinued and she remained in remission at 2 years of follow-up.[35]

MEDICATION-RELATED OSTEONECROSIS OF THE JAW AND OSTEORADIONECROSIS OF THE JAW

MRONJ and osteoradionecrosis of the jaw (ORN) are 2 conditions of the jaw whereby a jaw bone with a decreased capacity to heal develops necrosis after a traumatic injury, most commonly after dental extractions. In ORN, the offending insult is from radiation damage for the treatment of head and neck cancers to bone marrow and soft tissue supplying blood to the bone. The resulting bone becomes hypovascular, hypoxic, and hypocellular[36] and has a decreased capacity to heal in response to stress, resulting in necrosis. In MRONJ, the compromised bony healing is from antiresorptive medications, including bisphosphonates and denosumab.[37] The strengthened bone resulting from decreased osteoclastic activity also limits bone turnover in response to trauma, which results in a chronic nonhealing wound and then develops necrosis. The treatment of the necrotic jaw is difficult and without consensus.[36,37] Marx[38] has been at the forefront of understanding and treating both conditions. Marx[38] (1983) proposed a treatment protocol that

recommends hyperbaric oxygen (30 preoperative dives and 10 postoperative dives) to all ORN patients and surgery corresponding with the staging of the disease. The hyperbaric oxygen acts to promote vascular infiltration and angiogenesis to the hypovascular, hypoxic jaw and surgery removes necrotic bone. Marx[39] (2003) was also the first to describe osteonecrosis related to bisphosphonate use. He recommended avoiding tooth removals when possible and to treat established cases with palliation and control of overlying osteomyelitis. Unlike ORN, there is no hypoxic state, and hyperbaric oxygen has not been shown to be effective in treatment of MRONJ.[40] In both conditions, the role of surgery must be evaluated judiciously because it is difficult to obtain healthy bony margins in an unhealthy bone. Surgical trauma has the potential to create more osteonecrosis, the same condition it aims to address. This factor creates a need to a find nonsurgical treatment in the management of necrosis of the jaw.

Pentoxifylline, Tocopherol, and Clodronate for Osteoradionecrosis of the Jaw

After Marx described ORN, it was proposed that radiation causes vascular damage by inducing fibrosis of the bone marrow.[36] Pentoxifylline, tocopherol, and clodronate (PENTOCLO) was proposed to treat ORN medically without surgery. Pentoxifylline is a xanthine derivative used for the management of peripheral vascular disease.[41] It increases red blood cell deformability through second messenger cascades, thereby promoting flow of blood to the tissues, in the case of ORN, necrotic bone. Tocopherol is a free radical scavenger that limits oxidative stress damage in necrotic bone. Clodronate is a bisphosphonate that acted to strengthen irradiated bone. Patel and associates[36] showed in a large cohort of 169 cases that this triple therapy achieved an overall healing rate of 54.4% and achieved a stabilization and healing rate of 85.8%. Severe ORN cases that presented with pathologic fractures, extraoral fistulas, or full-thickness soft tissue defects responded less favorably with a stabilization rate of 53.7%. In this subpopulation, Patel and colleagues recommended surgery, although some were not surgical candidates for other reasons. The mean time to achieve healing was 13 months. The PENTOCLO regimen described by Patel and associates started with treating any active infection before initiating PENTOCLO with broad spectrum antibiotics followed by 30 days of doxycycline 100 mg/d. Pentoxifylline was given 400 mg twice daily with 1000 IU tocopherol daily. Clodronate was given 800 mg twice daily.

Common adverse events include nausea and vomiting. PENTOCLO is contraindicated in patients who have an increased bleeding risk, have a known allergy to xanthine (eg, caffeine, theophylline), severe kidney or liver disease, and acute myocardial infarction or severe coronary artery disease owing to risk of increased myocardial demand.[41]

Pentoxifylline and Tocopherol for Medication-Related Osteonecrosis of the Jaw

Owing to the success of PENTOCLO therapy in ORN, the same formulation has been adopted to MRONJ, with the modification to omit the bisphosphonate clodronate. Cavalcante and Tomasetti[37] reviewed 23 patients from 4 studies. All 23 patients developed MRONJ after dental extractions. After PENTO treatment, bone lesion size was reported to be smaller in all patients. Sixty-one percent had completed eliminated bone exposure. Thirty percent had partially eliminated bone exposure. Fifty-two percent had medical therapy only. The remaining patients had some form of surgery including saucerization or sequestrectomy. No patients required resection. The mean follow-up was 10.6 months. All patients before therapy had pain; none of the patients after therapy had pain. From these data, it seems that PENTO therapy has clinical and measurable benefits in MRONJ patients with or without surgery.

DISCLOSURE

The authors have nothing to disclose.

REFERENCES

1. Ogle OE, Santosh AB. Medication management of jaw lesions for dental patients. Dent Clin North Am 2016;60(2):483–95.
2. de Lange J, van den Akker HP, van den Berg H. Central giant cell granuloma of the jaw: a review of the literature with emphasis on therapy options. Oral Surg Oral Med Oral Pathol Oral Radiol Endod 2007;104(5):603–15.
3. Jaffe HL. Giant-cell reparative granuloma, traumatic bone cyst, and fibrous (fibro-oseous) dysplasia of the jawbones. Oral Surg Oral Med Oral Pathol 1953;6(1):159–75.
4. Ahmed A, Naidu A. Towards better understanding of giant cell granulomas of the oral cavity. J Clin Pathol 2021. https://doi.org/10.1136/jclinpath-2020-206858. jclinpath-2020-206858.
5. Chuong R, Kaban LB, Kozakewich H, et al. Central giant cell lesions of the jaws: a clinicopathologic study. J Oral Maxillofac Surg 1986;44(9):708–13. https://doi.org/10.1016/0278-2391(86)90040-6.
6. About Noonan Syndrome. National Human Genome Research Institute. 2013. Available at: https://www.genome.gov/Genetic-Disorders/Noonan-Syndrome#:~:text=is%20Noonan%20Syndrome%3F-,Noonan%20syndrome%20is%20a%20disorder%20that%20involves%20unusual%20facial%20characteristics,of%20several%20autosomal%20dominant%20genes. Accessed April 23, 2021.
7. Bataineh AB, Al-Khateeb T, Rawashdeh MA. The surgical treatment of central giant cell granuloma of the mandible. J Oral Maxillofac Surg 2002;60(7):756–61.
8. Osterne RL, Araújo PM, de Souza-Carvalho AC, et al. Intralesional corticosteroid injections in the treatment of central giant cell lesions of the jaws: a meta-analytic study. Med Oral Patol Oral Cir Bucal 2013;18(2):e226–32.
9. Vered M, Buchner A, Dayan D. Immunohistochemical expression of glucocorticoid and calcitonin receptors as a tool for selecting therapeutic approach in central giant cell granuloma of the jawbones. Int J Oral Maxillofac Surg 2006;35(8):756–60.
10. Hirayama T, Sabokbar A, Athanasou NA. Effect of corticosteroids on human osteoclast formation and activity. J Endocrinol 2002;175(1):155–63.
11. Dempster DW, Moonga BS, Stein LS, et al. Glucocorticoids inhibit bone resorption by isolated rat osteoclasts by enhancing apoptosis. J Endocrinol 1997;154(3):397–406.
12. Lin C. Intralesional steroid injection. DermNet NZ. 2021. Available at: https://dermnetnz.org/topics/intralesional-steroid-injection/. Accessed April 31, 2021.
13. Pondel M. Calcitonin and calcitonin receptors: bone and beyond. Int J Exp Pathol 2000;81(6):405–22.
14. Flanagan AM, Nui B, Tinkler SM, et al. The multinucleate cells in giant cell granulomas of the jaw are osteoclasts. Cancer 1988;62(6):1139–45.
15. Iida S, Kakudo S, Mori Y, et al. Human calcitonin has the same inhibitory effect on osteoclastic bone resorption by human giant cell tumor cells as salmon calcitonin. Calcif Tissue Int 1996;59(2):100–4.
16. Harris M. Central giant cell granulomas of the jaws regress with calcitonin therapy. Br J Oral Maxillofac Surg 1993;31(2):89–94.
17. Calcitonin salmon injection: MedlinePlus drug information. 2021. Available at: https://medlineplus.gov/druginfo/meds/a682788.html. Accessed April 31, 2021.
18. Baron R, Ferrari S, Russell RG. Denosumab and bisphosphonates: different mechanisms of action and effects. Bone 2011;48(4):677–92.
19. Landesberg R, Eisig S, Fennoy I, et al. Alternative indications for bisphosphonate therapy. J Oral Maxillofac Surg 2009;67(5 Suppl):27–34.
20. Chien MC, Mascarenhas L, Hammoudeh JA, et al. Zoledronic acid for the treatment of children with

refractory central giant cell granuloma. J Pediatr Hematol Oncol 2015;37(6):e399–401.

21. Choe M, Smith V, Okcu MF, et al. Treatment of central giant cell granuloma in children with denosumab. Pediatr Blood Cancer 2021;68(3):e28778.

22. Hebbale M, Munde A, Maria A, et al. Giant aneurysmal bone cyst of the mandible. J Craniofac Surg 2011;22(2):745–8.

23. Struthers PJ, Shear M. Aneurysmal bone cyst of the jaws. (II). Pathogenesis. Int J Oral Surg 1984;13(2): 92–100.

24. Sun ZJ, Sun HL, Yang RL, et al. Aneurysmal bone cysts of the jaws. Int J Surg Pathol 2009;17(4): 311–22.

25. George HL, Unnikrishnan PN, Garg NK, et al. Long-term follow-up of Ethibloc injection in aneurysmal bone cysts. J Pediatr Orthop B 2009;18(6):375–80.

26. Baldo TO, Kihara Filho EN, Dominguez GC. Percutaneous embolization of aneurysmal bone cyst of the mandible: a 3-year follow-up. Oral Maxillofacial Surg Cases 2019;5(4):100121.

27. Delloye C, De Nayer P, Malghem J, et al. Induced healing of aneurysmal bone cysts by demineralized bone particles. A report of two cases. Arch Orthop Trauma Surg 1996;115(3–4):141–5.

28. Clayer M. Injectable form of calcium sulphate as treatment of aneurysmal bone cysts. ANZ J Surg 2008;78(5):366–70.

29. Hullar TE, Lustig LR. Paget's disease and fibrous dysplasia. Otolaryngol Clin North Am 2003;36(4): 707–32.

30. Ralston SH, Corral-Gudino L, Cooper C, et al. Diagnosis and management of Paget's disease of bone in adults: a clinical guideline. J Bone Miner Res 2019;34(4):579–604.

31. Liens D, Delmas PD, Meunier PJ. Long-term effects of intravenous pamidronate in fibrous dysplasia of bone. Lancet 1994;343(8903):953–4.

32. Chapurlat RD, Delmas PD, Liens D, et al. Long-term effects of intravenous pamidronate in fibrous dysplasia of bone. J Bone Miner Res 1997;12(10): 1746–52.

33. Kos M, Luczak K, Godzinski J, et al. Treatment of monostotic fibrous dysplasia with pamidronate. J Craniomaxillofac Surg 2004;32(1):10–5.

34. Egner-Höbarth S, Welkerling H, Windhager R. Bisphosphonate in der Therapie der fibrösen Dysplasie. Relevante Daten und praktische Aspekte [Bisphosphonates in the therapy of fibrous dysplasia. Relevant data and practical aspects]. Orthopade 2007;36(2):124–30.

35. Raborn LN, Burke AB, Ebb DH, et al. Denosumab for craniofacial fibrous dysplasia: duration of efficacy and post-treatment effects [published online ahead of print, 2021 Mar 27]. Osteoporos Int 2021. https://doi.org/10.1007/s00198-021-05895-6.

36. Patel S, Patel N, Sassoon I, et al. The use of pentoxifylline, tocopherol and clodronate in the management of osteoradionecrosis of the jaws. Radiother Oncol 2021;156:209–16.

37. Cavalcante RC, Tomasetti G. Pentoxifylline and tocopherol protocol to treat medication-related osteonecrosis of the jaw: a systematic literature review. J Craniomaxillofac Surg 2020;48(11):1080–6.

38. Marx RE. Osteoradionecrosis: a new concept of its pathophysiology. J Oral Maxillofac Surg 1983; 41(5):283–8.

39. Marx RE. Pamidronate (Aredia) and zoledronate (Zometa) induced avascular necrosis of the jaws: a growing epidemic. J Oral Maxillofac Surg 2003; 61(9):1115–7.

40. Beth-Tasdogan NH, Mayer B, Hussein H, et al. Interventions for managing medication-related osteonecrosis of the jaw. Cochrane Database Syst Rev 2017; 10(10):CD012432.

41. Annamaraju P, Baradhi KM. Pentoxifylline. In: StatPearls. Treasure Island (FL): StatPearls Publishing; 2020.

Pharmacology of Aesthetic Medicines

Natalie Dunlop, DDS, MD[a], Shelly Abramowicz, DMD, MPH[b], Elda Fisher, MD[c],*

KEYWORDS

- Filler • Neurotoxin • Botox • Chemical peel • Aesthetic pharmacology

KEY POINTS

- Botulinum toxin functions by paralyzing or weakening muscles of facial expression and thereby diminishing the appearance of mimetic lines.
- Hyaluronic acid fillers have a wide variety of clinical applications in facial aesthetic medicine, and variation in filler density determines indication for location and depth of injection.
- Chemical peels predictably rejuvenate the face and vary in depth of penetration from superficial to deep; chemoexfoliation coagulates proteins in the skin and induces regeneration of collagen and keratinocytes.
- Topical aesthetic medicines are gaining popularity for treatment of acne, photodamage, fine rhytids, and dyschromia.

The realm of aesthetic medicine is broad, and there are now countless medications and topical agents used in the practice of aesthetic medicine. This chapter examines the most commonly used injectable and topical medications for aesthetic medicine.

BOTULINUM TOXINS

Since the 1990s botulinum toxins have been used in aesthetic medicine. Botulinum toxin is a neurotoxin produced by the bacteria Clostridium botulinum. Originally used for the medical purpose of treating blepharospasm, botulinum toxins are now approved by Food and Drug Administration (FDA) for a wide range of indications. The first use in aesthetic medicine was noted when treatment of blepharospasm resulted in the additional benefit of reducing crow's feet lines produced by constriction of the vertical portion (lateral aspect) of the orbicularis oculi muscle. Interestingly,

botulinum toxins were not approved to treat crow's feet lines until 2013. In its first use as an aesthetic medicine, botulinus toxins were used to treat vertical glabellar lines and horizontal forehead rhytids.

Mimetic lines are produced by the contraction of facial muscles. Mimetic lines are commonly seen in the forehead, glabella, and lateral orbicularis (crow's feet areas) but can also be identified in other facial subunits such as the lower face and midface (**Fig. 1**). Mimetic lines are amenable to treatment with botulinum toxins because the mechanism of action of botulinum toxins is to paralyze or weaken muscles by inhibiting the release of acetylcholine from the neuromuscular junction (**Fig. 2**).

The botulinum toxin polypeptide chain has a heavy (H) chain and a light (L) chain linked by a disulfide bond. Intramuscular injection of botulinum toxins acts at the neuromuscular junction to cause

[a] Oral and Maxillofacial Surgery, Division of Craniofacial and Surgical Care, University of North Carolina at Chapel Hill, 149 Brauer Hall, CB #7450, Chapel Hill, NC 27599, USA; [b] Division of Oral and Maxillofacial Surgery, Section of Oral and Maxillofacial Surgery, Emory University School of Medicine, Children's Healthcare of Atlanta, Emory University, 1365 Clifton Road, Northeast, Building B, Suite 2300, Atlanta, GA 30322, USA; [c] Division of Craniofacial and Surgical Care, Residency Program in Oral and Maxillofacial Surgery, University of North Carolina at Chapel Hill, 149 Brauer Hall, CB #7450, Chapel Hill, NC 27599, USA
* Corresponding author.
E-mail address: elda.fisher@unc.edu
Twitter: @fisherelda (E.F.)

Oral Maxillofacial Surg Clin N Am 34 (2022) 189–200
https://doi.org/10.1016/j.coms.2021.08.017

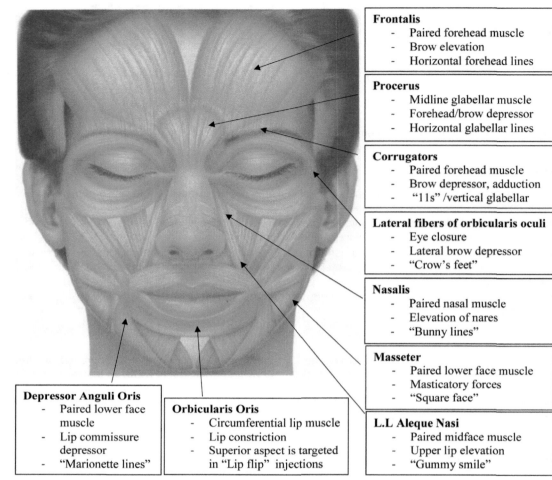

Frontalis
- Paired forehead muscle
- Brow elevation
- Horizontal forehead lines

Procerus
- Midline glabellar muscle
- Forehead/brow depressor
- Horizontal glabellar lines

Corrugators
- Paired forehead muscle
- Brow depressor, adduction
- "11s" /vertical glabellar

Lateral fibers of orbicularis oculi
- Eye closure
- Lateral brow depressor
- "Crow's feet"

Nasalis
- Paired nasal muscle
- Elevation of nares
- "Bunny lines"

Masseter
- Paired lower face muscle
- Masticatory forces
- "Square face"

L.L Aleque Nasi
- Paired midface muscle
- Upper lip elevation
- "Gummy smile"

Depressor Anguli Oris
- Paired lower face muscle
- Lip commissure depressor
- "Marionette lines"

Orbicularis Oris
- Circumferential lip muscle
- Lip constriction
- Superior aspect is targeted in "Lip flip" injections

Fig. 1. Facial musculature for neurotoxin injection sites.

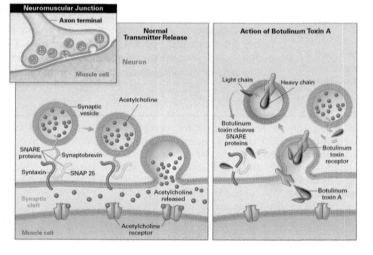

Fig. 2. Mechanism of action of botulinum toxin. (*From* Rowland LP. Stroke, spasticity, and botulinum toxin. N Engl J Med. 2002 Aug 8;347(6):382-3. doi: 10.1056/NEJMp020071; with permission.)

muscle paralysis by inhibiting the release of acetylcholine from presynaptic motor neurons. The heavy (H) chain of the toxin is an irreversible binder to high-affinity receptors at the presynaptic surface of cholinergic neurons. The toxin-receptor complex is endocytosed into the cell, and the disulfide bond between the 2 chains is cleaved. The toxin is then released into the cytoplasm. The light (L) chain interacts with different proteins (SNAP 25, vesicle-associated membrane protein and syntaxin) in the nerve terminals and prevents fusion of acetylcholine vesicles with the cell membrane.[1,2] The peak of the effect occurs approximately 7 days after injection. Doses of all commercially available botulinum toxins are expressed in terms of units of biological activity. One unit of botulinum toxin corresponds to the calculated median intraperitoneal lethal dose (LD50) in female Swiss-Webster mice.[1] The affected nerve terminals do not degenerate, but the blockage of neurotransmitter release is irreversible. Function is recovered by the sprouting of nerve terminals and formation of new synaptic contacts; this usually takes approximately 3 months.

Commercially Available Types of Neurotoxins for Aesthetic Use

There are now on the market several brands of neurotoxins using different formulations of botulinum toxin. Several are FDA approved for nonaesthetic uses (eg, Myobloc), whereas others (Botox, Dysport, Xeomin, Jeuveau) are FDA approved for use to treat mimetic rhytids.

Botox (onabotulinum A)

Botox (Allergan) is the most commonly used neurotoxin for treatment of facial mimetic rhytids. Botox is FDA approved for glabellar, forehead, and lateral canthal ("crow's feet") lines. Botox cosmetic is packaged in vials of 50U and 100U of lyophilized white powder with human albumin. It is freezer packaged for delivery and is reconstituted with sterile preservative-free 0.9% sodium chloride. Once reconstituted, package safety instructions direct that the Botox should be used or discarded after 24 hours and kept refrigerated when not in use.

Dysport (abobotulinum A)

Dysport (Galderma) is a commonly used botulinum neurotoxin in aesthetic medicine and for these purposes is FDA approved for treatment of glabellar lines. Dysport is also packaged as a lyophilized white powder with human albumin, bovine protein, and lactose. Unlike Botox, Dysport comes in vials of 300U and 500U. Per package insert, Dysport is reconstituted with 0.6 mL to 5 mL of preservative-free saline. The reconstituted product is stored in the refrigerator and should be discarded after one use or after 24 hours (whichever is first). Studies have demonstrated 2.5U to 3U of Dysport is approximately equivalent in potency and efficacy to 1U of Botox.[3]

Jeuveau (prabotulinum toxin A)

Jeuveau (Evolus) is a newer formulation of botulinum toxin An FDA approved for treatment of glabellar lines. Jeuveau is supplied as a vacuum-dried vial of 100U of toxin. It is reconstituted with preservative-free 0.9% saline and can be kept refrigerated up to 24 hours.

Xeomin (incobotulinum toxin A)

Xeomin (Merz) botulinum toxin complex is purified from the culture supernatant and then the active neurotoxin is separated from the proteins (hemagglutinins and nonhemagglutinins) through a series of steps yielding the active neurotoxin with molecular weight of 150 kDa, without accessory proteins in 50U, 100U, and 200U vials. Xeomin is packaged as a sterile white to off-white lyophilized powder that is unrefrigerated. It is reconstituted with preservative-free 0.9% sodium chloride injection and requires refrigeration up to 24 hours after reconstitution.

Current Practical Use of Neurotoxins

Although individual neurotoxins are approved for specific areas and indications, all formulations listed earlier are widely used throughout the upper face, lower face, and neck for aesthetic purposes. Off-label uses range from "bunny lines," "gummy smile," masseter reduction, and treatment of platysmal bands. Neurotoxin may be used at all regions illustrated in **Fig.1**, as well as in additional areas such as platysma, temporalis, and labii inferioris. Xeomin does not require refrigeration before reconstitution, which makes it easier to store. Recommended dosing for neurotoxins is also at the discretion of the surgeon/physician, and in this author's (E. F.) experience, manufacturer recommends dosing guides far exceed necessary doses to achieve the desired effect. Following manufacturer dosing guidelines particularly in the frontalis can predispose to unwanted effects, such as brow ptosis. Initial treatment dosing should start at half to one-third recommended dosing and increase as necessary at the 3-month follow-up appointment to achieve the desired result. Reconstitution recommendations on package inserts are routinely modified by practitioners to produce more concentrated solutions. For example, this author routinely uses a 0.9% saline with preservative as diluent and reconstitutes Botox to 1U/0.01 mL diluent, and Dysport to 3U/0.01 mL diluent. This reconstitution method reduces injection site spread and diminishes the risk of dispersion to unwanted regions. Finally, although package inserts indicate products should be discarded 24 hours after reconstitution, most practitioners will use reconstituted neurotoxins for up to a week when properly refrigerated.

Contraindications to Neurotoxin Use for Aesthetic Purposes

Contraindications to neurotoxin treatment of cosmetic purposes are active infection in the area (pustules, active acne), allergy to neurotoxin or its reconstitution constituents (eg, cow's milk allergy for Dysport injections), or known neuromuscular disorders such as amyotrophic lateral sclerosis, Lambert-Eaton syndrome, and other myopathies. Relative contraindications include pregnancy and breastfeeding, history of keloid formation, unrealistic expectations, immunocompromised state, or body dysmorphic disorder.[4–6]

Adverse Effect of Neurotoxin Treatment

There are few complications associated with the cosmetic use of neurotoxins, and most adverse reactions are mild and temporary. Most common adverse event is bruising at the injection site. Other complications include postinjection headache. Most adverse reactions to neurotoxins are secondary to poor injection technique or inadequately understanding the associated anatomy. Neurotoxin may disperse up to 3 cm from the injection site depending on the dilution.[2] Higher concentrations of neurotoxin (less diluent) can help prevent spread after injection. This author routinely uses a concentration of 1U/0.01 mL preservative containing 0.9% normal saline. Avoidance of additional swelling in the area is helpful to minimize this dispersion; for example, laser treatment should be avoided in the same week as neurotoxin injection. Injection site reactions such a pain, bruising, and erythema are mitigated by using proper injection technique including smaller gauge needles and avoidance of touch the periosteum during injection. This author uses 31-gauge needles with 8 mm length for injection. In addition, using a normal saline diluent with preservative has been demonstrated to reduce pain on injection. Incidence of severe headache following neurotoxin injection is approximately 1%, and resolution is typically within 24 hours, with complete resolution in all patient by 2 to 4 weeks.[3]

Several adverse effects are the result of poor injection technique of various muscle groups. For example, in the treatment of glabellar lines and corrugators, diffusion of neurotoxin into the levator palpebrae muscle causes true eyelid ptosis. Although this is self-limiting, it is very disconcerting for patients who experience this complication because it is aesthetically unpleasing, limits the superior visual field, and also makes it difficult to apply eye makeup. This complication is generally avoidable by keeping injection into the corrugator muscles superficial. Brow ptosis is also a common adverse outcome of neurotoxin injection. Because the frontalis elevates the brows, injection into this muscle group is expected to result in some limitations of brow elevation. Patient with significant horizontal forehead rhytids often has standing static elevation of the brows and activation of the frontalis. The inclination to injecting more neurotoxin in patients with deep horizontal rhytids should be tempered by the understanding that this may cause significant brow ptosis in these patients. Additional techniques to limit brow ptosis in addition to limiting total frontalis dose of neurotoxin is avoiding injection within 1.5 cm of the orbital rim. Injection of brow depressors (corrugators, procerus, lateral orbicularis oculi) will help decrease the risk of brow ptosis. A final potential complication of administration of neurotoxin to the forehead is inadequate weakening of the lateral portion of the frontalis, leading to a lateral arching ("peaking") of the brow (**Fig. 3**). Injecting a small amount of neurotoxin (eg, 1–2U Botox) into the lateral frontalis should reduce this effect.

Complications resulting from injection into the lower face are more common because uses here are off label. There is also more variation in soft tissue anatomy in the lower face requiring more expertise in anatomic understanding of muscle function in this area. Common treatments such as neurotoxin injection into the orbicularis oris ("lip flip") and treatment of gummy smile or nasal "bunny lines" produced by alaeque nasi muscles can result in upper lip incompetence and difficulty using straws. Similarly, injection to depressor anguli oris for improvement in commissure position can result in inadvertent injection of the depressor labii muscles, resulting in asymmetry and lower lip malfunction. Treatment of neck platysmal banding should be executed with minimal dosing (8–12U Botox or equivalent per band), and injection should be superficial to avoid injection of the sternocleidomastoid or diffusion to the laryngeal muscles.

HYALURONIC ACID FILLERS

Injectable fillers have a wide range of applications in aesthetic medicine. They can be injected in the

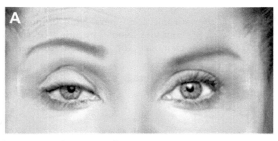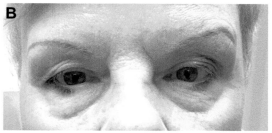

Fig. 3. Complications of neurotoxins. (*A*) Eyelid ptosis. Treat with 0.5% apraclonidine drops, 1 to 2 drops tid. (*B*) Brow ptosis. Add 1 to 3 units of neurotoxin above superiorly placed lateral brow to decrease activity of the vertical fibers of the orbicularis oculi, which depresses the lateral brow.

superficial to middle dermis for fine rhytids, in the middle to deep dermis for moderate to severe volume loss, in the submucosal plane for lip volumization and in a subcutaneous, supraperiosteal, or subperiosteal plane for cheek or jawline augmentation.[7,8] Hyaluronic acid (HA) is by far the most common filler material used for injectable facial rejuvenation, consisting of about 80% of the soft tissue fillers administered in 2019.[9] HA fillers volumize the face by occupying space as well as inducing the synthesis of collagen.[10] There are many brands and formulations of HA fillers approved by the FDA in the United States, but the most commonly used brands in clinical practice are Juvéderm, Restylane, and Belotero.

HA is native to all mammalian species in the extracellular matrix of the dermis.[10] It is abundantly present in human skin and aids in soft tissue resilience and lubrication. The amount of HA present in human tissue decreases with age, leading to reduced dermal hydration and increased skin folding: common signs of aging.[11] HA is a biodegradable glycosaminoglycan molecule that functions by binding to water molecules. Dermal fillers are made of HA modified to have specific physicochemical properties related to their tissue stability, viscosity, and elasticity. This allows the clinician to choose the most appropriate filler for a given indication.[8] Cross-linking of the HA molecules gives mechanical strength to the gel and improves product longevity by deterring degradation.[8,10,12] The elastic modulus (or G′) is primarily used to characterize filler products based on multiple factors that affect gel strength, such as HA concentration and degree of cross-linking. A higher G′ value is associated with better ability for a substance to rebound to its original shape when acted on by a dynamic force; in the world of dermal fillers, a higher G′ correlates to a firmer gel.[8] A lower G′ value may be more appropriate for a patient with thinner skin or for performing more superficial injections.[8] Fillers such as Juvéderm Volbella that are cross-linked and

fragmented into smaller pieces are used for superficial facial planes, whereas fillers such as Restylane Lyft and Juvéderm Voluma with larger fragments are used in deeper planes.[8,12]

Once injected, HA is slowly degraded by naturally occurring hyaluronidase and free radicals in the skin. Factors that influence how quickly the modified HA in filler dissolves include particle size, HA concentration, type of cross-linking agent, and G′ value.[13] Each brand and type of HA filler boasts their own estimation of duration, but typically HA fillers are quoted to last around 12 to 24 months. A key advantage of HA fillers as opposed to non-HA fillers is the ability to reverse the effects with injectable hyaluronidase if complications or overtreatment occurs.[14]

Technique for Injection

Each filler is packaged in a sterile syringe with 2 Luer-lock needles of appropriate dimension for the filler. Lower G′ filler can be delivered through smaller gauge needles, whereas high G′ filler must be injected through larger bore needles. The use of cannulas for injection is highly popular and is associated with lower incidence of bruising and intravascular injections (**Fig. 4**). Injection sites should be cleaned thoroughly before injection with chlorhexidine or other preparation. Once the needle or canula is in the desired location for filler placement, the injector should create mild negative pressure by aspiration on the syringe for verification that the placement is not intravascular. Injection of filler material should be slow and not exceed 0.1 mL per site before reaspiration and injection.

In general, most practitioners become comfortable with a complement of filler products that ranges from lower to higher G′ and can use the products in various facial areas. This author uses high G′ materials for supra- or subperiosteal augmentation of malar regions, temporal regions, and jawline. Lower G′ fillers are ideal for tear

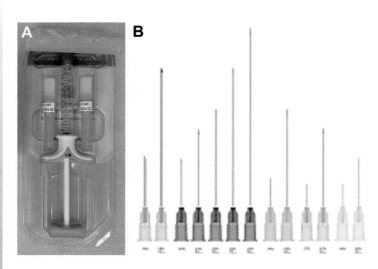

Fig. 4. (*A*) Typical packaging for hyaluronic acid fillers. Note syringe and Luer-lock needles included. (*B*) Microcannulas for injection of dermal fillers.

trough regions—for example, in these areas Belotero can be placed superficially and Restylane can be placed in the subdermal region. Lip and perioral augmentation is variable, ranging from medium to higher G′ fillers for nasolabial fold, marionette lines, and offering structure and support to these areas. Lips are tailored to the desires of the patient; younger patients often desire fuller, plumper lips (Juvéderm Ultra, Juvéderm Ultra Plus, Prollenium Versa, Restylane), whereas older patients desire correction of vertical lip rhytids and mild more natural lip augmentation (Juvéderm Ultra, Juvéderm Volbella, Restylane).

Contraindications

Contraindications for the use of HA filler include history of allergy or anaphylaxis to HA, hypersensitivity to lidocaine or gram-positive bacterial proteins (for products that contain or are derived from these), active infection near the site of injection, and bleeding disorders. The safety of HA filler in pregnant or lactating patients and pediatric patients has not been reliably established.[15,16]

Adverse Reactions and Complications

Complications associated with soft tissue filler injection can be divided into early and late reactions. Early reactions include inflammatory reactions, such as infection or allergic reaction, injection-related events, such as pain, bleeding, or bruising, and vascular infarction leading to tissue necrosis or blindness. Late reactions include granuloma formation, nodules, or displacement of the filler material.[14]

Filler-associated blindness is exceedingly rare but can be caused by accidental intraarterial injection and retrograde flow of filler particles into the arteries supplying the eye, most common with nose, glabella, and forehead injections.[17,18]

Granulomatous reactions are treated with hyaluronidase, with or without antibiotic therapy if infection is on the differential diagnosis. Oral steroids or intralesional steroid injections can be considered for persistent granulomas or malar edema, which is a common complication of filler placement for tear trough correction.[14] Delayed hypersensitivity can manifest weeks to months after HA filler injection. There have been case reports of immunologic interactions between dermal fillers and influenza infection causing delayed hypersensitivity, as well as case reports of delayed inflammatory reactions to HA fillers after exposure to COVID-19 spike protein by either direct virus exposure or vaccine inoculation.[19,20] The most common adverse events are local reactions at injection site such as bruising. True allergic or granulomatous reactions are rare.[21] Serious adverse events are uncommon[22] **Fig. 5**.

In practice, HA fillers are a ubiquitous tool for the oral and maxillofacial surgeon to rejuvenate the face and decrease the signs of aging. The appropriate filler choice for each patient is based on the physicochemical properties of the filler, the specific indication for its use, and clinician preference.

NONHYALURONIC ACID FILLERS
Calcium Hydroxylapatite—Radiesse

Calcium hydroxylapatite (CaHA) is an injectable implant material composed of CaHA microspheres (30%) in an aqueous gel made of sodium carboxymethylcellulose, glycerin, and water.[23] Calcium hydroxylapatite is biocompatible, as it is the same mineral found in bones and teeth. As a filler,

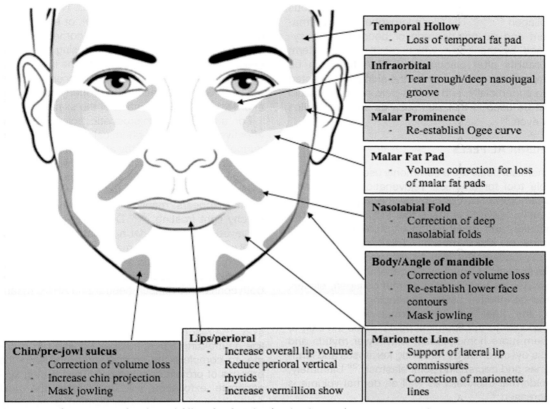

Fig. 5. Sites for injection for dermal fillers for facial volumization and contour correction.

CaHA is effective by providing both immediate correction of volume deficiencies as well as induction of collagen formation in the dermis.[24,25] The aqueous gel is phagocytosed and degraded within 4 to 12 weeks, leaving behind just the CaHA microspheres that remain in the tissue and induce fibroblast proliferation. The CaHA microspheres are then slowly broken down into their composite ions calcium and phosphate[26]; this takes about 12 to 18 months in dynamic areas of the face and can last up to 18 to 24 months in more static areas.[25] The filler is generally injected subdermally and is considered high viscosity and high elasticity.[27] As such, CaHA filler is best indicated for deeper rhytids in areas such as the nasolabial folds, marionette lines, and infraorbital rim.[28]

Poly-L-Lactic-Acid Filler—Sculptra

As calcium hydroxylapatite fillers, poly-L-lactic acid (PLLA) fillers are composed of microspheres of PLLA in an aqueous gel with carboxymethylcellulose and mannitol.[29] When injected, PLLA microspheres induce subclinical inflammation within the skin that causes a mild foreign body reaction and promotes gradual collagen synthesis,[29] and this results in a natural, progressive increase in dermal thickness and volumization over 1 year that can last up to 2 to 3 years.[24,30] The microspheres are eventually degraded by the body through the same pathway as lactic acid.[31] PLLA fillers are injected subcutaneously and are indicated for loss of temporal fat pads, moderate facial wrinkles, and contour deficiencies. As the results of the filler are gradual with the new synthesis of collagen, this filler can be used in conjunction with other fillers that have immediate results.[27]

Polymethylmethacrylate Fillers—Bellafill, ArteFill

Polymethylmethacrylate (PMMA) is a synthetic filler that has been used for various medical purposes over 30 years. It is composed of small microspheres suspended in a bovine collagen solution.[32] Injection of PMMA fillers requires a skin test before treatment to test for hypersensitivity, as there is a 3% prevalence of hypersensitivity in the general population to bovine collagen.[33] PMMA fillers function by progressively increasing the production of natural collagen to surround the microspheres. The resultant volume increase is composed of 20% PMMA and 80% autologous collagen.[27,34,35] The filler microspheres are permanent and do not degrade or become phagocytosed by the body, which results in long term durability after placement. PMMA filler can be palpated as nodules under the skin if it is injected too superficially, and as it is permanent, it should not be used in thin skin such as around the lips or eyes.[33]

CHEMICAL PEELS

Chemical peels are a commonly used and predictable tool for chemical rejuvenation of the face. Chemoexfoliation occurs by the application of a caustic agent to the face that induces keratocoagulation and denaturation of proteins within the epidermis and dermis.[36,37] This type of controlled injury causes the skin to respond by sloughing the superficial layers and regenerating new keratinocytes as well as new dermal collagen, elastin, and connective tissue, depending on the depth of the peel.[36,38] The normal wound healing response to the chemical peel causes the skin to seem more homogenous, with fewer rhytids and less dyschromia, by removing keratoses and lentigines and decreasing solar elastosis.[39] Ultimately, epidermal thickness as well as dermal volume is increased.[36]

Chemical peels are classified by the depth of their tissue penetration into superficial, medium, and deep. The chemoexfoliative agents can generally be categorized into these depths, but the actual depth of the chemical peel is determined by a combination of factors including the agent, the concentration, the skin type, the number of layers applied to the skin, and the time in contact with the skin. Superficial peels penetrate only the epidermis, medium-depth peels reach the papillary dermis, and deep peels reach the midreticular dermis.[36,40] There are many chemoexfoliative agents available; the most used agents in clinical practice are discussed here.

Superficial Peeling Agents

The most common superficial peeling agents in practice today are 30% to 50% glycolic acid (GA) and 10% to 30% lactic acid. GA and lactic acid are both keratolytic alpha-hydroxy acids (AHAs) that induce desquamation of epidermal cells and cell-cycle acceleration.[40] The increased desquamation enhances skin light reflection and radiance. Specifically, these chemicals treat photoaging by decreasing the appearance of fine lines, freckles, lentigines, and surface roughness. Depth of the GA peel depends on the concentration of the acid used, the number of coats applied,

and the time for which it is applied. Hence, it can be used as a very superficial peel, or even a medium depth peel. GA targets the corneosome by enhancing breakdown and decreasing cohesiveness, causing desquamation.[41,42] The intensity of GA peel is determined by the concentration of the acid. GA peels need to be properly neutralized in order to stop acidification of the skin.

For superficial trichloroacetic acid peels, the effective depth of the chemical peel is observed during the procedure by the appearance of a white frost, signifying the denaturation of the keratin and collagen. During superficial chemical peels with AHAs, the peel should be left on only until level I frosting appears, manifesting as erythema with a patchy light frosting.[36,38] Deeper peeling can be achieved with additional applications to achieve level II–III frosting, which manifests as a hard white frosting. Trichloroacetic acid peels do not require neutralization. Glycolic acid and lactic acid are both considered nonself-neutralizing AHAs, meaning their keratocoagulation will continue to occur for the duration the acid is in contact with the skin. The reaction requires application of an alkaline neutralizing agent, such as sodium bicarbonate, to complete the neutralization and stop the process of protein denaturation. The ensuing keratinocyte exfoliation will occur over the next several days, and reepithelialization is complete within 7 to 10 days.[36] Thirty percent (30%) salicylic acid, a beta-hydroxy acid, is an example of a superficial peel that is self-neutralizing by the lipoproteins of the skin. It is less commonly used for photorejuvenation and hyperpigmentation, but it is the gold standard for the treatment of acne. Although the acid is self-neutralizing, excessive keratocoagulation can occur past the epidermis into the papillary dermis if multiple layers are applied or the dose application is too long.

Medium Depth Agents

Medium depth agents include 70% glycolic acid and 35% to 50% trichloroacetic acid (TCA) with or without adjuvant combination products such as Jessner solution. The penetration of the peel through the epidermis and into the papillary dermis allows treatment of deeper pathology such as fine rhytids, actinic photodamage, melasma, and acne scars.[39] Skin is reepithelialized by migration from adnexal structures and stimulation of new collagen.[43] GA, as described earlier, can be used at a higher concentration of 70% for deeper chemoexfoliation, or a lower concentration such as 50% can be paired with a pretreatment agent to facilitate deeper penetration into the papillary dermis.

Jessner solution is a common chemoexfoliation agent and is composed of 14 g resorcinol, 14 g salicylic acid, and 14 mL lactic acid in ethanol constituted to 100 mL. Jessner solution functions to disrupt the epidermal barrier in a homogenous manner and thoroughly cleanse the skin from natural oils to allow the following chemoexfoliant to more homogenously penetrate the skin and decrease the likelihood of chemical burns in particular areas. For medium-depth peels, level II–III frosting signifies that the agent has reached the papillary dermis; this will be evident as a uniform, white-coated frosting with underlying erythema showing through (level II) or a solid white enamel frosting with no background erythema (level III).

Deep Peel Agents

The most common deep peeling agents are TCA greater than 50% and the Baker-Gordon phenol peel, and these agents are indicated to treat heavy rhytids due to chronic photodamage and solar lentigines.[39] High-concentration TCA carries a risk of hypertrophic scarring and difficulty predicting the depth of the peel. The Baker-Gordon phenol peel is composed of a detergent, croton oil, 45% to 50% phenol, and water, which allows for uniform chemoexfoliation to the level of the midreticular dermis. At higher concentrations, phenol denatures proteins and creates a barrier that prevents its deep penetration into the dermis, but at lower concentrations around 50%, the phenol is keratolytic and therefore has an increased peel depth.[39] The Baker-Gordon phenol peel can be applied in an occluded method, wherein an occlusive dressing such as petroleum jelly is applied over the treatment area after application, or unoccluded, which does not provide as deep a penetration. Deep peels containing any phenol must be used with caution due to their arrhythmogenic properties, hepatic metabolism, and renal clearance and require pretreatment with herpes simplex virus and bacterial prophylaxis. After a deep peel, the patient will experience full-thickness epidermal necrosis with resultant crusting, and reepithelialization will commence after 3 to 4 days and continue for 14 days. Deep peel agents have recently fallen out of favor due to the risks associated with phenol and the increasing popularity of laser resurfacing with similar results.[44]

TOPICAL AESTHETIC MEDICATIONS

Extrinsic and intrinsic aging of the skin due to sun exposure, environmental stressors, and progressive, age-related decline in the antioxidizing capacity of the skin result in breakdown of collagen and elastin in dermis, and this leads to a loss of skin elasticity, collagen atrophy, dyschromia, and rhytids. Topical treatments for skin rejuvenation that are effective, safe, and noninvasive are in high demand.

Tretinoin

Tretinoin, or all transretinoic acid, is a synthetic derivative of vitamin A. It is widely used to treat moderate acne by reducing comedogenesis and normalizing keratinization of the facial skin.[45] The mechanism is by increasing the follicular epithelial turnover and accelerating the shedding of corneocytes, thereby ridding the skin of mature comedones and suppressing the formation of microcomedones, and this promotes an inhospitable and anaerobic environment for the bacteria that causes acne, Propionibacterium acnes.[46] Tretinoin is also widely used for treating rhytids, dyschromia, and roughness associated with photodamaged skin. This rejuvenation occurs due to thickening of the epidermis, compaction of the stratum corneum, increased collagen synthesis in the dermis, and promotion of epidermal hyperplasia and angiogenesis.[47] Tretinoin is available in 0.01% or 0.05% cream and is typically applied once daily. The most common adverse effect is dermatitis, which can persist up to 3 months but is typically mild. Tretinoin should not be used during pregnancy due to known teratogenic effects.[47] Isotretinoin (Accutane) is an oral prescription medication for the treatment of severe acne. Isotretinoin has broad systemic effects that require monitoring before and during use and is a known teratogen. As a result, prescriptions for the isotretinoin (Accutane) are limited to those physician practitioners participating in the iPLEDGE Registry. The use of isotretinoin in the setting of concomitant cosmetic surgical and nonsurgical skin procedures has been associated with severe scarring. Typically, patients who are taking isotretinoin are instructed to wait at least 6 to 12 months after completing the treatment course before undergoing cosmetic surgical or nonsurgical procedures (such as ablative laser treatments or chemical peeling).

Hydroquinone

Hydroquinone has been used in a topical fashion for skin lightning since the 1950s.[48,49] It is now the standard depigmentation agent for treating dyschromias including melasma, solar lentigines, freckles, and postinflammatory hyperpigmentation after laser treatment.[50] The mechanism of action of hydroquinone is by inhibition of melanin synthesis, blocking the conversion of L-DOPA to melanin.

It is available in 2% topical formula over the counter or 4% as prescription. Evidence has shown that patients can achieve maximum results when using a combination product of hydroquinone 4%, tretinoin 0.05%, and fluocinolone acetonide 0.01%.[51] Hydroquinone is a known carcinogen and can induce exogenous ochronosis in the skin, and this author limits duration of treatment with the prescription strength formulations for 6 months.[52]

Growth Factors

Topical application of growth factors is a relatively new field of research for treatment of visual signs of skin aging. Growth factors regulate cell replication, collagen production, and reduction of inflammation by attaching to cell surface receptors and serving as chemical messengers to mediate signaling pathways.[53] They can be applied topically or injected in autologous platelet-rich plasma, and they function locally to increase dermal collagen synthesis and decrease collagen degradation, which reduces the appearance of fine lines and wrinkles. Growth factors can be derived from humans, animals, plants, bacteria, and yeast. The topical application of growth factors regulate immune processing by promoting fibroblast and keratinocyte formations. Growth factors are now a common accompaniment to skin treatments such as microneedling and have demonstrated clinical improvement in treatment of rhytids and sun-damaged skin.[53]

Vitamin C

Vitamin C, or ascorbic acid, is a potent antioxidant and, when used as a topical agent, has been shown to prevent and treat photodamage as well as treat melasma and dyschromia.[54,55] The mechanism of action of topical vitamin C is through stimulation of type I procollagen synthesis and free radical scavenging of reactive oxygen species, classically caused by ultraviolet (UV) damage.[54] Vitamin C, when combined with UVA or UVB sunscreen, improves sun protection when compared with sunscreen alone.[56] Daily application of 5% vitamin C has been shown to significantly reduce deep furrows of the skin and increase the levels of procollagen types I and III[55,57]; this stimulates fibroblast proliferation and collagen production in the dermis, leading to reduction in the appearance of rhytids.[52] Oral ingestion of vitamin c does not increase cutaneous levels to the same extent that topical application does; the standard dosage is 5% vitamin C topical application once to twice daily.[54]

CLINICS CARE POINTS

- Patients with significant horizontal forehead rhytids often have standing static elevation of the brow by activation of the frontalis—be judicious with neurotoxin injection to avoid brow ptosis.
- Inadequate weakening of the lateral frontalis can result in lateral brow "peaking" and can be corrected with a small amount of neurotoxin in the lateral frontalis.
- The depth of penetration of a chemical peel depends on the mechanism of chemoexfoliation.
- Nonself-neutralizing peels such as GA will continue to keratocoagulate for the duration of their contact with the skin and can reach deeper layers by prolonged skin contact.
- Self-neutralizing chemical peels, such as salicylic acid, reach an endpoint after which they no longer penetrate the dermis.
- Patients should wait 6 to 12 months after stopping isotretinoin (Accutane) before undergoing surgical or nonsurgical cosmetic procedures such as laser resurfacing or chemical peels.

DISCLOSURE

The authors have nothing to disclose.

REFERENCES

1. Nigam PK, Nigam A. Botulinum toxin. Indian J Dermatol 2010;55(1):8–14.
2. Sellin LC. The pharmacological mechanism of botulism. Trends Pharmacol Sci 1985;6:80–2.
3. Scaglione F. Conversion ratio between Botox®, Dysport®, and Xeomin® in clinical practice. Toxins (Basel) 2016;8(3):65.
4. Small R. Botulinum toxin injection for facial wrinkles. Am Fam Physician 2014;90(3):168–75.
5. Hirsch R, Stier M. Complications and their management in cosmetic dermatology. Dermatol Clin 2009;27(4):507–20, vii.
6. Krishtul A, Waldorf HA, Blitzer A. Complications of cosmetic botulinum toxin therapy. In: Carruthers A, editor. Botulinum toxin. Philadelphia, PA: W.B. Sanders; 2007. p. 111–21.
7. Rohrich RJ, Ghavami A, Crosby MA. The role of hyaluronic acid fillers (Restylane) in facial cosmetic

surgery: review and technical considerations. Plast Reconstr Surg 2007;120(6 Suppl):41S–54S.

8. Fagien S, Bertucci V, von Grote E, et al. Rheologic and physicochemical properties used to differentiate injectable hyaluronic acid filler products. Plast Reconstr Surg 2019;143(4):707e–20e.

9. American society of plastic surgeons plastic surgery statistics report. Available at: https://www.plasticsurgery.org/news/plastic-surgery-statistics. Accessed April 5, 2021.

10. Bacos JT, Dayan SH. Superficial dermal fillers with hyaluronic acid. Facial Plast Surg 2019;35(3):219–23.

11. Duranti F, Salti G, Bovani B, et al. Injectable hyaluronic acid gel for soft tissue augmentation. A clinical and histological study. Dermatol Surg 1998;24(12):1317–25.

12. Kablik J, Monheit GD, Yu L, et al. Comparative physical properties of hyaluronic acid dermal fillers. Dermatol Surg 2009;35(Suppl 1):302–12.

13. Bogdan Allemann I, Baumann L. Hyaluronic acid gel (Juvéderm) preparations in the treatment of facial wrinkles and folds. Clin Interv Aging 2008;3(4):629–34.

14. Signorini M, Liew S, Sundaram H, et al. Global aesthetics consensus: avoidance and management of complications from hyaluronic acid fillers-evidence- and opinion-based review and consensus recommendations. Plast Reconstr Surg 2016;137(6):961e–71e.

15. Walker K, Basehore BM, Goyal A, et al. Hyaluronic acid. In: StatPearls [Internet]. Treasure Island (FL): StatPearls Publishing; 2021. Available at: https://www.ncbi.nlm.nih.gov/books/NBK482440/.

16. Lafaille P, Benedetto A. Fillers: contraindications, side effects and precautions. J Cutan Aesthet Surg 2010;3(1):16–9.

17. Sorensen EP, Council ML. Update in soft-tissue filler–associated blindness. Dermatol Surg 2020;46(5):671–7.

18. McCleve DE, Goldstein JC. Blindness secondary to injections in the nose, mouth, and face: cause and prevention. Ear Nose Throat J 1995;74:182–8.

19. Turkmani MG, De Boulle K, Philipp-Dormston WG. Delayed hypersensitivity reaction to hyaluronic acid dermal filler following influenza-like illness. Clin Cosmet Investig Dermatol 2019;12:277–83.

20. Munavalli GG, Guthridge R, Knutsen-Larson S, et al. COVID-19/SARS-CoV-2 virus spike protein-related delayed inflammatory reaction to hyaluronic acid dermal fillers: a challenging clinical conundrum in diagnosis and treatment" [published online ahead of print, 2021 Feb 9]. Arch Dermatol Res 2021;1–15.

21. Niamtu J 3rd. Complications in fillers and Botox. Oral Maxillofac Surg Clin North Am 2009;21(1):13–21.

22. Stojanovič L, Majdič N. Effectiveness and safety of hyaluronic acid fillers used to enhance overall lip fullness: a systematic review of clinical studies. J Cosmet Dermatol 2019;18(2):436–43.

23. Ahn MS. Calcium hydroxylapatite: Radiesse. Facial Plast Surg Clin North Am 2007;15(1):85, vii.

24. Trinh LN, Gupta A. Non-hyaluronic acid fillers for midface augmentation: a systematic review [published online ahead of print, 2021 Mar 1]. Facial Plast Surg 2021. https://doi.org/10.1055/s-0041-1725164.

25. Busso M, Karlsberg PL. Cheek augmentation and rejuvenation using injectable calcium hydroxylapatite (Radiesse®). Cosmet Dermatol 2006;19:583–8.

26. Marmur ES, Phelps R, Goldberg DJ. Clinical, histologic and electron microscopic findings after injection of a calcium hydroxylapatite filler. J Cosmet Laser Ther 2004;6:223–6.

27. Attenello NH, Maas CS. Injectable fillers: review of material and properties. Facial Plast Surg 2015;31(1):29–34.

28. Sklar JA, White SM. Radiance FN: a new soft tissue filler. Dermatol Surg 2004;30:764–8.

29. Fitzgerald R, Bass LM, Goldberg DJ, et al. Physiochemical characteristics of Poly-L-Lactic Acid (PLLA). Aesthet Surg J 2018;38(suppl_1):S13–7.

30. Ezzat WH, Keller GS. The use of poly-L-lactic acid filler in facial aesthetics. Facial Plast Surg 2011;27(06):503–9.

31. Chen HH, Javadi P, Daines SM, et al. Quantitative assessment of the longevity of poly-L-lactic acid as a volumizing filler using 3-dimensional photography. JAMA Facial Plast Surg 2015;17(01):39–43.

32. Cohen SR, Berner CF, Busso M, et al. Five-year safety and efficacy of a novel polymethylmethacrylate aesthetic soft tissue filler for the correction of nasolabial folds. Dermatol Surg 2007;33(Suppl 2):S222–30.

33. Greco TM, Antunes MB, Yellin SA. Injectable fillers for volume replacement in the aging face. Facial Plast Surg 2012;28(1):8–20.

34. Lemperle G, Romano JJ, Busso M. Soft tissue augmentation with artecoll: 10-year history, indications, techniques, and complications. Dermatol Surg 2003;29(6):573–87 [discussion 587].

35. Paulucci BP. PMMA safety for facial filling: review of rates of granuloma occurrence and treatment methods. Aesthet Plast Surg 2020;44(1):148–59.

36. Soleymani T, Lanoue J, Rahman Z. A practical approach to chemical peels: a review of fundamentals and step-by-step algorithmic protocol for treatment. J Clin Aesthet Dermatol 2018;11(8):21–8. Chemical rejuvenation of the face.

37. Baumann L, Baumann L. Hydroxy acids. In: Cosmeceuticals and cosmetic ingredients. New York, NY: McGraw-Hill Education/Medical; 2015. p. 322–7.

38. Glogau RG, Matarasso SL. Chemical peels. Trichloroacetic acid and phenol. Dermatol Clin 1995; 13(2):263–76.

39. Tse Y, Ostad A, Lee HS, et al. A clinical and histologic evaluation of two medium-depth peels. Glycolic acid versus Jessner's trichloroacetic acid. Dermatol Surg 1996;22(9):781–6.

40. Kotler R. Chemical rejuvenation of the face. St. Louis, Mo: Mosby Year Book; 1992. p. 60–70.

41. Sharad J. Glycolic acid peel therapy - a current review. Clin Cosmet Investig Dermatol 2013;6:281–8.

42. Fartasch M, Teal J, Menon GK. Mode of action of glycolic acid on human stratum corneum: ultrastructural and functional evaluation of the epidermal barrier. Arch Dermatol Res 1997;289(7):404–9.

43. Niamtu J. Cosmetic facial surgery. Second Edition. Edinburgh: Elsevier; 2018. p. 732–55.

44. Deprez P. Textbook of chemical peels: superficial, medium and deep peels in cosmetic practice. London: Informa Healthcare; 2007.

45. Baumann L, Baumann L. Retinol, retinyl esters, and retinoic acid. In: Cosmeceuticals and cosmetic ingredients. New York, NY: McGraw-Hill Education/Medical; 2015. p. 306–10.

46. Thielitz A, Abdel-Naser MB, Fluhr JW, et al. Topical retinoids in acne–an evidence-based overview. J Dtsch Dermatol Ges 2008;6(12):1023–31.

47. Baumann L, Baumann L. Hydroquinone. In: Cosmeceuticals and cosmetic Ingredients. New York, NY: McGraw-Hill Education/Medical; 2015. p. 100–4.

48. Schwartz C, Jan A, Zito PM. Hydroquinone. In: StatPearls. Treasure Island (FL): StatPearls Publishing; 2020.

49. Sofen B, Prado G, Emer J. Melasma and post inflammatory hyperpigmentation: management update and expert opinion. Skin Ther Lett 2016;21(1):1–7.

50. Baumann L, Baumann L. Ascorbic acid (Vitamin C). In: Cosmeceuticals and cosmetic ingredients. New York, NY: McGraw-Hill Education/Medical; 2015. p. 176–81.

51. Humbert PG, Haftek M, Creidi P, et al. Topical ascorbic acid on photoaged skin. Clinical, topographical and ultrastructural evaluation: double-blind study vs. placebo. Exp Dermatol 2003;12(3):237–44.

52. Tse TW. Hydroquinone for skin lightning: safety profile, duration of use and when should we stop? J Dermatolog Treat 2010;21(5):272–5.

53. Pamela RD. Topical growth factors for the treatment of facial photoaging: a clinical experience of eight cases. J Clin Aesthet Dermatol 2018;11(12):28–9.

54. Darr D, Dunston S, Faust H, et al. Effectiveness of antioxidants (vitamin C and E) with and without sunscreens as topical photoprotectants. Acta Derm Venereol 1996;76(4):264–8.

55. Stamford NP. Stability, transdermal penetration, and cutaneous effects of ascorbic acid and its derivatives. J Cosmet Dermatol 2012;11(4):310–7.

56. Fabi S, Sundaram H. The potential of topical and injectable growth factors and cytokines for skin rejuvenation. Facial Plast Surg 2014;30(2):157–71.

57. Wu DC, Goldman MP. A prospective, randomized, double-blind, split-face clinical trial comparing the efficacy of two topical human growth factors for the rejuvenation of the aging face. J Clin Aesthet Dermatol 2017;10(5):31–5.

Medication for Gravid and Nursing Oral and Maxillofacial Surgery Patients

Yoav Nudell, DDS, MS[a],*, Jared Miller, DDS[b]

KEYWORDS

- Medications • Dentistry • Maxillofacial surgery • Pregnancy • Nursing • Drugs • Lactating • Risk

KEY POINTS

- The new FDA labeling system for the safety of medications in pregnant and lactating patients provides a nuanced array of data and risks
- Available data related to the safe use of medications in pregnant and lactating patients are complex and incomplete.
- Before prescribing any drug to a nursing mother or pregnant patient, the maxillofacial surgeon and other dental and medical providers should consider the available evidence, benefits, and risk for that particular drug.

INTRODUCTION

In the United States, there are more than 6 million pregnancies every year. It is estimated that a pregnant woman receives 3 to 5 prescription drugs during pregnancy.[1] The purpose of this article is to clarify clinically impactful features of the perioperative and postoperative pharmacologic management of pregnant and lactating patients in the maxillofacial or dental setting.

We hope to provide you with concise, memorable, and actionable information to use in your clinical practice. We will also discuss the relevant physiologic changes of the gravid and postpartum patient, and the recent changes to the federal safety labeling guidelines. We will focus on the pharmacologic strategies that will minimize the risk to the mother, fetus, and child. This is not intended to be a comprehensive resource; we will direct you to helpful and comprehensive resources for further reading and reference.

FDA CATEGORIES: OLD AND NEW

Patients, along with their medical and dental providers, rely on evidence-based safeguards and guidelines to make informed decisions about which medication choices are the safest (**Table 1**). It is critical for the safety and wellbeing of the mother, fetus, and child to have a functional classification or labeling system that can guide pharmacologic management. In 1979, the US Food and Drug Administration (FDA) published *Labeling for Prescription Drugs Used in Man Regulations* which instituted a letter labeling system that categorized medications in an attempt to emphasize the risk a medication may have to a fetus (categories A, B, C, D, and X).[2]

The letter system was established to create guidance for safely prescribing medication for pregnant patient. However, over time the letter categorization system presented significant shortcomings. The system can oversimplify decision-making for prescription medications for pregnant

[a] 155 Ashland Place, Brooklyn, NY 11201, USA; [b] Department of Dentistry/Oral and Maxillofacial Surgery, The Brooklyn Hospital Center, Brooklyn, 155 Ashland Place, NY 11201, USA
* Corresponding author.
E-mail address: ynudell@gmail.com

Oral Maxillofacial Surg Clin N Am 34 (2022) 201–212
https://doi.org/10.1016/j.coms.2021.08.012
1042-3699/22/© 2021 Elsevier Inc. All rights reserved.

Table 1
Old and new FDA categories for medication use in pregnant patients

FDA Pregnancy Risk Categories	
FDA Category	
Category A	Adequate and well-controlled studies in pregnant women have failed to demonstrate a risk to the fetus in the first trimester of pregnancy (and there is no evidence of a risk in later trimesters)
Category B	Animal reproduction studies have failed to demonstrate a risk to the fetus and there are no adequate and well-controlled studies in pregnant women
Category C	Animal reproduction studies have shown an adverse effect on the fetus, if there are no adequate and well-controlled studies in humans, and if the benefits from the use of the drug in pregnant women may be acceptable despite its potential risks
Category D	There is positive evidence of human fetal risk based on adverse reaction data from investigational or marketing experience or studies in humans, but the potential benefits from the use of the drug in pregnant women may be acceptable despite its potential risks
Category X	Studies in animals or humans have demonstrated fetal abnormalities or if there is positive evidence of fetal risk based on adverse reaction reports from investigational or marketing experience, or both, and the risk of the use of the drug in a pregnant woman clearly outweighs any possible benefit

Adapted from Content and Format of Labeling for Human Prescription Drug and Biological Products; Requirements for Pregnancy and Lactation Labeling. Federal Register/Vol. 73, No. 104/Thursday, May 29, 2008.

patients. To illustrate this issue, consider that 60% of all medications fall into the category C. Category C medications have data supporting adverse effects in animals, yet they also include medications with no data from animal studies. This results in drugs with evidence of potential risk and those without evidence of risk being grouped together in the same category. In addition, the reductionist A-B-C-D-X labels may be misinterpreted or misused and often the labeling lacked clarity of specific risks. Furthermore, the categories did not include meaningful evidence-based clinical information as it relates to exposure during pregnancy and lactation. The consequences to the mother and fetus of discontinuing a drug therapy needed during pregnancy were also not included. There is a potential bias toward choosing A and B medications, pressuring providers toward medicolegal defensive medicine and unnecessary obstetrician consultations causing delays in treatment. Importantly, the letter categories focus on the quality and quantity of data available, and not the severity or incidence of risk.[1,2]

To respond to the need for updated risk categories, the FDA published a rule entitled *Content and format of labeling for human prescription drug and biological products; requirements for pregnancy and lactation labeling; Final Rule.* These

new FDA labeling guidelines for prescribing to pregnant and lactating patients went into effect on June 30, 2015. Pregnancy Lactation Labeling Rule (PLLR) replaced the previous letter system eliminating the A, B, C, D, and X risk categories. Pertinent details of the PLLR will be discussed next.[3]

Labels now have a section with information on the available pregnancy exposure registry, risk summary, clinical considerations, and data. The pregnancy exposure registry is a voluntary study where data are collected from pregnant patients who are taking certain medications or vaccines during pregnancy. These data may inform future guidelines on the use of the medication during pregnancy and lactation. Within the portion of the clinical consideration, subsections include disease-associated maternal and fetal risk, relevant dose adjustments during pregnancy and the postpartum period, maternal and fetal adverse reactions, and labor or delivery information (when this information is available).

The previous "Nursing mother" section will become the "Lactation" section including a "Risk summary," "Clinical considerations," and "Data." The lactation label will include information such as the presence of the drug in breast milk, effects on milk production, any potential risk for the child, and a statement on the risk-versus-benefit analysis for its use. There will also be a new section addressing females' and males' reproductive prudential risk including pregnancy testing, contraception, and infertility.[2–4]

The PLLR hopes to deliver concise, standardized summaries of the available evidence. This will provide the provider with up-to-date data. Though this system is more complex and potentially more time-consuming, it does provide an evidence-based tool for clinical decision-making.

NEW PREGNANCY-RISK CATEGORIES

These include subset categories.

- *Pregnancy (including labor and delivery)*
  1. Pregnancy exposure registry
  2. Risk summary
  3. Clinical considerations
  4. Data
- *Lactation*
  1. Risk summary
  2. Clinical considerations
  3. Data
- *Females and Males of Reproductive Potential*
  1. Pregnancy testing
  2. Contraception
  3. Infertility

The FDA online Drug Safety-related Labeling Changes can be accessed (https://www.accessdata.fda.gov/scripts/cder/safetylabelingchanges/)

PHARMACOLOGY IN LACTATING PATIENTS

It is the position of the American Academy of Pediatrics (AAP) that "breastfeeding and human milk is the normative standard for infant nutrition (**Table 2**)." In addition, the World Health Organization subscribes to the same ideal. There are well-documented medical and neurodevelopmental advantages to breastfeeding infants for the first 6 months of life, followed by continued breastfeeding as foods are introduced. They go on to support continued breastfeeding for 1 year or longer.[5] During that period, a lactating individual may require medication. Therefore, as a clinician, it is critical to understand the implications that medications may have on the mother and child. Ideally, a clinician's therapeutic choices should limit the negative effects that medications may have on the mother, child, and milk production. Generally, there are a limited number of medications that are contraindicated, and a suitable replacement can typically be found. Adherence to medications may also improve if the mother is fully informed of the risks, benefits, and alternatives for her and her child when she takes them. This portion of the text will review common medications found in the dental setting and also how these medications may impact the individual who is lactating and the infant receiving the milk.

LactMed (https://www.ncbi.nlm.nih.gov/books/NBK501922/), an online source published by the National Library of Medicine/National Institutes of Health, is a powerful reference for the most up-to-date information on the safety of drugs and other chemicals to which breastfeeding mothers may be exposed.

PHARMACOKINETICS IN LACTATING PATIENTS

Molecular transfer into breast milk can occur passively, down a concentration gradient or actively against a concentration gradient, through carrier-mediated transport or diffusion. Drug features such as molecular weight, ionization, protein binding, lipophilicity, and pharmacokinetics in the mother can influence how they enter breast milk. Biochemically, milk tends to have lower pH and higher lipid content as compared with plasma, thus drugs with chemical attributes that are conducive for transfer are more likely to be found in milk. These attributes include low plasma protein binding, low molecular weight, high lipophilicity, and positively charged drugs.[6]

DRUG SAFETY MEASUREMENTS

The milk-to-plasma ratio (M/P) of a drug is determined by dividing the concentration of drug in the milk by the drug level in the plasma. M/P is usually derived from experimental data; it can vary with time and maternal drug dose. Using the M/P, we can start to understand an infant's exposure to a drug. However, the process of determining the amount of drug that an infant is truly exposed to is influenced by several factors beyond the M/P. For instance, with the M/P, we can estimate the propensity of a drug to pass to a unit of breast milk, yet the actual dose can vary with the elimination half-life of the drug, the number of feeds, amount of milk ingested, and time from maternal intake of the drug to feeding time. Furthermore, the clearance and bioavailability of the drug to the infant will play a role in a drug's potential for toxicity.

A second well-accepted estimation of infant drug exposure with breast milk consumption is the relative infant dose (RID). The RID uses a known breast milk concentration of the drug and compares it to the therapeutic infant dose or the weight-adjusted adult dose when an infant dose is not known. Understanding drug exposure, we must also consider

204   Nudell & Miller

Table 2
Commonly used medications in oral and maxillofacial surgery practice and their use during pregnancy and lactation

Table	Medication	Use During Pregnancy	Use During Breastfeeding	Previous Letter Classification	Hale Lactation Risk Category	Comments
Local Anesthetics	Lidocaine	Yes	Yes	B	L2	No evidence of harm
	Mepivacaine	Yes	Yes	C	L3	Risk of methemoglobinemia
	Prilocaine	Yes	Yes	B	Unknown	Risk of methemoglobinemia
	Bupivacaine	No, may cause hypotension	Yes	C	L2	—
	Benzocaine	(Avoid)	Avoid	C	Unknown	Risk of methemoglobinemia
	Articaine	(Avoid)	Avoid	C	Unknown	—
	Epinephrine			C	L1	Reports of fetal malformations with intravenous doses no significant documented risk when used in association with a local anesthetic
Antibiotics	Amoxicillin	Yes	Yes	B	L1	—
	Penicillin	Yes	Yes	B	L1	—
	Amoxicillin and clavulanate potassium (Augmentin)	Yes	Yes	B	L1	—
	Clindamycin	Yes	Yes	B	L2	Use in the first trimester only if clearly needed
	Azithromycin	(Yes)	Yes, caution (risk-benefit analysis)	B	L2	Avoid in the first trimester
	Erythromycin	Yes	Yes, caution (risk-benefit analysis)	B	L2 / L3 early postnatal (pylorus-stenosis!)	Avoid in the first trimester
	Metronidazole (Flagyl)	(Yes)	Yes, caution (risk-benefit analysis)	B	L2	Fetal carcinogen in nonhuman mammals; no proven risk in humans; contraindicated for use in the first trimester as per manufacturer

Category	Drug				Comments
Analgesics	Ibuprofen	Avoid in the third trimester; may close PDA	Yes	B	L1	Associated with ductus arteriosus constriction when used during the first trimester
	Aspirin	No, associated with IUGR	Yes	C/D	L3	—
	COX-2 inhibitor	Avoid in the third trimester; may close PDA	Yes	C	L2	—
	Acetaminophen	Yes	Yes	B	L1	Associated with pulmonary hypertension when used in the third trimester
	Opioids (oxycodone, hydrocodone, codeine)	Yes	Yes, caution (risk-benefit analysis), monitor baby	B/C	L3	Frequent use may be associated with a fetal abnormality. First trimester use: low risk of neural tube defects. Third trimester use: risk of fetal dependence and newborn respiratory depression
	Morphine	Yes	Yes	C	L3	Breastfeeding can be resumed when the mother recovers from anesthesia.
	Fentanyl	Yes	Yes	B	L2	
Anxiolytics/ Sedatives	Diazepam (Valium)	No	No	D	L3; L4 if used chronically	Associated with fetal craniofacial and thoracic abnormalities in the first/second trimester
	Triazolam	No	No	X	L3	No known association with fetal abnormalities
	Midazolam	No, risk for fetal craniofacial anomalies	(No)	D	L3	Use near birth associated with adverse neonatal neurobehavior
	Barbiturates	No, risk for fetal craniofacial anomalies	No	D	L3	—
	Nitrous Oxide	Controversial, avoid in the first trimester	Yes, after recovery from anesthesia	Not assigned	L3	It is generally considered safe in pregnant and nursing patients as long as there is <50% of N_2O with supplemental oxygen coadministration.

(continued on next page)

Table 2
(continued)

Table	Medication	Use During Pregnancy	Use During Breastfeeding	Previous Letter Classification	Hale Lactation Risk Category	Comments
						Theoretically, these patients may benefit from prophylactic folic acid, methionine, and vitamin B12. However, it should be avoided in the first trimester.
Steroids						Systemically administered corticosteroids appear in human milk and could suppress growth, interfere with endogenous corticosteroid production, or cause other untoward effects
	Dexamethasone	Avoid in the first trimester	Avoid	NA	L3	Low risk of oral clefts during the first trimester
	Triamcinolone	Avoid in the first trimester	Yes, lack of evidence, alternative preferred	C	L3	Pregnancy: First-trimester risk of oral clefts; continued use may restrict fetal growth; Lactation: As a nasal spray or local injections, such as for tendinitis, it would not be expected to cause any adverse effects.
	Prednisone	Avoid in the first trimester	Yes	NA	L2	Low risk of oral clefts during the first trimester No adverse effect has been reported in breastfed infants with maternal use of any corticosteroid during breastfeeding. With high maternal doses, the use of prednisolone instead of prednisone and avoiding breastfeeding for 4 h after a dose.

Muscle relaxant	Cyclobenzaprine	Yes	Yes, caution (risk-benefit analysis), monitor baby	B	L3	May continue breastfeeding. Monitor the infant for drowsiness, adequate weight gain, and developmental milestones, particularly in neonates and preterm infants.

Hale Lactation risk Category	Safety	Description
L1	Safest	Drug that has been taken by a large number of breastfeeding mothers without any observed increase in adverse effects in the infant. Controlled studies in breastfeeding women fail to demonstrate a risk to the infant and the possibility of harm to the breastfeeding infant is remote, or the product is not orally bioavailable in an infant.
L2	Safer	Drug that has been studied in a limited number of breastfeeding women without an increase in adverse effects in the infant, and/or the evidence of a demonstrated risk which is likely to follow the use of this medication in a breastfeeding woman is remote.
L3	Moderately safe	There are no controlled studies in breastfeeding women; however, the risk of untoward effects to a breastfed infant is possible, or controlled studies show only minimal nonthreatening adverse effects. Drugs should be given only if the potential benefit justifies the potential risk to the infant.
L4	Possibly hazardous	There is positive evidence of risk to a breastfed infant or breast milk production, but the benefits of use in breastfeeding mothers may be acceptable despite the risk to the infant (eg, if the drug is needed in a life-threatening situation or for a serious disease for which safer drugs cannot be used or are ineffective).
L5	Contraindicated	Studies in breastfeeding mothers have demonstrated that there is a significant and documented risk to the infant based on human experience, or it is a medication that has a high risk of causing significant damage to an infant. The risk of using the drug in breastfeeding women clearly outweighs any possible benefit from breastfeeding. The drug is contraindicated in women who are breastfeeding an infant.

Data from Refs.[4,8,11,16,27–29], and Adapted from Hale, TW. Medications and mothers' milk: a manual of lactational pharmacology. 19th edition. Springer Publishing Company; 2019.

the gestational and postnatal age of the infant, other medications the infant may be receiving, properties of the maternal medication, and medical conditions of the mother and infant.[4,7]

LOCAL ANESTHETICS

Local anesthetics have their primary effects locally, though they inevitably enter the systemic circulation via diffusion or intravascular injection. Local anesthetics are known to cross the blood-placental barrier; thus, care must be taken to avoid toxicities in a developing fetus.

Common amide local anesthetics such as lidocaine, mepivacaine, or bupivacaine bind orosomucoid (alpha-1-acid glycoprotein). Levels of orosomucoid decrease during pregnancy and therefore possibly increase unbound plasma concentrations. Theoretically, an increased plasma concentration could lead to increased fetal exposure. Despite this, neonatal exposure to local anesthetics appears generally safe even at higher doses.[8]

The American College of Obstetricians and Gynecologists, FDA, American Dental Association, among others, consider lidocaine to be compatible with pregnancy and breastfeeding.[9,10]

As animal reproduction studies in rats have shown, doses up to 6.6 times the human dose have revealed no evidence of harm to the fetus caused by lidocaine. There are no high-powered and well-controlled studies in pregnant women. The most common local anesthetic used in the dental setting is lidocaine 2% with epinephrine 1:100,000. Much of the safety data from lidocaine is found in the obstetrics and pediatric literature. There are low concentrations of lidocaine in milk even after continuous high-dose intravenous and epidural infusions of local anesthesia. Lidocaine is also poorly absorbed by the infant. Therefore, lidocaine is not thought to have significant adverse effects on breastfed infants.[11]

When evaluating the use of epinephrine separately, limited studies have also been performed. One should be cautious when administering local anesthesia with epinephrine due to the theoretic potential for cardiovascular effects. Especially if injected intravenously, there could be vasoconstrictive or altered hemodynamic consequences within the mother that may reduce oxygenation of the fetus.[11]

Interestingly, an Egyptian study compared surgical infiltration with 2% lidocaine without epinephrine versus 2% lidocaine with epinephrine during C-section surgery and found an approximate 1-hour delay in breastfeeding initiation in patients who received lidocaine without epinephrine.

The authors posited the benefits of using vasoconstrictor enhanced the effects of the local anesthetic, thus reducing the need for additional opioids, consequently enhancing the mother's chances of earlier mobilization and breastfeeding, resulting in better potential outcomes for the mother and child. This article demonstrates the safety of lidocaine with epinephrine, and also makes the case for the importance of thoughtful choice of medication. The risk of epinephrine was outweighed by the benefits of its use with lidocaine.[11]

As plain lidocaine is not readily available in dental carpules, plain prilocaine is used as a safe alternative. Animal studies have shown that 30 times the human dose of prilocaine demonstrated no evidence of impaired fertility or damage to the fetus, in rats.[12]

The safety of mepivacaine hydrochloride (Carbocaine), articaine (Septocaine), and bupivacaine (Marcaine) are unknown.[4,13]

ANTIBIOTICS

Several physiologic changes occur during pregnancy, which may affect the pharmacokinetics of antibiotic medications taken by the mother. Circulating blood volume increases anywhere from 30% to 50%, and the glomerular filtration rate can increase by as much as 50%. The increased volume of distribution and increased drug filtration may impact the peak antibiotic concentrations. It is possible that this may impact the effectiveness of certain antibiotics; however, this has not been directly studied to our knowledge.[8,14]

Most antibiotics cross the blood-placenta barrier and are excreted in breast milk. Within the drug class of penicillins, amoxicillin and ampicillin have been approved by the AAP to be compatible during breastfeeding. Generally, penicillins are not contraindicated while breastfeeding.[7] Clavulanic acid, often used in combination with amoxicillin to combat beta-lactamase-producing bacteria, is well-absorbed orally and transfers to breast milk, yet no harmful effects have been reported.

Cephalosporins are considered to be safe during pregnancy. Though there are no large human clinical trials studying their safety, they are presumed safe. Animal reproduction studies have been performed on mice and rats using oral cephalexin monohydrate up to 1.5 times the maximum daily human dose and no harm to the fetus was found. Cephalosporins have been found in breast milk and are compatible with breastfeeding.[15]

Macrolide antibiotics, specifically clindamycin, are often chosen for patients with orofacial infections who are allergic to penicillin, or when the bacteria causing the orofacial infection is resistant to first-line penicillins. Macrolide antibiotics such as erythromycin, clindamycin, and azithromycin do not cross the placenta readily. They are considered safe during pregnancy and lactation. There is clinical data to support a low risk of increased congenital abnormalities when administered in the second and third trimesters of pregnancy. Risk for the first trimester also appears low, but with less convincing clinical data. Therefore, avoiding macrolides such as clindamycin in the first trimester is recommended, unless clearly needed.

The use of metronidazole (Flagyl) during pregnancy is controversial. There does not appear to be a risk of congenital anomalies for women who had first-trimester exposure to metronidazole. In vitro studies have shown mutagenicity; however, in vivo experiments have not demonstrated genetic damage. Furthermore, although mouse and rat studies have demonstrated tumorigenicity, hamster studies have not. Human data have not convincingly shown metronidazole to be carcinogenic. Metronidazole is generally considered safe during the second and third trimesters, and caution should be taken when used while breastfeeding. A risk-benefit analysis should be performed in consultation with the obstetrician for its use if deemed essential.[8,16]

Tetracyclines are a group of broad-spectrum antibiotics that reversibly bind the 30S ribosome, inhibit the initiation of translation, and consequently inhibit bacterial protein synthesis. Tetracyclines cross the placenta and form a stable calcium complex in any bone-forming tissue, such as fetal teeth and bone, causing yellow-grey-brown discoloration if given after the fifth month of gestation. Enamel hypoplasia has also been reported, but it appears to be rare. A decrease in fibular growth rate has been observed in premature human infants given oral tetracycline; however, this reaction was shown to be reversible when the drug was discontinued. Animal studies demonstrated that tetracyclines can delay fetal skeletal development. Also, embryotoxicity has been noted in animals treated early in pregnancy. In summary, to prevent intrinsic tooth staining, tetracycline drugs should not be used during tooth development, unless other drugs are contraindicated or are suspected to be ineffective. Although tetracycline is compatible with breastfeeding, other antibiotics are preferred. Doxycycline and minocycline should be avoided because of higher absorption by infants and toxicity in children, causing dental staining and potentially decreased bone growth.

Trimethoprim/sulfamethoxazole (TMP/SMX, or Bactrim) has the potential to cause damage to the developing fetus. There is potential for neural tube defects, cardiovascular defects, and facial clefts. Theoretically, some risks could be mitigated with folic acid supplementation. There is not enough clinical data to support TMP/SMX's potential safety or harm. In a nested, case-control study within the Quebec Pregnancy Cohort, sulfonamide use during the first trimester was associated with an increased risk of spontaneous abortion. Its use during pregnancy should only be considered if there are no effective alternative therapies available. Small quantities have been found in breast milk. There is an increased risk for hyperbilirubinemia in premature neonates and neonates with glucose-6-phosphate dehydrogenase (G6PD) deficiency. It is recommended that care be taken when giving the drug to neonates, and it should be avoided in preterm neonates and neonates who have hyperbilirubinemia. The AAP approves TMP/SMX for use in lactating women.[16]

When a child consumes milk potentially containing antibiotics, it is wise to recommend monitoring the child for possible disturbances to the gastrointestinal flora microbiome resulting in diarrhea, candidiasis, or bloody stool suggestive of antibiotic-associated colitis.

PAIN MANAGEMENT

Analgesics are an important class of medication for the maxillofacial surgeon and other dental professionals. Nonsteroidal anti-inflammatory drugs (NSAIDs) are given routinely and are often the first-line therapies for the treatment of pain.

ANALGESICS

NSAIDs and aspirin are used commonly by pregnant and lactating women. They are used for pain, but low-dose aspirin is often additionally prescribed for the prevention of preeclampsia and recurrent miscarriage in antiphospholipid syndrome.

There is evidence for NSAIDs and aspirin increasing the risk of early pregnancy loss. Their use in the second trimester is considered safer than the first, but there is an association with fetal testicular abnormalities. In the third trimester, NSAIDs and aspirin are usually avoided because of significant risks to the fetus such as renal injury, oligohydramnios, constriction or premature closure of the ductus arteriosus, necrotizing enterocolitis, and intracranial hemorrhage. Lactating mothers who take NSAIDs usually have low infant exposure through breast milk;

consequently, cyclooxygenase-1 and cyclooxygenase-2 inhibitors are considered safe, and higher-dose analgesic levels of aspirin should be avoided. Short-term use of ibuprofen, naproxen, diclofenac, indomethacin, and ketorolac are considered compatible with breastfeeding by the AAP. Ibuprofen is considered more compatible with long-term use in a breastfeeding mother.[17]

Of the NSAIDs, ibuprofen is the preferred choice because it has poor transfer into milk and has been well-studied in children. NSAIDs with a long half-life such as naproxen can accumulate in the infant with prolonged use and are therefore less desirable.

Acetaminophen (paracetamol or Tylenol) is the recommended medication for pregnant women with pain, and most women use this medication at some point during pregnancy. Only approximately 0.04% to 0.23% of the maternal dose is excreted in breast milk, with peak levels at 1 to 2 hours after ingestion and a half-life of 2.7 hours. The AAP considers this drug compatible with breastfeeding.[7]

Morphine, meperidine, and oxycodone are considered safe analgesic agents for use any time during pregnancy. There is insufficient data available for codeine sulfate to inform a drug-linked risk for major birth defects and/or miscarriage. Notably, animal studies have linked codeine to delayed ossification without structural malformations in mice, cranial malformations in hamsters, and fetotoxic effects in rats and hamsters. Nevertheless, the use of codeine is considered safe to administer to pregnant patients. As with all opioid narcotics, chronic use can cause neonatal withdrawal symptoms.[7]

Meperidine is not a preferred analgesic for use in breastfeeding women because of the long half-life of its active metabolite in infants. Infant sedation is strongly associated with oxycodone in particular, and other agents are preferred.

Morphine, codeine, and hydrocodone are considered compatible with breastfeeding by the AAP. Opioid narcotics during breastfeeding can cause infant drowsiness, central nervous system depression, and possible death. Infant sedation can occur with maternal use of agents such as hydrocodone and codeine. Newborn infants may be especially sensitive to the effects of small doses of opioid narcotic analgesics. Therefore, it is recommended to monitor the infant closely for drowsiness, adequate weight gain, and developmental milestones.[8]

HYPNOTICS

Benzodiazepines such as diazepam and midazolam have been associated with various congenital malformations. Cleft palate, central nervous system dysfunction, and dysmorphism have been found to be associated with in utero exposure to benzodiazepines. Neurotransmitters such as gamma-aminobutyric acid (GABA) are important regulators of palatal shelf reorientation during maxillofacial development. Theoretically, benzodiazepines can mimic GABA and disrupt the proper signaling necessary for proper palatal closure. Barbiturates have been shown to cause congenital defects in animal models; however, human defects have not been consistently reported. Generally, it is recommended that benzodiazepines and barbiturates should be avoided during pregnancy, and propofol is the preferred alternative. In a mother who has recovered from anesthesia, the quantity of propofol found in breast milk is thought to be low. Most experts recommend that a mother can resume breastfeeding an infant after she is fully recovered from general anesthesia. There is evidence that propofol can delay the onset of lactation. Another study found that mothers who breastfeed prior to general anesthesia induction have lower requirements of sevoflurane and propofol. There are reports of blue-green discoloration to breastmilk after receiving propofol, and mothers should be informed of this possibility.[18-20]

INHALATIONAL AGENTS

The most common inhalational agent used in the dental setting is nitrous oxide (N_2O). The potential teratogenic effects of N_2O are linked to its oxidative inactivation of methionine synthetase. Methionine synthetase converts homocysteine and methyltetrahydrofolate to methionine and tetrahydrofolate. Regenerating methionine is important as it is an essential amino acid, and tetrahydrofolate is important for DNA synthesis. Animal studies show N_2O to trigger spontaneous abortion and birth defects. Human correlation has not been definitely demonstrated. Theoretically, supplementation of folic acid, methionine, and cobalamin (vitamin B12) could mitigate some of the adverse molecular effects of N_2O. There has been a report of chronic nonscavenged exposure of N_2O, for more than or equal to 3 hours per week, causing spontaneous abortion in female dental assistants. It is generally considered safe in a pregnant patient as long as there is less than 50% of N_2O with supplemental oxygen coadministration. In addition, these patients should receive prophylactic folic acid, methionine, and vitamin B12.

Sevoflurane is considered to be safe during pregnancy. There are animal studies that suggest a single exposure to sevoflurane 3% does not produce long-term cognitive impairment in rat offspring; however, repeated exposure is sufficient to cause long-term cognitive impairment. Sevoflurane may cause inflammatory damage in the hippocampus and parietal cortex. There is minimal published data on the effects of sevoflurane during breastfeeding. Owing to the extremely short serum half-life of the drug, a recovered mother is not expected to transfer sevoflurane to the infant via breast milk. No waiting period before breastfeeding is required, and the mother does not need to discard her milk.[21–27]

SUMMARY

Many of the common drugs used by dentists have been found to be safe for pregnant and breastfeeding women, the notable exceptions above notwithstanding. Before prescribing any drug to a nursing mother or pregnant patient, the maxillofacial surgeon and other dental and medical providers should consider the available evidence and risk for that particular drug. It is always wise to have open communication with your patient's obstetricians and appropriate consultation may also be indicated.

The new PLLR guidelines are a necessarily more sophisticated guide than the old letter category system. The letter categories were more a measure of the quality of evidence rather than the level of specific risk. There are many complex factors to consider when prescribing in order to maintain the safety of the pregnant individual, fetus, and infant. The new labeling rule allows detailed safety and specific risk information to be more easily accessible to prescribers. As the FDA states, "prescribing decisions during pregnancy and lactation are individualized and involve complex maternal, fetal, and infant risk-benefit considerations." (Food and Drug Administration. FDA issues final rule on changes to pregnancy and lactation labeling information for prescription drug and biological products. December 3, 2014. Available at: www.fda.gov/NewsEvents/Newsroom/PressAnnouncements/ucm425317.htm. Accessed February 13, 2016.)

CLINICS CARE POINTS

- The A-B-C-D-X categories focus on the quality and quantity of data available, and not the severity or incidence of risk. The letter labels may be misinterpreted or misused and often the labeling lacked clarity of specific risks.

- Many of the common drugs used have been found to be safe for pregnant and breast feeding women. Consider the available evidence and risk for that particular drug. It is wise to have open communication with your patient's obstetricians and appropriate consultation may be indicated.

DISCLOSURE

The authors have nothing to disclose.

REFERENCES

1. Whyte J. FDA implements new labeling for medications used during pregnancy and lactation. Am Fam Physician 2016;94(1):12–5.
2. Pernia S, DeMaagd G. The new pregnancy and lactation labeling rule. P T 2016;41(11):713–5.
3. Food and Drug Administration HHS. Content and format of labeling for human prescription drug and biological products; requirements for pregnancy and lactation labeling. Final rule. Fed Regist 2014; 79(233):72063–103.
4. Stern A, Elmore J. Medication for gravid and nursing dental patients. Dent Clin North Am 2016;60(2):523–31.
5. Eidelman AI. Breastfeeding and the use of human milk: an analysis of the American Academy of Pediatrics 2012 Breastfeeding Policy Statement. Breastfeed Med 2012;7(5):323–4.
6. Ito S, Lee A. Drug excretion into breast milk–overview. Adv Drug Deliv Rev 2003;55(5):617–27.
7. Bar-Oz B, Bulkowstein M, Benyamini L, et al. Use of antibiotic and analgesic drugs during lactation. Drug Saf 2003;26(13):925–35.
8. Turner MD, Singh F, Glickman RS. Dental management of the gravid patient. N Y State Dent J 2006; 72(6):22–7.
9. Committee Opinion No. 569: oral health care during pregnancy and through the lifespan. Obstet Gynecol 2013;122(2 Pt 1):417–22.
10. American Dental Association. ADA current policies, 1954-2020 2021. Available at:. https://www.ada.org/~/media/ADA/Member%20Center/Members/current_policies.pdf. Accessed May 20, 2021.
11. Drugs and lactation database (LactMed) [Internet]. Bethesda (MD): National Library of Medicine (US); 2006. Lidocaine. Available at: https://www.ncbi.nlm.nih.gov/books/NBK501230/. Accessed May 20, 2021.
12. AstraZeneca Group. 4% Citanest Plain Dental® (Prilocaine Hydrochloride Injection, USP) [package insert]. U.S. Food and Drug Administration; 2018. Available at: https://www.accessdata.fda.gov/

drugsatfda_docs/label/2018/021382s008lbl.pdf. Accessed May 20, 2021.

13. Septodont. SEPTOCAINE® (articaine hydrochloride and epinephrine injection) [package insert]. U.S. Food and Drug Administration; 2018. Available at: https://www.accessdata.fda.gov/drugsatfda_docs/label/2018/020971s042lbl.pdf. Accessed May 20, 2021.

14. Cheung KL, Lafayette RA. Renal physiology of pregnancy. Adv Chronic Kidney Dis 2013;20(3): 209–14.

15. Pragma Pharmaceuticals, LLC. KEFLEX® (CAPSULES CEPHALEXIN, USP) [package insert]. U.S. Food and Drug Administration; 2018. Available at: https://www.accessdata.fda.gov/drugsatfda_docs/label/2018/050405s107lbl.pdf. Accessed May 20, 2021.

16. Libecco JA, Powell KR. Trimethoprim/sulfamethoxazole: clinical update. Pediatr Rev 2004;25(11): 375–80.

17. Bloor M, Paech M. Nonsteroidal anti-inflammatory drugs during pregnancy and the initiation of lactation. Anesth Analg 2013;116(5):1063–75.

18. Drugs and Lactation Database (LactMed) [Internet]. Bethesda (MD): National Library of Medicine (US); 2006. Propofol. [Updated 2021, Feb 15]. Available from: https://www.ncbi.nlm.nih.gov/books/NBK501298/.

19. Fresenius Kabi. DIPRIVAN® (propofol) Injectable Emulsion [package insert]. U.S. Food and Drug Administration; 2017. Available at: https://www.accessdata.fda.gov/drugsatfda_docs/label/2017/019627s066lbl.pdf. Accessed May 20, 2021.

20. Drugs and Lactation Database (LactMed) [Internet]. Bethesda (MD): National Library of Medicine (US); 2006. Nitrous Oxide. [Updated 2020, Nov 16].

Available from: https://www.ncbi.nlm.nih.gov/books/NBK501501/.

21. Wu Z, Li X, Zhang Y, et al. Effects of sevoflurane exposure during mid-pregnancy on learning and memory in offspring rats: beneficial effects of maternal exercise. Front Cell Neurosci 2018;12:122.

22. Zhu Y, Lv C, Liu J, et al. Effects of sevoflurane general anesthesia during early pregnancy on AIM2 expression in the hippocampus and parietal cortex of Sprague-Dawley offspring rats. Exp Ther Med 2021;21(5):469.

23. Kurien S, Kattimani VS, Sriram RR, et al. Management of pregnant patient in dentistry. J Int Oral Health 2013;5(1):88–97.

24. Briggs GG, Freeman RK, Towers CV, et al. Drugs in pregnancy and lactation. 11th edition. Philadelphia, PA, USA: Lippincott Williams & Wilkins; 2017. Available at: http://ovidsp.ovid.com. Accessed April 27, 2021.

25. Section on Breastfeeding. Breastfeeding and the use of human milk. Pediatrics 2012;129(3):e827–41.

26. Drugs and Lactation Database (LactMed) [Internet]. Bethesda (MD): National Library of Medicine (US); 2006. Sevoflurane. [Updated 2020, Nov 16]. Available from: https://www.ncbi.nlm.nih.gov/books/NBK501504/

27. Drugs and Lactation Database (LactMed) [Internet]. Bethesda (MD): National Library of Medicine (US); 2006. Metronidazole. [Updated 2021, Mar 17]. Available from: https://www.ncbi.nlm.nih.gov/books/NBK501315/.

28. Armstrong C. ACOG guidelines on psychiatric medication use during pregnancy and lactation. Am Fam Physician 2008;78(6):772.

29. Hale TW. Medications and mothers' milk: a manual of lactational pharmacology. 19th edition. New York: Springer Publishing Company; 2019.

Moving?

Make sure your subscription moves with you!

To notify us of your new address, find your **Clinics Account Number** (located on your mailing label above your name), and contact customer service at:

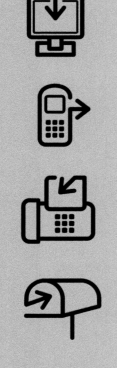

Email: journalscustomerservice-usa@elsevier.com

800-654-2452 (subscribers in the U.S. & Canada)
314-447-8871 (subscribers outside of the U.S. & Canada)

Fax number: 314-447-8029

Elsevier Health Sciences Division
Subscription Customer Service
3251 Riverport Lane
Maryland Heights, MO 63043

ELSEVIER